Fred F. Ferri, MD, FACP

Ferri's
FAST
FACT

Clinical Professor
Brown Medical Sc
Providence, Rhod

ELSEVIER
MOSBY

ELSEVIER
MOSBY

1600 John F. Kennedy Blvd., Ste 1800
Philadelphia, PA 19103-2899

FERRI'S FAST FACTS   ISBN 0-323-03592-2
Copyright © 2005, Elsevier Inc.

NOTICE

Knowledge and best practice in this field are constantly changing.
As new research and experience broaden our knowledge, changes
in practice, treatment and drug therapy may become necessary or
appropriate. Readers are advised to check the most current
information provided (i) on procedures featured or (ii) by the
manufacturer of each product to be administered, to verify the
recommended dose or formula, the method and duration of
administration, and contraindications. It is the responsibility of the
practitioner, relying on their own experience and knowledge of
the patient, to make diagnoses, to determine dosages and the best
treatment for each individual patient, and to take all appropriate
safety precautions. To the fullest extent of the law, neither the
Publisher nor the Author assumes any liability for any injury
and/or damage to persons or property arising out or related to
any use of the material contained in this book.

Library of Congress Cataloging-in-Publication Data

Ferri, Fred F.
    Ferri's fast facts / Fred F. Ferri.
        p. cm.
    ISBN 13: 978-0-323-03592-7
    1. Internal medicine—Handbooks, manuals, etc. I. Title: Fast facts.
II. Title.
RC55.F467 2005
616—dc22   2005041518

Printed in China
Last digit is the print number: 9 8 7 6 5

Preface

The purpose of this handbook is to provide the clinician with a quick reference covering a broad spectrum of inpatient and outpatient medicine that is small enough to fit easily in a pocket. Its focus is on key points in the diagnosis and treatment of disorders that are likely to be encountered in a medical service. For ease of retrieval, each disorder is listed alphabetically. This handbook is not meant to replace the many texts that form the cornerstone of one's medical education, but rather is a "peripheral brain" to be used when time to explore a medical topic fully is limited and there is a need to rapidly review essential facts on diagnosis and treatment.

Fred F. Ferri, MD, FACP

Acknowledgments

The author wishes to acknowledge the following physicians who have contributed to several of the topics in this book and to my other books: *Ferri's Clinical Advisor* and *Practical Guide to the Care of the Medical Patient.*

SONYA S. ABDEL-RAZEQ, M.D., Department of Obstetrics and Gynecology/Resident Education, State University of New York at Buffalo, Buffalo, New York ● PHILIP J. ALIOTTA, M.D., M.S.H.A., F.A.C.S., Department of Urology, School of Medicine and Biomedical Sciences, State University of New York at Buffalo, Buffalo, New York ● GEORGE O. ALONSO, M.D., Department of Medicine, Mount Sinai School of Medicine, New York, New York ● MEL L. ANDERSON, M.D., F.A.C.P., Department of Medicine, Brown Medical School, Providence, Rhode Island ● ETSUKO AOKI, M.D., PH.D., Internal Medicine Department, Rhode Island Hospital, Providence, Rhode Island ● VASANTHI ARUMUGAM, M.D., Department of Medicine, Mount Sinai School of Medicine, New York, New York ● AMAAR ASHRAF, M.D., Department of Medicine, Mount Sinai School of Medicine, New York, New York ● SUDEEP KAUR AULAKH, M.D., C.M., F.R.C.P.C., Department of Medicine, Albany Medical College, Albany, New York ● MICHAEL BENATAR, M.B.Ch.B., D. Phil., Department of Neurology, Emory University, Atlanta, Georgia ● LYNN BOWLBY, M.D., Division of General Internal Medicine, Rhode Island Hospital, Providence, Rhode Island ● WILLIAM F. BOYD, M.D., M.P.H., Internal Medicine, Rhode Island Hospital/The Miriam Hospital, Providence, Rhode Island ● MANDEEP K. BRAR, M.D., Department of Obstetrics and Gynecology, State University of New York at Buffalo, Buffalo, New York ● REBECCA S. BRIENZA, M.D., M.P.H., Department of Internal Medicine, Yale University School of Medicine, New Haven, Connecticut ● JENNIFER CLARKE, M.D., Departments of Medicine and Obstetrics and Gynecology, Brown Medical School, Rhode Island Hospital, Providence, Rhode Island ● MARIA A. CORIGLIANO, M.D., F.A.C.O.G., Department of Obstetrics and Gynecology, State University of New York at Buffalo, Buffalo, New York ● KAROLL CORTEZ, M.D., Division of Infectious Disease, Rhode Island Hospital, Providence, Rhode Island ● JOHN E. CROOM M.D., Ph.D., Neurology Department, Harvard Medical School, Boston, Massachusetts ● CLAUDIA L. DADE, M.D., Division of Infectious Diseases, Mount Sinai School of Medicine, New York, New York ● GEORGE T. DANAKAS, M.D., F.A.C.O.G., Department of Obstetrics and Gynecology, State University of New York at Buffalo, Buffalo, New York ● ALEXANDRA DEGENHARDT, M.D., Department of Neurology, Beth Israel Deaconess Medical Center, Boston, Massachusetts ● JOSEPH DIAZ, M.D., Department of Medicine, Brown Medical School, Providence, Rhode Island ● CHRISTINE M. DUFFY, M.D., M.P.H.,

Center for Gerontology and Health Care Research, Brown University, Providence, Rhode Island ● JEFFREY S. DURMER, M.D., PH.D., Department of Neurology, Emory University School of Medicine, Atlanta, Georgia ● JANE EVASON, M.D., Division of Infectious Diseases, Elmhurst Hospital Center, Mount Sinai School of Medicine, New York, New York ● RIF S. EL-MALLAKH, M.D., Department of Psychiatry and Behavioral Sciences, University of Louisville School of Medicine, Louisville, Kentucky ● MARILYN FABRI, M.D., Department of Medicine, Mount Sinai School of Medicine, New York, New York ● MARK J. FAGAN, M.D., Department of Medicine, Brown Medical School, Providence, Rhode Island ● GIL FARKASH, M.D., Department of Obstetrics and Gynecology, State University of New York at Buffalo, Buffalo, New York ● TAMARA G. FONG, M.D., PH.D., Neurology Department, Beth Israel Deaconess Medical Center, Harvard Medical School, Boston, Massachusetts ● GLENN G. FORT, M.D., Ph.D., Department of Medicine, Brown Medical School, Providence, Rhode Island ● TIFFANY B. GLENWICK, M.D., Department of Obstetrics and Gynecology, State University of New York at Buffalo, Buffalo, New York ● DAVID R. GIFFORD, M.D., M.PH., Department of Community Health and Medicine, Brown Medical School, Providence, Rhode Island ● GEETHA GOPALAKRISHNAN, M.D., Department of Endocrinology, Brown Medical School, Providence, Rhode Island ● REBECCA J. GRIFFITH, M.D., Department of Medicine, Morristown Memorial Hospital, Morristown, New Jersey ● JOSEPH GRILLO, M.D., Infectious Diseases Department, Roger Williams Medical Center, Providence, Rhode Island ● MICHAEL GRUENTHAL, M.D., Ph.D., Department of Neurology, University of Louisville School of Medicine, Louisville, Kentucky ● MICHELE HALPERN, M.D., Department of Medicine, New York Medical College, Valhalla, New York ● SAJEEV HANDA, M.D., Division of Hospitalist Medicine, Brown Medical School, Providence, Rhode Island ● TAYLOR HARRISON, M.D., Department of Neurology, Emory University, Atlanta, Georgia ● SHARON S. HARTMAN, M.D., Ph.D., Department of Neurology, Emory University, Atlanta, Georgia ● JENNIFER ROH HUR, M.D., Department of Medicine, Brown Medical School, Providence, Rhode Island ● RICHARD S. ISAACSON, M.D., Department of Medicine, Beth Israel Deaconess Medical Center, Harvard Medical School, Boston, Massachusetts ● JENNIFER JEREMIAH, M.D., Department of Medicine, Brown Medical School, Providence, Rhode Island ● MICHAEL P. JOHNSON, M.D., Department of Medicine, Brown Medical School, Providence, Rhode Island ● POWELL KAZANJIAN, M.D., Department of Internal Medicine, University of Michigan Medical School, Ann Arbor, Michigan ● WAN J. KIM, M.D., Department of Obstetrics and Gynecology, State University of New York at Buffalo, Buffalo, New York ● MELVYN KOBY, M.D., Department of Ophthalmology, University of Louisville School of Medicine, Louisville, Kentucky ● DAVID KURSS, M.D., E.A.C.O.G., Department of

Obstetrics and Gynecology, State University of New York at Buffalo, Buffalo, New York ● JOSEPH J. LIEBER, M.D., Department of Medicine, Mount Sinai School of Medicine, New York, New York ● CHUN LIM, M.D., PH.D., Department of Neurology, Beth Israel Deaconess Medical Center, Boston, Massachusetts ● ZEENA LOBO, M.D., Division of Infectious Diseases, Elmhurst Hospital Center, Elmhurst, New York ● EUGENE J. LOUIE-NG, M.D., Department of Obstetrics and Gynecology, State University of New York at Buffalo, Buffalo, New York ● JOSEPH R. MASCI, M.D., Department of Medicine, Mount Sinai School of Medicine, New York, New York ● DANIEL T. MATTSON, M.D., M.SC.(MED.), Department of Neurology, Beth Israel Deaconess Medical Center, Harvard Medical School, Boston, Massachusetts ● MAITREYI MAZUMDAR, M.D., M.P.H., Department of Medicine, Harvard Medical School, Children's Hospital of Boston, Boston, Massachusetts ● KELLY McGARRY, M.D., Department of Medicine, Brown Medical School, Providence, Rhode Island ● LYNN McNICOLL, M.D., Department of Medicine, Brown Medical School, Providence, Rhode Island ● LONNIE R. MERCIER, M.D., Department of Orthopedic Surgery, Creighton University School of Medicine, Omaha, Nebraska ● DENNIS J. MIKOLICH, M.D., Department of Medicine, Brown Medical School, Providence, Rhode Island ● TAKUMA NEMOTO, M.D., Department of Surgery, State University of New York at Buffalo, Buffalo, New York ● JAMES J. NG, M.D., Department of Obstetrics and Gynecology, The Vancouver Clinic, Vancouver, Washington ● GAIL M. O'BRIEN, M.D., Department of Medicine, Department of Medicine Brown Medical School, Providence, Rhode Island ● CAROLYN J. O'CONNOR, M.D., Department of Internal Medicine, Danbury Hospital, Southbury, Connecticut ● LAURA OFSTEAD, M.D., Department of Medicine, Brown Medical School, Rhode Island Hospital, Providence, Rhode Island ● ALEXANDER OLAWAIYE, M.D., Department of Obstetrics and Gynecology/Resident Education, State University of New York at Buffalo, Women's and Children's Hospital, Buffalo, New York ● JEANNE M. OLIVA, M.D., Division of General Internal Medicine, Rhode Island Hospital, Providence, Rhode Island ● MINA B. PANTCHEVA M.D., Internal Medicine, Roger Williams Medical Center, Providence, Rhode Island ● PETER PETROPOULOS, M.D., F.A.C.C., Internal Medicine, Brown Medical School, Providence, Rhode Island ● MICHAEL PICCHIONI, M.D., Department of Medicine, Tufts University School of Medicine, Springfield, Massachusetts ● PAUL A. PIRRAGLIA, M.D. M.P.H., Department of Medicine, Brown University, Rhode Island Hospital, Providence, Rhode Island ● MAURICE POLICAR, M.D., Department of Medicine, Mount Sinai School of Medicine, New York, New York ● HEMCHAND RAMBERAN, M.D., Internal Medicine, Memorial Hospital of Rhode Island, Brown Medical School, Providence, Rhode Island ● HARLAN G. RICH, M.D., Department of Medicine, Brown Medical School, Providence, Rhode Island ● LUTHER K. ROBINSON,

SEAN I. SAVITZ, M.D., Department of Pediatrics, Dysmorphology and Clinical Genetics, State University of New York at Buffalo, Buffalo, New York ● JACK L. SCHWARTZWALD, M.D., Neurology Department, Harvard Medical School, Beth Israel Deaconess Medical Center, Boston, Massachusetts ● HARVEY M. SHANIES, M.D., Ph.D., Critical Care Medicine, Vassar Brothers Medical Center, Poughkeepsie, New York ● DEBORAH L. SHAPIRO, M.D., Department of Medicine, Mount Sinai School of Medicine, New York, New York ● I. SHIRAVI SOHUR, M.D., Ph.D., Neurology Department, Harvard Medical School, Beth Israel Deaconess Medical Center, Boston, Massachusetts ● JENNIFER SOUTHER, M.D., Department of Family Practice, Memorial Hospital of Rhode Island, Pawtucket, Rhode Island ● ANNE SPAULDING, M.D., Centers for Disease Control and Prevention, Atlanta, Georgia ● MICHELLE STOZEK, M.D., Division of General Internal Medicine, Brown Medical School, Rhode Island Hospital, Providence, Rhode Island ● JULIE ANNE SZUMIGALA, M.D., Department of Obstetrics and Gynecology, State University of New York at Buffalo, Buffalo, New York ● DOMINICK TAMMARO, M.D., Department of Medicine, Brown Medical School, Providence, Rhode Island ● PETER E. TANGUAY, M.D., Department of Psychiatry and Behavioral Sciences, University of Louisville School of Medicine, Louisville, Kentucky ● IRIS TONG, M.D., Department of Medicine, Brown Medical School, Providence, Rhode Island ● EROBOGHENE E. UBOGU, M.B.B.S. (HONS), Department of Neurology, Emory University School of Medicine, Atlanta, Georgia ● NICOLE ULLRICH M.D., Ph.D., Department of Neurology/Neurooncology, Children's Hospital Boston, Boston, Massachusetts ● TOM J. WACHTEL, M.D., Department of Community Health and Medicine, Brown Medical School, Providence, Rhode Island ● DENNIS M. WEPPNER, M.D., F.A.C.O.G., Department of Clinical Gynecology/Obstetrics, State University of New York at Buffalo, Buffalo, New York ● LAUREL W. WHITE, M.D., Department of Obstetrics and Gynecology Division of Maternal Fetal Medicine, State University of New York at Buffalo, Buffalo, New York ● MATTHEW I. WITHIAMFLETCH, M.D., Department of Obstetrics and Gynecology, State University of New York at Buffalo, Buffalo, New York ● WEN-CHIH WU, M.D., Department of Medicine, Brown Medical School, Providence, Rhode Island ● BETH L WUTZ, M.D., Department of Medicine, State University of New York at Buffalo, Buffalo, New York ● MADHAVI YERNENI, M.D., Academic Medical Center, Miriam Hospital, Pawtucket, Rhode Island ● CINDY ZADIKOFF M.D., Movement Disorders, Morton and Gloria Shulman Movement Disorders Center, Toronto Western Hospital, Toronto, Ontario ● SCOTT J. ZUCCALA, D.O., F.A.C.O.G., Department of Obstetrics and Gynecology, Mercy Hospital of Buffalo, Buffalo, New York

Contents

Abscess, brain

Definition: Focal collection of pus surrounded by a well-vascularized capsule

DIAGNOSIS
- Classic triad—fever, headache, and focal neurologic deficit—is present in 50% of cases.
- Focal neurologic findings are seen in 30% to 50% of cases and depend on location of abscess.
- Papilledema is present in 25% of cases.
- MRI is diagnostic procedure of choice.
- CT scan with intravenous contrast administration is alternative imaging choice when MRI is unavailable or contraindicated (sensitivity 95-99%).

ETIOLOGY
- **Contiguous focus of infection (55% of cases):** paranasal sinus infection (*Streptococcus, Bacteroides, Haemophilus, Fusobacterium*); otitis media/mastoiditis (Streptococcus, Enterobacteriaceae, *Bacteroides, Pseudomonas*); dental sepsis (*Fusobacterium, Bacteroides, Streptococcus*); penetrating head injury (*Staphylococcus aureus, Clostridium*); postoperative (*Staphylococcus epidermidis, S. aureus*)
- **Hematogenous spread (25% of cases):** endocarditis (*S. aureus*, viridans streptococci); congenital heart disease (*Streptococcus, Haemophilus*); urinary tract infection (Enterobacteriaceae, Pseudomonadaceae); lung (*Streptococcus, Actinomyces, Fusobacterium*); intraabdominal (*Streptococcus*, Enterobacteriaceae, anaerobes)
- **Immunocompromised host:** *Toxoplasma*, fungi, *Nocardia, Listeria monocytogenes*, Enterobacteriaceae

TREATMENT
- **Empiric antibiotic therapy:** varies with suspected source
- **Otitis media/mastoiditis:** cefotaxime 2 g IV q6h or ceftriaxone 2 g IV q12h) plus metronidazole 7.5 mg/kg IV q6h or 15 mg/kg IV q12h
- **Dental infection:** penicillin G 6 million U IV q6h plus metronidazole 7.5 mg/kg IV q6h
- **Head trauma or post cranial surgery:** third-generation cephalosporin plus metronidazole and nafcillin or vancomycin
- **Hematogenous spread:** nafcillin or vancomycin plus metronidazole plus third-generation cephalosporin

- If evidence of edema or mass effect, treatment of elevated intracranial pressure is paramount: mannitol, dexamethasone, hyperventilation of mechanically ventilated patient

CLINICAL PEARL

- Lumbar puncture is contraindicated in patients with suspected abscess (20% die or experience neurologic decline).
- Stereotactic biopsy or aspirate of abscess if surgically feasible
- Medical therapy is never a substitute for surgical intervention to relieve increased intracranial pressure.

Abscess, breast

Definition: Acute inflammatory process resulting in the formation of a collection of pus

DIAGNOSIS

- Painful erythematous induration is present occasionally with draining through the overlying skin or nipple opening.
- Incision and drainage and culture and sensitivity of abscess content are diagnostic procedures.
- Ten percent to 30% of breast abscesses are lactational.
- Acute mastitis occurs in 2.5% of nursing mothers.

ETIOLOGY

- **Lactational abscess:** *Staphylococcus aureus*
- **Subareolar abscess:** anaerobes, *Staphylococcus*, *Streptococcus*

TREATMENT

- **If lactational abscess:** nafcillin or oxacillin 2 g IV q4h or cefazolin 1 g IV q8h
  - **If nonpuerperal abscess:** clindamycin 300 mg PO/IV q6h plus metronidazole 7.5 mg/kg IV q6h. May substitute nafcillin, oxacillin, or cefazolin for clindamycin

CLINICAL PEARL

- If mammogram or ultrasound is prevented by discomfort, imaging should be performed after resolution.

Abscess, liver

Definition: Necrotic infection of the liver usually classified as pyogenic or amebic

DIAGNOSIS
- Right upper quadrant abdominal pain, fever, nausea, cough with pleuritic chest pain, anorexia, jaundice are often present.
- CT scan of abdomen is imaging study of choice.
- Ultrasound has 80% to 95% sensitivity.
- Laboratory results include leukocytosis, positive blood cultures (50%), prolonged international normalized ratio (70%), elevated alkaline phosphatase >90%, elevated alanine aminotransferase/aspartate aminotransferase (50%), positive stool samples for *Entamoeba histolytica* (10-15%). Serologic testing for *E. histolytica* does not differentiate acute from prior infection.
- CT-guided or ultrasound-guided aspiration (50% sterile) should be performed in suspected pyogenic abscess.

ETIOLOGY
- **Pyogenic abscess:** usually polymicrobial (*Streptococcus* [37%], *Escherichia coli* [33%], *Klebsiella pneumoniae* [18%], *Pseudomonas*, *Proteus*, *Bacteroides*)
- **Sources of pyogenic abscess:** biliary disease with cholangitis, gall-bladder disease, diverticulitis, appendicitis, penetrating wounds, hematogenous
- **Amebic abscess:** *E. histolytica*; transmission usually due to fecal-oral contamination with invasion of intestinal mucosa and portal system

TREATMENT
- Medical management is the cornerstone of therapy in amebic abscess, whereas early intervention in the form of surgical therapy or catheter drainage and parenteral antibiotics is the rule in pyogenic liver abscess.
- **Pyogenic abscess:** cefotaxime or piperacillin/tazobactam and metronidazole administered intravenously for 2 weeks followed by oral administration for 4 to 6 weeks
- **Amebic abscess:** metronidazole 750 mg PO tid for 10 days

CLINICAL PEARLS
- Most patients with pyogenic abscess defervesce within 10 days; with amebic abscess, defervescence occurs within 4 to 5 days.
- Persistent fever for 2 weeks is an indication for surgery.
- In the United States, pyogenic abscess is more common than amebic abscess. The opposite is true worldwide.

Abscess, lung

Definition: Infection of the lung parenchyma resulting in a necrotic cavity containing pus

DIAGNOSIS

- Chest x-ray reveals the cavitary lesion with an air-fluid level.
- Chest CT scan can localize and size the lesion and assist in differentiating lung abscess from other processes.
- Blood tests are not specific and rarely helpful; complete blood count with leukocytosis, blood cultures, and sputum Gram stain and culture are usually ordered.
- Fiberoptic bronchoscopy using bronchial brushings or bronchoalveolar lavage is the most widely used intervention when trying to obtain diagnostic bacteriologic cultures.
- Symptoms are generally insidious and prolonged and include fever, cough, sputum production (purulent with foul odor), and hemoptysis.
- Dullness to percussion, whispered pectoriloquy and bronchophony are helpful in diagnosis.

ETIOLOGY

- Aspiration is most common factor.
- Anaerobic microorganisms (*Bacteroides fragilis, Fusobacterium, Peptostreptococcus*) cause 90% of abscesses.
- In most cases, anaerobic infection is mixed with aerobic or facultative anaerobic organisms (*Staphylococcus aureus, Escherichia coli, Klebsiella pneumoniae, Pseudomonas aeruginosa*).
- Immunocompromised hosts may become infected with *Aspergillus, Mycobacterium, Nocardia,* and *Rhodococcus equi.*

TREATMENT

- Penicillin 1-2 million U IV q4h until improvement, followed by penicillin V potassium 500 mg qid for at least 3 weeks
- Metronidazole 7.5 mg/kg IV q6h followed by 500 mg PO bid-qid given with penicillin
- Alternative choice if penicillin resistance is a concern: clindamycin 600 mg IV q8h followed by 300 mg PO q6h

- Chest x-ray is abnormal in 50% of cases, showing elevated right hemidiaphragm, pleural effusion, and subdiaphragmatic air-fluid levels.

- Risk factors include alcoholism, seizure disorder, cerebrovascular accident with dysphagia, poor oral hygiene, bronchiectasis, obstructive lung lesions, esophageal disorders, and drug abuse.
- Cure rate is >95% with appropriate antibiotics.
- Necrotizing pneumonia is similar to lung abscess but differs in size (<2 cm in diameter) and number (usually multiple suppurative cavitary lesions).

Abscess, pelvic

Definition: Localized infection involving the pelvic viscera

DIAGNOSIS
- Clinical presentation includes abdominal or pelvic pain, fever, nausea, abnormal bleeding, and vaginal discharge.
- CT scan of pelvis is best imaging study.
- Ultrasound also is excellent (>90% sensitivity) diagnostic modality.
- Surgical diagnostic options include CT-guided drainage, laparoscopy with drainage and irrigation, transvaginal colpotomy (midline abscess), and laparotomy.
- Laboratory studies include complete blood count with differential and aerobic and anaerobic cultures of blood, cervix, urine, and peritoneal cavity (if entered) before starting antibiotics. A pregnancy test is indicated in all women of childbearing age.

ETIOLOGY
- Mixed flora of anaerobes, aerobes, and facultative anaerobes (*Escherichia coli, Bacteroides fragilis, Prevotella,* aerobic streptococci, *Peptococcus, Peptostreptococcus*)

TREATMENT
- Decision as to whether patient requires immediate surgery (uncertain diagnosis or suspicion of rupture) or management with intravenous antibiotics, reserving surgery for patients with inadequate clinical response
- Clindamycin 900 mg IV q8h or metronidazole 500 mg IV q6-8h plus gentamicin 5-7 mg/kg q24h or 1.5 mg/kg q8h
- **Alternatives:** ampicillin/sulbactam 3 g IV q6h or cefoxitin 2 g IV q6h or cefotetan 2 g IV q12h plus doxycycline 100 mg IV q12h

CLINICAL PEARLS

- *Neisseria gonorrhoeae* and *Chlamydia* are the major etiologic factors in cervicitis and salpingitis, but are rarely found in abscess cavity cultures.
- Pelvic abscess occurs in 34% of hospitalized patients with pelvic inflammatory disease.

Abscess, perirectal

Definition: Localized inflammatory process associated with infections of soft tissue and anal glands

DIAGNOSIS

- Clinical presentation includes localized perirectal or anal pain, often worsened with movement or straining; perirectal erythema or mass is found by inspection or palpation
- Laboratory studies include complete blood count with differential, local aerobic and anaerobic cultures, and blood cultures if toxic, febrile, or immunocompromised.
- Sigmoidoscopy is indicated in selected cases.
- Imaging studies (pelvic CT) usually are not indicated, unless patient has extensive disease or is immunocompromised.

ETIOLOGY

- Polymicrobial aerobic (*Staphylococcus aureus, Streptococcus, Escherichia coli*) and anaerobic (*Bacteroides fragilis, Peptostreptococcus, Prevotella, Fusobacterium*) bacteria

TREATMENT

- Incision and drainage of abscess, débridement of necrotic tissue
- **Outpatient (oral):** amoxicillin/clavulanic acid, ciprofloxacin plus metronidazole or clindamycin
- **Inpatient (intravenous):** ampicillin/sulbactam, cefotetan, piperacillin/tazobactam, imipenem

CLINICAL PEARL

- Many patients have predisposing underlying conditions (e.g., diabetes mellitus, malignancy or leukemia, immune deficiency, steroid therapy, recent surgery).

Acetaminophen poisoning

Definition: Disorder secondary to excessive acetaminophen ingestion manifested by hepatic necrosis, jaundice, somnolence, and potential death if not treated appropriately

DIAGNOSIS
- Initial laboratory evaluation consists of a plasma acetaminophen level with a second level drawn 4 to 6 hours after the initial level. Subsequent levels can be drawn every 2 to 4 hours until the levels stabilize or decline. These levels can be plotted using the Rumack-Matthew nomogram (Fig. 1) to calculate potential hepatic toxicity.
- Alanine aminotransferase, aspartate aminotransferase, prothrombin time (international normalized ratio), blood urea nitrogen, and creatinine should be obtained initially on all patients.
- Serum and urine toxicology screen for other potential toxic substances also is recommended on admission to emergency department.
- Clinical presentation varies depending on dose ingested and time from ingestion. Initially presentation includes malaise, nausea, vomiting, and diaphoresis, followed by somnolence, coma, and jaundice. After the initial 12 to 24 hours, patients also may complain of right upper quadrant pain.

TREATMENT
- Perform gastric lavage and administration of activated charcoal if the patient is seen within 1 hour of ingestion or polydrug ingestion is suspected.
- Determine blood acetaminophen level 4 hours after ingestion; if in toxic range, start N-acetyl cysteine (Mucomyst) 140 mg/kg as a loading dose followed by 70 mg/kg PO q4h for 48 hours.
- N-acetyl cysteine therapy should be started within 24 hours of acetaminophen overdose. If charcoal therapy was instituted initially, lavage the stomach and recover as much charcoal as possible, then instill N-acetyl cysteine, increasing the loading dose by 40%.
- Provide adequate intravenous hydration (e.g., dextrose 5% in half-normal saline at 150 mL/hr).
- If acetaminophen level is nontoxic, N-acetyl cysteine therapy may be discontinued.

CLINICAL PEARL
- The amount of acetaminophen necessary for hepatic toxicity varies with the patient's body size and hepatic function. A toxic dose of acetaminophen usually is >7.5 g or >140 mg/kg in adults.

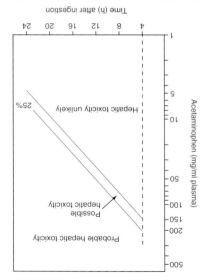

FIGURE 1. Rumack-Matthew nomogram for acetaminophen poisoning. (From Rumack BH, Matthew H: Pediatrics 1975;55:871.)

Achalasia

Definition: Motility disorder of the esophagus characterized by inadequate relaxation of the lower esophageal sphincter (LES) and ineffective peristalsis of esophageal smooth muscle, resulting in functional obstruction of the esophagus

DIAGNOSIS

- Barium swallow with fluoroscopy reveals uncoordinated or absent esophageal contractions, an acutely tapered contrast column ("bird's beak"), dilation of the distal (smooth muscle) portion of the esophagus, and esophageal air-fluid level.
- Manometry may be indicated if barium swallow is inconclusive. Manometry reveals low amplitude, disorganized contractions, high intraesophageal resting pressure, high LES pressure, and inadequate LES relaxation after swallow.
- Direct visualization by endoscopy can rule out other causes of dysphagia.
- Clinical presentation may include dysphagia to solids and liquids, difficulty belching, chest pain/heartburn, frequent hiccups, weight loss, vomiting of undigested food, and symptoms of aspiration (cough, wheezing).

ETIOLOGY

- Etiology is poorly understood; it may be due to autoimmune degeneration of the esophageal myenteric plexus. An association with the HLA class II antigen DQw1 has been noted.

TREATMENT

- **Medical:** Smooth muscle relaxants, including nitrates and calcium channel blockers, are effective in 70% of patients. Botulinum toxin injection benefits 90% of patients, but repeat injections are required.
- **Mechanical dilation:** Fixed or pneumatic dilators may benefit 90% of patients. Esophageal rupture or perforation is a rare complication.
- **Surgical:** Open and thoracoscopic esophagomyotomy are available and effective (90%). This approach currently offers the most durable symptom relief.

CLINICAL PEARL

- About 10% of patients undergoing surgery have symptomatic reflux disease. Chronic gastroesophageal reflux disease as a result of treatment may be complicated by Barrett's esophagus and malignant transformation.

Acidosis, metabolic

Definition: Disturbance of acid-base homeostasis; primary change is a decrease in serum bicarbonate secondary to factors described in etiology section

DIAGNOSIS

- **Evaluation of serum electrolytes and arterial blood gases:** Draw arterial blood gas and electrolyte samples concomitantly; evaluate the following:
  - Plasma bicarbonate (HCO_3^-)
    - Increased in metabolic alkalosis or respiratory acidosis (compensated)
    - Decreased in metabolic acidosis or respiratory alkalosis (compensated)
  - Serum potassium (K^+) ($\Delta pH\ 0.1 = \Delta K^+\ 0.6$)
    - Increased in acidemia
    - Decreased in alkalemia
  - Serum chloride (Cl^-)—compare with plasma sodium (Na^+) concentration; they should be proportionately increased or decreased if the change in Cl^- concentration is the result of a change in the hydration of the patient
    - If Cl^- is disproportionately increased, consider metabolic acidosis or respiratory alkalosis
    - If the Cl^- is disproportionately decreased, consider metabolic alkalosis or respiratory acidosis
  - Evaluate type of disturbance present by examining pH, Pco_2, and HCO_3^- (Fig. 2).
- **Calculation of the degree of compensation:** The degree of compensation is calculated to distinguish the following:
  - Simple acid-base disorders (metabolic acidosis, metabolic alkalosis, respiratory acidosis, respiratory alkalosis)—adequate compensation.
  - Mixed acid-base disorders—simultaneous presence of two or more abnormalities
  - The following formulas are used to calculate if the degree of compensation is adequate:
    - If adequate compensation, in metabolic acidosis, decrease from normal $Paco_2$ should equal 1.3 times decrease from normal HCO_3^-; usually $Paco_2$ = last 2 digits of the pH.
    - If actual $Paco_2$ is greater than calculated, metabolic acidosis and respiratory acidosis are present.

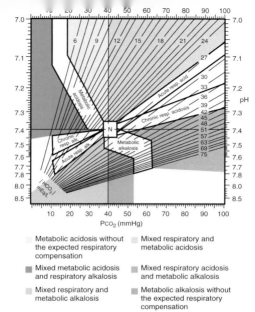

FIGURE 2. Map for acid-base disorders. (From Pulmonary Disease Section, University of Oklahoma Health Sciences Center, Oklahoma City, Oklahoma, as reprinted in Williamson JO: Acid-base disorders: Classification and management strategies. Am Fam Physician 1995;52:584-590.)

- If actual Paco₂ is less than calculated, metabolic acidosis and respiratory alkalosis are present.

ETIOLOGY

- Metabolic acidosis with increased anion gap (AG) (AG acidosis):
  - Lactic acidosis
  - Ketoacidosis (diabetes mellitus, alcoholic ketoacidosis)
  - Uremia (chronic renal failure)
  - Ingestion of toxins (paraldehyde, methanol, salicylate, ethylene glycol)
  - High-fat diet (mild acidosis)
- Metabolic acidosis with normal AG (hyperchloremic acidosis):
  - Renal tubular acidosis (including acidosis of aldosterone deficiency)
  - Intestinal loss of HCO_3^- (diarrhea, pancreatic fistula)
  - Carbonic anhydrase inhibitors (e.g., acetazolamide)
  - Dilutional acidosis (as a result of rapid infusion of bicarbonate-free isotonic saline)
  - Ingestion of exogenous acids (ammonium chloride, methionine, cystine, calcium chloride)
  - Ileostomy
  - Ureterosigmoidostomy
  - Drugs (amiloride, triamterene, spironolactone, β-blockers)

TREATMENT

- Correct underlying cause (e.g., diabetic ketoacidosis, diarrhea, uremia).
- Sodium bicarbonate (NaHCO₃) therapy generally has been given for most cases of life-threatening metabolic acidosis. Its use has become controversial, and its further administration is no longer recommended for cardiopulmonary arrest therapy or other causes of metabolic acidosis except for cases associated with severe HCO_3^- loss from gastrointestinal or genitourinary tract.

CLINICAL PEARLS

- Measurement of urinary AG ($U_{Na}^+ + U_K^+ - U_{Cl}^-$) and urinary pH is useful in the differential diagnosis of hyperchloremic metabolic acidosis:
  - Negative urinary AG suggests gastrointestinal loss of HCO_3^-.
  - Positive urinary AG suggests altered distal urinary acidification.
  - Low urinary pH and elevated plasma K⁺ in patients with positive urinary AG suggest selective aldosterone deficiency.
  - Urinary pH <5.5 and elevated plasma K⁺ suggest hyperkalemic distal renal tubular acidosis.

• Urinary pH >5.5 and normal or decreased plasma K$^+$ indicate classic renal tubular acidosis.

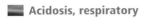 Acidosis, respiratory

Definition: Disturbance of acid-base homeostasis characterized by a primary elevation in P_{CO_2} secondary to factors described in etiology section

DIAGNOSIS

- **Evaluation of serum electrolytes and arterial blood gases:** Draw arterial blood gas and electrolyte samples concomitantly; evaluate the following:
  - Plasma bicarbonate (HCO_3^-)
    - Increased in metabolic alkalosis or respiratory acidosis (compensated)
    - Decreased in metabolic acidosis or respiratory alkalosis (compensated)
  - Serum potassium (K^+) ($\Delta pH\ 0.1 = \Delta K^+\ 0.6$).
    - Increased in acidemia
    - Decreased in alkalemia
  - Serum chloride (Cl^-)—compare with plasma sodium (Na^+) concentration; they should be proportionately increased or decreased if the change in Cl^- concentration is the result of a change in the hydration of the patient.
    - If the Cl^- is disproportionately increased, consider metabolic acidosis or respiratory alkalosis.
    - If the Cl^- is disproportionately decreased, consider metabolic alkalosis or respiratory acidosis.
  - Evaluate type of disturbance present by examining pH, P_{CO_2}, and HCO_3^-.
- **Calculation of the degree of compensation:** The degree of compensation is calculated to distinguish the following:
  - Simple acid-base disorders (metabolic acidosis, metabolic alkalosis, respiratory acidosis, respiratory alkalosis)—adequate compensation
  - Mixed acid-base disorders—simultaneous presence of two or more abnormalities
  - The following formulas are used to calculate if the degree of compensation is adequate:

- Acute—an increase in $Paco_2$ by 10 mm Hg decreases pH by 0.08 and increases HCO_3^- by 1 mEq/L; usual upper limit of compensation is $HCO_3^- = 30$ mEq/L.
- Chronic—an increase in $Paco_2$ by 10 mm Hg decreases pH by 0.03 and increases HCO_3^- by 3.5 mEq/L; usual upper limit of compensation is $HCO_3^- = 55$ mEq/L.
- Evaluation of type of disturbance present by examining pH, Pco_2, and HCO_3^- is illustrated in Figure 2 on Page 11.

ETIOLOGY

- Pulmonary disease (chronic obstructive pulmonary disease, severe pneumonia, pulmonary edema, interstitial fibrosis)
- Airway obstruction (foreign body, severe bronchospasm, laryngospasm)
- Thoracic cage disorders (pneumothorax, flail chest, kyphoscoliosis)
- Defects in muscles of respiration (myasthenia gravis, hypokalemia, muscular dystrophy)
- Defects in peripheral nervous system (amyotrophic lateral sclerosis, poliomyelitis, Guillain-Barré syndrome, botulism, tetanus, organophosphate poisoning, spinal cord injury)
- Depression of respiratory center (anesthesia, narcotics, sedatives, vertebral artery embolism or thrombosis, increased intracranial pressure)
- Failure of mechanical ventilator

TREATMENT

- Correction of underlying etiology

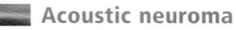 **Acoustic neuroma**

Definition: Benign proliferation of Schwann cells that cover the vestibular branch of the eighth cranial nerve

DIAGNOSIS

- Clinical presentation includes unilateral hearing loss or tinnitus or both, balance problems, vertigo, facial pain (trigeminal neuralgia) and weakness, difficulty swallowing, and fullness or pain of the involved ear.
- MRI with gadolinium is best imaging test.

ETIOLOGY

- Etiology is poorly understood, but long-term exposure to acoustic trauma has been implicated.

neuromas may be inherited in an autosomal dominant manner as part of neurofibromatosis type 2.

TREATMENT
- Treatment decisions vary with size of tumor, rate of growth, degree of neurologic deficit, life expectancy, age of patient, and surgical risk.
- Surgery is the definitive treatment.
- Proton-beam radiotherapy can be used for tumors <3 cm in diameter.

CLINICAL PEARL
- Hearing loss is the most common presenting complaint and is usually high frequency.

▨ Acquired immunodeficiency syndrome (AIDS)

Definition: Disorder caused by infection with human immunodeficiency virus type 1 (HIV-1) and marked by progressive deterioration of the cellular immune system, leading to secondary infections and malignancies

DIAGNOSIS
- Three HIV viral antibody screening tests currently are in use:
  - ELISA:
    - Bound anti-HIV antibody is detected by antihuman antibody labeled with an enzyme. The use of recombinant proteins has reduced false-positive results (specificity 99.9%).
    - False-negative test may result when measured in the acute infection period (sensitivity 99.9%).
  - New rapid serologic-screening assays include HIV antigen–coated gelatin or latex particle agglutination assays. The single-use test can be performed rapidly, but may be less sensitive and specific than standard ELISA tests.
  - A Food and Drug Administration–approved oral salivary test called OraSure (sensitivity 99.9%) is sent to a reference laboratory after being inserted into the mouth for 2 minutes.
- Western blot confirmatory test is performed when ELISA is positive. This test identifies specific viral antigens; it is positive when core and envelope antigens are present. The result is indeterminate when either antigen is present; if unchanged when repeated in 6 months in more than one laboratory, this is considered a false-positive result.

- The 1993 Centers for Disease Control and Prevention case definition of AIDS includes HIV-infected people with a CD4 cell count <200/mm^3 or <14% of the total lymphocytes and an indicator illness.

ETIOLOGY

- Infection with HIV-1

TREATMENT

- **Management strategies for asymptomatic patients:**
  - **Initial testing:** CD4 cell count and HIV viral load measured every 3 to 6 months to guide decisions regarding antiretroviral use and prophylaxis against *Pneumocystis carinii* pneumonia (PCP) and *Mycobacterium avium* complex (MAC) infection.
  - **Other testing:** identifies previously acquired latent infections that may become reactivated because of loss of T-cell function but can be prevented by the use of specific agents.
    - Serology to *Toxoplasma gondii* (IgG)
      - Clinical infection may be prevented by trimethoprim-sulfamethoxazole (TMP-SMZ) used as prophylaxis for PCP.
    - Venereal Disease Research Laboratories (VDRL) test
      - Lumbar puncture should be performed in patients with a confirmatory specific test (fluorescent treponemal antibody).
      - Treat with intramuscular benzathine penicillin if the cerebrospinal fluid (CSF) formula is normal and intravenous penicillin for 10 days if there is reactive CSF VDRL, pleocytosis, protein elevation, or hypoglycorrhachia.
    - Purified protein derivative (PPD) skin test showing induration of ≥5 mm, or patients with exposure to someone with active tuberculosis
      - Treat with isoniazid 300 mg/day for 9 months or, if isoniazid-induced hepatitis, rifampin 600 mg PO qd (only for patients not receiving (protease inhibitors [PIs] or nonnucleotide reverse transcriptase inhibitors [NNRTI]) for 4 months.
  - Immunizations
    - Patients should receive an annual influenza vaccine in the fall.
    - Pneumococcal polysaccharide vaccine (Pneumovax) is recommended for all persons with HIV infection and is most effective in patients with CD4 counts >200/mm^3.
    - Hepatitis B virus vaccine is recommended for persons who have no evidence of prior infection with hepatitis B and who are at risk for acquiring it. They also should receive hepatitis A vaccine.
    - Tetanus-diphtheria vaccine boosters should be given every 10 years.
    - Mumps and rubella vaccines are recommended for susceptible adults.

- Treatment for several opportunistic infections may be discontinued if there has been a sustained highly active antiretroviral therapy (HAART)–associated CD4 cell count elevation >200/mm³ (PCP, toxoplasmosis, cryptococcosis and >100/mm³ for MAC) for >3 to 6 months. Primary prophylaxis against each of these opportunistic infections should be reintroduced if the CD4 count decreases below this range.
  - PCP prophylaxis (CD4 count <200/mm³)
    - TMP-SMZ 1 double-strength qd is most effective agent; it also provides protection against infections due to *Toxoplasma gondii, Nocardia,* and enteric pathogens.
      - Adverse reactions to TMP-SMZ (gastrointestinal distress, fever, rash, and leukopenia) occur in 40% to 60%; discontinuation of drug may be necessary.
      - Oral dose escalating regimens may be tried in patients with TMP-SMZ-associated rash that is not Stevens-Johnson syndrome or toxic epidermal necrolysis.
    - Dapsone is indicated in patients with TMP-SMZ toxicity or who fail TMP-SMZ desensitization; 30% of persons with TMP-SMZ rash develop a reaction to dapsone.
    - Aerosolized pentamidine 300 mg/mo is less effective than TMP-SMZ or dapsone in reducing the incidence of PCP in persons with CD4 counts <100/mm³.
    - Atovaquone 750 mg bid may be considered if the patient is unable to tolerate other prophylactic regimens.
  - Prophylaxis against MAC in patients with CD4 cell counts <75/mm³
    - Azithromycin 1200 mg weekly is the most effective agent in preventing MAC. Emergence of resistant strains may occur with azithromycin (11%).
    - Mycobacterial blood culture for MAC should be drawn and return negative before initiating prophylaxis against MAC.
  - Prophylaxis against *Cryptococcus* (oral fluconazole) and cytomegalovirus (CMV) (oral ganciclovir) is not indicated because neither regimen reduces mortality, both are costly, and they may cause emergence of resistant strains.
- **Highly active antiretroviral therapy:**
  - Treatment goals are maximal and durable suppression of viral loads (<50 copies/mL), restoration of immunologic function (CD4 cell count), and reduction of HIV-related morbidity and mortality.
  - The accepted HAART regimens use 16 licensed agents in combination among three classes: nucleoside reverse transcriptase

inhibitors (NRTIs), NNRTIs, and PIs. HAART should be offered as initial therapy to asymptomatic, antiviral-naive patients with CD4 count <350/mm^3 or whose HIV viral load is >55,000. Before starting treatment, CD4 and HIV viral load values should be repeated because of variations in laboratory values. HAART is indicated for all symptomatic persons and patients with acute HIV infection. After initiating HAART, CD4 counts and viral loads should be measured at 1 and 4 months. The criteria used to assess initial HAART efficacy are:

- Greater than 1.0 log reduction in HIV viral load within 4 weeks
- An undetectable viral load (HIV RNA <50 copies/mL) within 4 months

- Subsequently, CD4 counts and viral loads should be measured every 3 to 4 months. The criteria used to assess the long-term durability of HAART are maintenance of an undetectable HIV viral load and prevention of CD4 deterioration.

- **Treatment of symptomatic patients with AIDS-defining illness:**
  - **Fungal disorders:**
    - ***Candida* (thrush):** Treat with clotrimazole troches five times per day for 10 days; refractory cases may require 10 days of oral fluconazole 100 mg/day.
    - **Esophagitis:** Treat with fluconazole 100 mg PO bid for 3 weeks.
    - ***Cryptococcus neoformans:*** Initial therapy is with amphotericin B 0.7 mg/kg/day for 2 weeks with adjunctive flucytosine 100 mg/kg/day, unless preexisting cytopenias prohibit its use. Serum flucytosine levels must be monitored. Oral fluconazole therapy 200-400 mg/day prevents relapse after initial management of infection with amphotericin B; fluconazole therapy is needed indefinitely.
  - **Coccidioidomycosis:**
    - Patients should avoid activities associated with increased risk (disturbed native soil, dust storms) in endemic areas.
    - After initial therapy for coccidioidomycosis, lifelong suppressive therapy is recommended with fluconazole 400 mg PO qd or itraconazole 200 mg PO bid.
    - Fluconazole and itraconazole have potential teratogenicity in pregnant women. Consider amphotericin B (preferred), especially during the first trimester. All HIV-positive women on azole therapy for coccidioidomycosis should maintain birth control precautions.
  - **Histoplasmosis:**
    - HIV-infected individuals living in or visiting areas endemic for histoplasmosis with CD4 count <200/mm^3 should avoid activities

... increased risks (surface soil dust, contact with chicken droppings, cave exposure).

- Initial therapy for histoplasmosis may include itraconazole rather than amphotericin in non–fulminantly ill patients; lifelong maintenance therapy is with itraconazole 200 mg PO bid.

- **PCP:**
  - **Oral regimens:** Treatment in mild cases can be given orally ($Po_2 > 70$ mm Hg, alveolar-arterial (A-a) gradient <35 mm Hg) for 3-week course.
    - TMP-SMZ (Bactrim DS, Septra DS)—TMP 15 mg/kg/day in three divided doses (5-7 tablets per day)
    - TMP/dapsone—trimethoprim 15 mg/kg/day and dapsone 100 mg/day (need to rule out glucose-6-phosphate dehydrogenase [G6PD] deficiency with dapsone)
    - Primaquine/clindamycin—primaquine 30 mg/day (also need to exclude G6PD deficiency) and clindamycin 450 mg PO qid
    - Atovaquone: 750 mg PO tid (may be less effective than TMP-SMZ)
  - **Intravenous regimens:** Treatment needs to be given intravenously in patients with moderate-to-severe infections ($Po_2 <70$ mm Hg, A-a gradient >35 mm Hg) or patients who cannot tolerate oral regimens.
    - TMP-SMZ—TMP 15 mg/kg/day in three individual doses
    - Pentamidine—3 mg/kg/day; may need to observe for hypotension, pancreatitis, and hypoglycemia
    - Trimetrexate—45 mg/m^2 once daily for patients intolerant or refractory to TMP-SMZ or pentamidine; must be given with leucovorin, which is given 72 hours beyond trimetrexate therapy to prevent potential bone marrow, gastrointestinal, renal, and hepatic dysfunction
    - Adjunctive corticosteroid therapy is indicated when Po_2 is <70 mm Hg or alveolar-arterial gradient is >35 mm Hg to prevent early deterioration of oxygenation by decreasing inflammation.
    - Other opportunistic infections (tuberculosis, fungal) must be excluded; prednisone is given, 40 mg bid days 1 to 5, 40 mg/day for 6 to 10 days, tapering over 21-day course of therapy.
    - There is a risk of reactivation of latent infection (CMV, histoplasmosis, tuberculosis) with steroid use.
- **Tuberculosis:**
  - Tuberculosis may cause pulmonary involvement or extrapulmonic involvement or both. Extrapulmonic involvement may

include meningitis, lymphadenitis, or peritonitis. With more advanced disease (CD4 <200/mm³), there may be atypical chest x-ray findings, possibly involving the lower lobes.

Caution is required for the use of tuberculosis medications and HAART. Rifampin should be substituted with rifabutin with the use of PIs and NRTIs. Saquinavir hard-gel should not be given with rifabutin. PIs (indinavir, nelfinavir, amprenavir) require dosage modifications; their use should be avoided with delavirdine.

HIV-infected pregnant women with positive PPD or exposure to active tuberculosis should be considered for chemoprophylaxis. Isoniazid with pyridoxine is recommended treatment. Starting treatment after the first trimester should be considered to avoid teratogenicity.

MAC:

- Combination therapy is with at least two agents. Addition of a third agent (rifabutin) may be considered.
- Clarithromycin 500 mg PO bid (azithromycin 500 mg/day PO is alternative)
- Ethambutol 15 mg/kg/day PO
- Medications to be considered in patients who have had relapsing disease are rifabutin, ciprofloxacin, and amikacin. Rifabutin 300 mg or ciprofloxacin 500–750 mg bid can be used as third agents. Intravenous amikacin 10–15 mg/kg/day and clofazimine 100 mg/day are alternatives for critically ill or nonresponding patients.
- *Salmonella* (species)—recurrent bacteremia: treat with ampicillin, TMP-SMZ, ciprofloxacin, or third-generation cephalosporin, based on sensitivities and clinical presentation. Gastrointestinal symptoms may not be present. Raw or undercooked eggs, poultry, meat, and seafood should be avoided.
- Listeriosis—in HIV-infected individuals who are severely immunosuppressed. Soft cheeses and ready-to-eat foods (hot dogs, cold cuts) should be avoided or heated until steaming hot.
- Sinusitis—may be routine bacterial infection or involve *Pseudomonas aeruginosa* or fungi.
- Bacillary angiomatosis—an infection involving skin, with red lesions that can be mistaken for Kaposi sarcoma (KS); can involve viscera (liver, spleen, bone); caused by *Rochalimaea henselae* or *Rochalimaea quintana*. Treatment is with erythromycin or doxycycline. Other potential bacterial pathogens in HIV are *Rhodococcus equi*, which may cause cavitating pneumonia, and *Nocardia*.

... **simplex virus (HSV):**

- HSV may involve mucous membranes, cause genital herpes, or cause rectal or perirectal infection, resulting in proctitis.
- Initial treatment is with acyclovir 200 mg PO five times per day for 7 to 10 days; recurrent episodes may need treatment with 400 mg PO three to five times a day for 5 to 7 days or until clinically resolved. Severe disease involving lung, bronchi, and esophagus may require intravenous acyclovir. Intravenous foscarnet or cidofovir can be used to treat infection caused by acyclovir-resistant isolates of HSV.

- **Hepatitis C virus (HCV):**
  - Patients with HIV infection should be tested for HCV by using enzyme immunoassay. If this test is positive, results should be confirmed with recombinant immunoblot assay or polymerase chain reaction for HCV RNA.
  - Patients with HCV and HIV should receive vaccination for hepatitis A if hepatitis A antibody negative.
  - Patients with HIV/HCV coinfection are at high risk for chronic liver disease and should be evaluated for treatment by providers with experience in treating HIV and HCV.

- **CMV:**
  - Infection from CMV may cause illness involving the retina, gastrointestinal tract (e.g., esophagus, colon), and central nervous system.
  - **Choreoretinitis:** This condition may develop in 25% of AIDS patients and may be unilateral, with viremia involving other organs; the patient usually complains of decreased vision or "floaters." Ophthalmologic evaluation may be necessary to confirm the diagnosis.
  - **Esophagitis:** Deep ulcerations are seen, confirmed by presence of inclusion bodies by biopsy.
  - **Colitis:** Colitis usually is associated with diarrhea, weight loss, and fever; it occurs in approximately 10% of AIDS patients.
  - **Central nervous system encephalitis or polyradiculopathy (areflexic paraplegia):** Three agents are available for treatment. Treatment may be discontinued if HAART-restored CD4 cell counts are >200.
    - Ganciclovir implant is effective in delaying progression of retinitis. Oral valganciclovir is used to prevent systemic manifestations of disease.
    - Ganciclovir induction dose, 5 mg/kg bid for 14 days, followed by 5 mg/kg/day indefinitely for retinitis; may cause granulocytopenia or neutropenia related to dose, which is compounded

by use of zidovudine and possibly by other antiretroviral medications.

- Foscarnet induction dose, 60 mg/kg IV q8h for 2 to 3 weeks; dosing depends on creatinine clearance and requires adjustment; maintenance therapy is 90–120 mg/kg q24h.
- Cidofovir 5 mg/kg weekly for 2 weeks, then every other week as maintenance.

Progressive multifocal leukoencephalopathy is a demyelinating disease most often involving the posterior cortex of the brain, resulting in slowly progressive cognitive impairments. Clinical and radiologic improvement or in some cases complete resolution may occur with HAART-associated restoration of CD4 cell counts.

- **Toxoplasmosis:**

  Pyrimethamine plus sulfadiazine—pyrimethamine 100–200 mg loading dose, followed by 50 mg/day PO; sulfadiazine 1–1.5 g PO q6h as initial treatment, followed by maintenance dose pyrimethamine 25 mg/day and sulfadiazine 500 mg q6h.
  Clindamycin 600–1200 mg IV or 600 mg PO q6 (2.4 g/day) and pyrimethamine 50 mg/day PO.
  Atovaquone, TMP-SMZ, and macrolides may have anti-*Toxoplasma* properties and can be considered as alternative treatments.

- **Additional parasites:**
  - **Cryptosporidiosis:** There is no effective therapy for this protozoal infection in HIV-infected patients, although nitazoxanide has been used in immunocompetent patients. Azithromycin, when taken for MAC prophylaxis, may reduce the risk for cryptosporidiosis.
  - **Isosporiasis:** Treatment with TMP-SMZ 1 double-strength tablet qid for 10 days is followed by maintenance.
  - **Microsporidiosis:** Treatment with albendazole 400 mg bid is effective only against certain species; atovaquone is effective against others.

- **Cancers associated with HIV infection:**
  - **KS:** KS is found most often in HIV-infected homosexual men and less frequently (<5%) in patients in other HIV risk groups. The lesions from KS may be multifocal, involving skin (79%), lymph nodes (70%), gastrointestinal tract (43%), and lungs (10%). Treatment is based on extent of involvement. Intralesional vinblastine and radiation is recommended for localized or small numbers of lesions, and chemotherapy with vincristine and vinblastine, etoposide, or bleomycin is

recommended for aggressive and disseminated disease. Use of many interleukins, tumor necrosis factor, and pentoxifylline is investigational.

- **Non-Hodgkin lymphoma:** Non-Hodgkin lymphoma is a B-cell tumor associated with Epstein-Barr virus; it is most often extra-nodal, and 30% may occur in patients with CD4 cell counts >200/mm³. The gastrointestinal tract, central nervous system, bone marrow, or liver (or other viscera in smaller percentages) may be affected. Regimens of M-BACOD (methotrexate, bleomycin, Adriamycin, cyclophosphamide, Oncovin, dexamethasone) have approximately 50% response. Dose-limiting multiagent therapy is myelosuppression.
- **Primary central nervous system lymphoma:** Most lymphomas occur in patients with a CD4 count <200/mm³, but one third occur with CD4 counts >200/mm³. Most are unifocal ring-enhancing mass lesions that cause focal neurologic deficits or seizures. Brain biopsy establishes diagnosis.
- **AIDS-related cervical cancer:** Cervical cancer is associated with human papillomavirus; it occurs often in patients with multiple sexual partners and possibly is related to primary association of HIV to cancer development.
- **Hodgkin's lymphoma:** Hodgkin's lymphoma may occur in a patient who is an intravenous drug abuser or who has sexually acquired disease. Epstein-Barr virus may be linked to Hodgkin's lymphoma; the virus usually is present with disseminated stage III or stage IV disease involving bone marrow (50%) or liver and lungs.
- **Anal carcinoma** is associated with human papillomavirus and impaired immunity; risk is increased in homosexual men.

Acromegaly

Definition: Chronic disorder resulting from the effects of either hypersecretion of growth hormone (GH) or increased amounts of insulin-like growth factor I (IGF-I)

DIAGNOSIS
- Elevated serum IGF-1 is best initial screening test.
- Failure to suppress serum GH to <2 ng/mL after 100 g of oral glucose is considered conclusive.
- GH-releasing hormone level >300 ng/mL indicates an ectopic source of GH.

- Baseline laboratory studies may reveal elevated serum phosphate and elevated urine calcium.
- MRI of pituitary and hypothalamus is the best diagnostic imaging study.
- Clinical presentation includes prognathism; history of increased hat, glove, and shoe size; coarse features resulting from growth of soft tissue; headache; arthralgias; muscle weakness; hypertension; visual field defects; and carpal tunnel syndrome.

ETIOLOGY

- Pituitary adenoma affecting anterior lobe
- Ectopic production of GH-releasing hormone from a carcinoid or other neuroendocrine tumor

TREATMENT

- Transsphenoidal microsurgical adenectomy is treatment of choice.
- Irradiation can be used to reduce tumor growth further.
- Medical therapy is indicated when patients have failed surgery, when surgery is contraindicated, or while waiting for effects of radiotherapy to begin.
- Medical therapy consists of the following agents: octreotide (somatostatin analogue), bromocriptine (dopamine analogue), or pegvisomant (GH receptor antagonist).

 Actinomycosis

Definition: Infection caused by anaerobic or microaerophilic bacteria that normally colonize the mouth, vagina, and colon, characterized by the formation of painful abscesses, soft tissue infiltration, and draining sinuses

DIAGNOSIS

- Diagnosis requires obtaining specimens by aspirating abscesses, excising sinus tracts, or performing tissue biopsies.
- Cervicofacial disease presents with painful soft tissue swelling at the angle of the mandible and generally occurs in the setting of poor dental hygiene, recent dental surgery or minor oral trauma.
- Thoracic disease can involve the lungs, pleura, mediastinum, or chest wall secondary to aspiration of Actinomyces organisms in patients with poor oral hygiene.
- Abdominal disease frequently affects the ileocecal valve and occurs most commonly after appendectomy, perforated bowel, diverticulitis, or surgery to the gastrointestinal tract.

lating nests of *Actinomyces* species ("sulfur granules") from tissue specimens or draining sinuses confirms the diagnosis.
- CT scan of head, chest, abdomen, and pelvic areas is useful in localizing site and spread of infection.

ETIOLOGY
- Most commonly *Actinomyces israelii*

TREATMENT
- Penicillin 10-20 million U/day IV in four divided doses for 4 to 6 weeks followed by oral penicillin V 500 mg PO qid for 6 to 12 months

CLINICAL PEARLS
- Actinomycosis infections are polymicrobial, usually associated with *Streptococcus, Bacteroides, Eikenella corrodens, Enterococcus,* and *Fusobacterium.*
- There is no person-to-person transmission of *Actinomyces.*

Acute respiratory distress syndrome (ARDS)

Definition: A form of noncardiogenic pulmonary edema that results from acute damage to the alveoli. The definition of ARDS includes the following components: a ratio of Pao_2 to fraction of inspired oxygen (Fio_2) ≤ 200, regardless of the level of positive end-expiratory pressure (PEEP); the detection of bilateral pulmonary infiltrates on the frontal chest x-ray; pulmonary artery wedge pressure ≤ 18 mm Hg or no clinical evidence of elevated left atrial pressure on the basis of the chest radiograph and other clinical data

DIAGNOSIS
- **Chest x-ray:** Bilateral interstitial infiltrates usually are seen within 24 hours; they often are more prominent in the bases and periphery. Near-total "whiteout" of both lung fields can be seen in advanced stages.
- **Arterial blood gases:** Initially: varying degrees of hypoxemia, generally resistant to supplemental oxygen, are present. Subsequently, respiratory alkalosis, decreased Pco_2, and widened alveolar-arterial gradient. Hypercapnia occurs as the disease progresses.
- **Hemodynamic monitoring (when indicated):** Although no hemodynamic profile is *diagnostic* of ARDS, the presence of pulmonary edema, a high cardiac output, and a low pulmonary artery wedge pressure are characteristic of ARDS.

ETIOLOGY

- Sepsis (>40% of cases)
- Aspiration (e.g., near-drowning, aspiration of gastric contents [>30% of cases])
- Trauma (>20% of cases)
- Multiple transfusions, blood products
- Drugs (e.g., overdose of morphine, methadone, heroin, reaction to nitrofurantoin)
- Noxious inhalation (e.g., chlorine gas, high oxygen concentration)
- Postresuscitation
- Cardiopulmonary bypass
- Pneumonia, tuberculosis
- Burns
- Pancreatitis

TREATMENT

- Identification and treatment of precipitating condition
  - Blood and urine cultures and trial of antibiotics in presumed sepsis (routine administration of antibiotics in all cases of ARDS is not recommended)
  - Stabilization of bone fractures in patients with major trauma
  - Bowel rest and crystalloid resuscitation in pancreatitis
- **Ventilatory support:** Mechanical ventilation generally is necessary to maintain adequate gas exchange. Assist-control generally is preferred initially with the following ventilator settings:
  - FIO_2—1.0 (until a lower value can be used to achieve adequate oxygenation). When possible, minimize oxygen toxicity by maintaining FIO_2 at <60%
  - Tidal volume—set initial tidal volume at 5 to 6 mL/kg of body weight. Aim to maintain plateau pressure at <30 mm Hg
- **PEEP:** ≥5 cm H_2O (to increase lung volume and keep alveoli open)
  - Inspiratory flow—60 L/min
  - Ventilatory rate—high ventilatory rates of >20 to 25 breaths/min are often necessary in patients with ARDS because of their increased physiologic dead space and smaller lung volumes
- **Fluid management:** Optimal fluid management is patient specific. Swan-Ganz catheterization may be indicated and is useful to guide fluid replacement. A pulmonary capillary wedge pressure of approximately 12 mm Hg is ideal.
- Deep venous thrombosis prophylaxis
- Stress ulcer prophylaxis with sucralfate suspension (via nasogastric tube) or intravenous proton-pump inhibitors or intravenous H_2 blockers

- A prior history of chronic alcohol abuse significantly increases the risk of developing ARDS in critically ill patients.

Acute tubular necrosis (ATN)

Definition: Acute injury to the tubules of the kidneys. The term *tubulointerstitial nephropathy* refers to damage to the tubules and interstitium. Because these structures are intimately related, initial damage to either one generally progresses to affect the other.

DIAGNOSIS

- Serial increases in creatinine (Cr) and blood urea nitrogen (BUN) vary with catabolic rate and protein intake.
- Oliguria or nonoliguria occurs, but outputs are relatively fixed.
- Response to high-dose furosemide is variable; it may allow diuresis but does not change the underlying lesion.
- Pulmonary vascular congestion and hyperkalemia are the most important parameters to monitor fluid status. A pulmonary artery catheter may be necessary to monitor fluid status.
- Urinary sodium is high (generally >30 mEq/day).
- Urinary osmolarity is <350 mOsm/kg and generally fixed (±300 mOsm/kg).
- Urinary Cr is low in relation to urinary volume, leading to a urine-to-plasma Cr ratio <20.
- Fractional excretion of sodium is >1.
- Urinary sediment contains "muddy-brown" renal tubular casts.
- Myoglobinuria and serum creatine phosphokinase are elevated in rhabdomyolysis.
- Polyuric phase often heralds healing.

ETIOLOGY

- **Perfusional deficits:** prolonged prerenal failure, shock, hypovolemia, sepsis, pancreatitis, low-output states, coronary artery bypass graft surgery, aortic aneurysm repair
- **Pigment nephropathy:** myoglobinuria (rhabdomyolysis), hemoglobinuria
- **Contrast-agent toxicity:**
  - **Drug toxicity:** aminoglycosides, cisplatin, pentamidine, lithium, amphotericin
  - **Crystal-induced acute renal failure:** acyclovir, sulfonamides, methotrexate, oxalate from ethylene glycol ingestion or high dose of vitamin C

- **Uric acid deposition:** in the tumor lysis syndrome
- The acute reduction in glomerular filtration rate lead to delta increases in Cr (2+ mg/day), a low urine-to-plasma Cr ratio (<20), oliguric or nonoliguric urinary volumes, threatening hyperkalemia, and pulmonary vascular congestion.

TREATMENT

- Most patients with acute renal failure recover with conservative management (fluid monitoring, protein restriction, drug adjustments, and dietary or Kayexalate potassium control).
- Dialysis, usually (fluid monitoring) may become necessary.
- Because the hemodynamic stress associated with hemodialysis can be additionally detrimental to renal function, the decision to start dialysis must weigh the acute needs against anticipated stabilization.
- Continuous hemofiltration or continuous hemodialysis conceptually is preferable to intermittent dialysis in an unstable renal failure patient in the ICU, but data are conflicting.
- Given an intact peritoneal surface, acute percutaneous peritoneal dialysis can stabilize BUN/Cr and control fluid balance in selected patients.

CLINICAL PEARLS

- Renal dopamine infusion (1.5 μg/kg/min) often is ordered, but acts primarily as an additional natriuretic agent and does not alter outcome of ATN.
- For prevention of ATN from radiocontrast agents, sodium chloride given before hydration is the best proven prophylactic measure. N-acetyl cysteine administration also reduces toxicity in high-risk patients.

■ Addison's disease (primary adrenocortical insufficiency)

Definition: Disorder characterized by inadequate secretion of corticosteroids resulting from partial or complete destruction of the adrenal glands

DIAGNOSIS

- Perform rapid adrenocorticotropin hormone (ACTH) (cosyntropin) test: Administer 250 μg of ACTH by intravenous push, and measure cortisol level at 0, 30, and 60 minutes. Cortisol level < 18 μg/dL at 30 minutes or 60 minutes suggests adrenal insufficiency. Measure plasma

...high level indicates primary adrenal insufficiency; a normal or low level indicates secondary adrenal insufficiency.

- Laboratory test results show increased potassium; decreased sodium and chloride; decreased glucose; increased blood urea nitrogen-to-creatinine ratio (prerenal azotemia); mild normocytic, normochromic anemia; neutropenia; lymphocytosis; eosinophilia (significant dehydration may mask the hyponatremia and anemia); decreased 24-hour urinary cortisol, 17-hydroxycorticosteroid, and 17-ketosteroid; and increased ACTH (if primary adrenocortical insufficiency).
- Clinical presentation includes hyperpigmentation, hypotension, generalized weakness, and amenorrhea and loss of axillary hair in women.

ETIOLOGY

- Autoimmune destruction of the adrenals (80% of cases)
- Tuberculosis (15% of cases)
- Carcinomatous destruction of the adrenals
- Adrenal hemorrhage (anticoagulants, trauma, coagulopathies, pregnancy, sepsis)
- Adrenal infarction (arteritis, thrombosis)
- AIDS (adrenal insufficiency develops in 30% of patients with advanced AIDS)
- **Other:** sarcoidosis, amyloidosis, postoperative, fungal infection, megestrol acetate therapy

TREATMENT

- Chronic adrenocortical insufficiency
  - Treat with hydrocortisone 15-20 mg PO every morning and 5-10 mg in late afternoon or prednisone 5 mg in morning and 2.5 mg at bedtime.
  - Mineralocorticoid replacement with oral fludrocortisone 0.05-0.20 mg/day is necessary if the patient has primary adrenocortical insufficiency. The dosage is adjusted based on the serum sodium level and the presence of postural hypotension or marked orthostasis.
  - Monitor serum electrolytes, vital signs, and body weight periodically; advise liberal sodium intake.
  - The administration of dehydroepiandrosterone 50 mg PO qd improves well-being and sexuality in women with adrenal insufficiency.
- **Addisonian crisis:** acute complications of adrenal insufficiency characterized by circulatory collapse, dehydration, nausea, vomiting, hypoglycemia, and hyperkalemia
  - Draw plasma cortisol level; do not delay therapy until confirming laboratory results are obtained.

- Administer hydrocortisone 50-100 mg IV q6h for 24 hours; if patient shows good clinical response, gradually taper dosage and change to oral maintenance dose (usually prednisone 7.5 mg/day).
- Provide adequate volume replacement with 5% dextrose in normal saline solution until hypotension, dehydration, and hypoglycemia are completely corrected. Large volumes (2-3 L) may be necessary in the first 2 to 3 hours to correct the volume deficit and hypoglycemia and to avoid further hyponatremia.
- Identify and correct any precipitating factor (e.g., sepsis, hemorrhage).

CLINICAL PEARL
- Patients should be instructed to increase glucocorticoid replacement in times of stress and to receive parenteral glucocorticoids if diarrhea or vomiting occurs.

Alcohol withdrawal

Definition: Syndrome that occurs when a person stops ingesting alcohol after prolonged consumption. Symptoms vary depending on the severity of the patient's alcohol abuse and the time interval from the patient's previous alcohol ingestion.

DIAGNOSIS
- **Tremulous state:** early alcohol withdrawal, "impending DTs," "shakes," "jitters"
  - **Time interval:** usually occurs 6 to 8 hours after the last drink or 12 to 48 hours after reduction of alcohol intake; becomes most pronounced at 24 to 36 hours.
  - **Manifestation:** tremors, mild agitation, insomnia, tachycardia; symptoms are relieved by alcohol.
- **Alcoholic hallucinosis:** usually auditory hallucinations, but occasionally hallucinations are visual, tactile, or olfactory; usually there is no clouding of sensorium as in delirium (clinical presentation may be mistaken for an acute schizophrenic episode). Disordered perceptions become most pronounced after 24 to 36 hours of abstinence.
- **Withdrawal seizures ("rum fits")**
  - **Time interval:** usually occurs 7 to 30 hours after cessation of drinking, with a peak incidence between 13 and 24 hours.
  - **Manifestations:** generalized convulsions with loss of consciousness; focal signs usually are absent; consider further investigation with CT scan of head and electroencephalogram if clearly indicated (e.g., presence of focal neurologic deficits, prolonged postic-

altered mental state, a lumbar puncture is necessary.

- **Delirium tremens (DTs)**
  - **Time interval:** variable; usually occurs within 1 week after reduction or cessation of heavy alcohol intake and persists for 1 to 3 days. Peak incidence is 72 to 96 hours after cessation of alcohol consumption.
  - **Manifestations:** profound confusion, tremors, vivid visual and tactile hallucinations, autonomic hyperactivity; this is the most serious clinical presentation of alcohol withdrawal (mortality is approximately 15% in untreated patients).

TREATMENT

- **Inpatient treatment:** Admit to medical floor (private room); monitor vital signs every 4 hours; institute seizure precautions; maintain adequate sedation.
- Administer lorazepam as follows:
  - In patients with DTs, lorazepam is administered initially, 2-5 mg IM or IV, and repeated as needed. In stable patients, oral administration may be sufficient:
    - Day 1—2 mg PO q4h while awake and not lethargic
    - Day 2—1 mg PO q4h while awake and not lethargic
    - Day 3—0.5 mg PO q4h while awake and not lethargic
  - In patients with mild-to-moderate withdrawal and without history of seizures, individualized benzodiazepine administration (rather than a fixed-dose regimen) results in lower benzodiazepine administration and avoids unnecessary sedation. The Clinical Institute Withdrawal Assessment–Alcohol (CIWA-A) scale can be used to measure the severity of alcohol withdrawal. It consists of the following items: nausea; tremor; autonomic hyperactivity; anxiety; agitation; tactile, visual, and auditory disturbances; headache; and disorientation. The maximum score is 67. When the CIWA-A score is ≥8, patients are usually given 2-4 mg of lorazepam hourly.
- **β-Adrenergic blockers:** β-Blockers are useful for controlling blood pressure and tachyarrhythmias. They do not prevent progression to more serious symptoms of withdrawal, however, and if used, they should not be administered alone but in conjunction with benzodiazepines. β-Blockers should be avoided in patients with contraindications to their use (e.g., bronchospasm, bradycardia).
- **Vitamin replacement:** thiamine 100 mg IV or IM for at least 5 days, plus oral multivitamins. The intravenous administration of glucose can precipitate Wernicke's encephalopathy in alcoholics with thiamine deficiency; thiamine administration should precede intravenous dextrose.

- **Hydration, oral or intravenous (high-caloric solution):** The intravenous solution should consist of glucose with sodium, potassium, magnesium, and phosphate replacement as needed.
- Withdrawal seizures can be treated with diazepam 2.5 mg/min IV until seizure is controlled (check for respiratory depression or hypotension); lorazepam 1-2 mg IV every 2 hours can be used in place of diazepam. Generally, withdrawal seizures are self-limited, and treatment is not required. The use of phenytoin or other anticonvulsants for short-term treatment of alcohol withdrawal seizures is not recommended.

CLINICAL PEARL

- Blood ethanol level decreases by 20 mg/dL/hr in a normal 70-kg person.

Alkalosis, metabolic

Definition: Disturbance of acid-base balance. The primary event is an elevation of the plasma bicarbonate concentration resulting from factors noted in etiology section.

DIAGNOSIS

Evaluate type of disturbance present by examining pH, PCO_2, and HCO_3^-. See Figure 2 on Page 11 for a map for acid-base disorders.

ETIOLOGY

Metabolic alkalosis is divided into chloride-responsive (urinary chloride <15 mEq/L) and chloride-resistant forms (urinary chloride level >15 mEq/L).

- **Chloride-responsive:**
  - Vomiting
  - Nasogastric suction
  - Diuretics
  - Posthypercapnic alkalosis
  - Stool losses (laxative abuse, cystic fibrosis, villous adenoma)
- **Chloride-resistant:**
  - Exogenous alkali administration
  - Massive blood transfusion
  - Hyperadrenocorticoid states (e.g., Cushing's syndrome, primary hyperaldosteronism, secondary mineralocorticoidism [licorice, chewing tobacco])
  - Hypomagnesemia
  - Hypokalemia
  - Bartter's syndrome

- Chloride-responsive forms are treated with saline administration and correction of accompanying hypokalemia.
- Chloride-resistant forms require correction of underlying cause and associated potassium depletion.

CLINICAL PEARL
- An increase in HCO_3^- by 1 increases pH by 0.015 and increases $Paco_2$ by 0.7. The compensatory response (increased $Paco_2$) usually is limited to a maximum $Paco_2$ of 55. There is an impaired compensatory response in patients with chronic obstructive pulmonary disease, heart failure, and hepatic coma.

 Alkalosis, respiratory

Definition: Disturbance of acid-base balance characterized by a primary decrease in Pco_2 resulting from factors noted in etiology section

DIAGNOSIS
- Evaluate type of disturbance present by examining pH, Pco_2, and HCO_3^-. See Figure 2 on Page 11 for a map for acid-base disorders.

ETIOLOGY
- **Hypoxemia:** pneumonia, pulmonary embolism, atelectasis, high-altitude living
- **Drugs:** salicylates, xanthines, progesterone, epinephrine, thyroxine, nicotine
- **Central nervous system disorders:** tumor, cerebrovascular accident, trauma, infections
- **Psychogenic hyperventilation:** anxiety, hysteria
- Hepatic encephalopathy
- Gram-negative sepsis
- Hyponatremia
- Sudden recovery from metabolic acidosis
- Assisted ventilation

TREATMENT
- Therapy of respiratory alkalosis is aimed at the underlying cause. Symptomatic patients with psychogenic hyperventilation often require some form of rebreathing apparatus (e.g., paper bag, breathing 5% carbon dioxide via mask).

CLINICAL PEARLS

- In acute respiratory alkalosis, a decrease in $Paco_2$ by 10 mm Hg increases pH by 0.08 and decreases HCO_3^- by 2.5.
- In chronic respiratory alkalosis, a decrease in $Paco_2$ by 10 mm Hg increases pH by 0.03 and decreases HCO_3^- by 5.

◼ α_1-Antitrypsin deficiency

Definition: Genetic deficiency of the protease inhibitor α_1-antitrypsin with resulting predisposition to pulmonary emphysema and hepatic cirrhosis

DIAGNOSIS

- Decreased serum level of α_1-antitrypsin is present.
- Chest x-ray reveals emphysematous changes at lung bases.
- High-resolution CT scan of chest confirms the lower lobe–predominant emphysema and may show significant bronchiectasis.
- Clinical presentation includes cough, dyspnea, and sputum production. Liver involvement includes neonatal hepatitis, cirrhosis in children and adults, and hepatocellular carcinoma. Panniculitis is the major dermatologic manifestation.

ETIOLOGY

- Degree of α_1-antitrypsin deficiency depends on phenotype. MM represents the normal genotype and is associated with α_1-antitrypsin deficiency in the normal range. The mutation most commonly associated with emphysema is Z, with homozygote (ZZ) resulting in approximately 85% deficit in plasma α_1-antitrypsin concentrations.

TREATMENT

- Acute exacerbations of chronic obstructive pulmonary disease (COPD) secondary to α_1-antitrypsin deficiency are treated in similar fashion to "typical" COPD exacerbations.
- Intravenous administration of pooled human α_1-antitrypsin can be used to increase α_1-antitrypsin levels above a minimum, "protective" threshold.
- Lung and liver transplantation are offered in suitable cases.

CLINICAL PEARL

- Consider α_1-antitrypsin deficiency in patients presenting with lower lobe–predominant emphysema because in most smokers without α_1-antitrypsin deficiency emphysema predominates in the upper lobes.

Altitude sickness

Definition: Spectrum of illnesses related to hypoxia occurring in people rapidly ascending to high altitudes

DIAGNOSIS
- Clinical presentation includes headache, dizziness, fatigue, sleep disturbance, dry cough, tachycardia, and tachypnea. Manifestations of high-altitude cerebral edema include delirium, ataxia, seizures, and coma.
- Laboratory tests are not useful in diagnosing altitude sickness.
- Chest x-ray reveals Kerley B lines and patchy edema in high-altitude pulmonary edema.
- CT scan of head reveals diffuse or patchy edema in high-altitude cerebral edema.

ETIOLOGY
- Hypoxia resulting from low Po_2

TREATMENT
- The person should stop ascent to allow acclimatization or start to descend until symptoms have resolved.
- Oxygen 4-6 L/min can be used for severe cases.
- Sublingual nifedipine 10 mg followed by long-acting nifedipine 30 mg bid can be used for patients who cannot descend immediately.
- Dexamethasone 4 mg PO q6h can be used in severe altitude sickness.
- Portable hyberbaric bags are useful if available at the site.
- Dehydration should be avoided.

CLINICAL PEARLS
- Prophylactic therapy with acetazolamide 750 mg daily or dexamethasone 8-16 mg/day decreases the risk of developing altitude sickness.
- Sildenafil (Viagra) may be useful for prophylactic therapy.

Amaurosis fugax

Definition: Temporary loss of monocular vision caused by transient retinal ischemia

DIAGNOSIS
- Because amaurosis is usually due to emboli, the workup should focus primarily on embolic sources. Also consider giant cell arteritis in an elderly patient.

- Examine retina for presence of embolus, auscultate carotids for bruits, evaluate for temporal artery tenderness, and examine for signs of hemispheric stroke (e.g., contralateral limb and face weakness or sensory loss, aphasia).
- Laboratory studies include complete blood count, erythrocyte sedimentation rate, and lipid panel. Hypercoagulation workup is discretionary based on younger age and history.

Diagnostic Imaging:

- Carotid Doppler imaging followed by magnetic resonance angiography or four-vessel angiography is performed as indicated.
- Transthoracic echocardiography is indicated to screen for embolization in patients with evidence of heart disease and in patients without an evident source for the transient neurologic deficit. Transesophageal echocardiography is more sensitive for detecting cardiac sources of embolization (e.g., ventricular mural thrombus, atrial appendage, patent foramen ovale, aortic arch).
- Consider MRI of the brain with diffusion-weighted imaging to look for ischemic injury.

ETIOLOGY

- Usually embolic from the internal carotid artery or the heart, but also may be due to vasculitis, such as giant cell arteritis, or hyperviscosity syndromes, such as sickle cell disease, which cause ischemia in the vascular territory of the ophthalmic artery

TREATMENT

- Treat with aspirin if etiology is presumed embolic.
- If giant cell arteritis is suspected, start prednisone, and refer for temporal artery biopsy within 48 hours.
- Reduce risks by carotid endarterectomy or stent if stenosis >70%.
- Control hypertension and manage vascular risk factors. Instruct patient to avoid tobacco.
- Begin antiplatelet therapy.
- Administer statin therapy in hyperlipidemic patients.

CLINICAL PEARL

- Among patients with >50% carotid stenosis who do not undergo carotid endarterectomy, patients who present with transient monocular blindness have about a 10% risk of stroke in 3 years compared with a 20% risk in patients who present with a hemispheric transient ischemic attack.

Amebiasis

Definition: An infection primarily of the colon caused by the protozoal parasite *Entamoeba histolytica*. Transmission is by the fecal-oral route. Infection usually is localized to the large bowel, particularly the cecum, where a localized mass lesion (ameboma) may form. Extraintestinal infection can occur, in which the organism invades the bowel mucosa and gains access to the portal circulation.

DIAGNOSIS

- Stool examination is generally reliable. Three stool specimens over 7 to 10 days exclude the diagnosis (sensitivity 50-80%).
- Mucosal biopsy is occasionally necessary.
- Serum antibody may be detected and is particularly sensitive and specific for extraintestinal infection or severe intestinal disease.
- Aspiration of abscess fluid is used to distinguish amebic from bacterial abscesses.
- Abdominal imaging studies (sonography or CT scan) are indicated to diagnose liver abscess.
- Clinical presentation is often nonspecific. Approximately 20% of cases are symptomatic.
  - Diarrhea, which may be bloody
  - Abdominal and back pain
  - Abdominal tenderness in 83% of severe cases
  - Fever in 38% of severe cases
  - Hepatomegaly, right upper quadrant tenderness, and fever in almost all patients with liver abscess (may be absent in fulminant cases)

TREATMENT

- Metronidazole (750 mg PO tid for 10 days) is used to treat mild to severe intestinal infection and amebic liver abscess; it may be administered intravenously when necessary.
- Follow with iodoquinol (650 mg PO tid for 20 days) to eradicate persistent cysts.
- For asymptomatic patients with amebic cysts on stool examination, use iodoquinol or paromomycin (500 mg PO tid for 7 days).
- Avoid antiperistaltic agents in severe intestinal infections to avoid risk of toxic megacolon.
- Liver abscess generally is responsive to medical management, but surgical intervention is indicated for extension of liver abscess into pericardium or, occasionally, for toxic megacolon.

Amyotrophic lateral sclerosis (ALS)

Definition: A progressive, degenerative neuromuscular condition of undetermined etiology affecting corticospinal tracts and anterior horn cells resulting in dysfunction of upper and lower motor neurons

DIAGNOSIS

- Lower motor neuron signs include weakness, hypotonia, wasting, fasciculations, and hyporeflexia or areflexia.
- Upper motor neuron signs include loss of fine motor dexterity, spasticity, extensor plantar responses, hyperreflexia, and clonus.
- Extraocular movements, sensation, and bowel and bladder function are preserved.
- Dysarthria, dysphagia, pseudobulbar affect, and frontal lobe dysfunction are present.
- **Workup:**
  - Electromyogram and nerve conduction studies
  - Lumbar puncture to assess protein and serum GM_1 antibody if multifocal motor neuropathy suspected
  - Assessment of respiratory function (force vital capacity, negative inspiratory force)
- **Laboratory studies:**
  - Vitamin B_{12}, thyroid function, parathyroid hormone; HIV may be considered
  - Serum protein and immunofixation electrophoresis
  - DNA studies for spinal muscular atrophy or bulbospinal atrophy, hexosaminidase levels in pure lower motor neuron syndrome
  - 24-hour urine for lead if indicated by history
- **Imaging:**
  - Craniospinal neuroimaging contingent on clinical scenario
  - Modified barium swallow to evaluate aspiration risk

ETIOLOGY

- Ninety percent to 95% of all cases of ALS are sporadic. Of the familial cases, approximately 20% are associated with a genetic defect in the copper-zinc superoxide dismutase enzyme (SOD1).

TREATMENT

- Noninvasive positive-pressure ventilation improves quality of life and increases tracheostomy-free survival.
- Percutaneous endoscopic gastrostomy (PEG) placement improves caloric and fluid status, eases medication administration, and may prolong life 1 to 4 months.

services should be offered.

- A suction device for sialorrhea is recommended.
- Communication may be eased with computerized assistive devices.
- Early discussion should occur of living will, resuscitation orders, desire for PEG and tracheostomy, and potential long-term care options.
- Consider use of riluzole (Rilutek), a glutamate antagonist, in selected patients.
- Relieve spasticity with baclofen or clonazepam.
- Treat pseudobulbar affect with amitriptyline, sertraline (Zoloft), or dextromethorphan.

CLINICAL PEARL

- Gastroenterology referral for PEG placement in ALS patients is recommended while forced vital capacity remains >50% to minimize the risks inherent to the procedure.

Anaphylaxis

Definition: Sudden-onset, life-threatening event characterized by bronchial contractions in conjunction with hemodynamic changes. Clinical presentation may include respiratory, cardiovascular, cutaneous, or gastrointestinal manifestations.

DIAGNOSIS

- Physical findings and clinical presentation include urticaria, pruritus, skin flushing, angioedema, weakness, dizziness, dyspnea, cough, malaise, difficulty swallowing, wheezing, tachycardia, diarrhea, hypotension, and vascular collapse.
- Workup is aimed mainly at eliminating other conditions that may mimic anaphylaxis (e.g., vasovagal syncope may be differentiated by the presence of bradycardia as opposed to tachycardia seen in anaphylaxis; the absence of hypoxemia in arterial blood gas analysis may be useful to exclude pulmonary embolism or foreign body aspiration).
- Laboratory evaluation is generally not helpful because the diagnosis of anaphylaxis is a clinical one.

ETIOLOGY

- Virtually any substance may induce anaphylaxis in a given individual.

- **Commonly implicated medications:** antibiotics, insulin, allergen extracts, opiates, vaccines, nonsteroidal antiinflammatory drugs, contrast media, streptokinase
- **Foods and food additives:** nuts, egg whites, shellfish, fish, milk, fruits, berries
- **Blood products:** plasma, immunoglobulin, cryoprecipitate, whole blood
- **Venoms:** snake, fire ant, bee (*Hymenoptera* stings)
- Latex

TREATMENT

- Epinephrine should be administered rapidly as a subcutaneous or intramuscular injection at a dose of 0.01 mL/kg of aqueous epinephrine 1 : 1000 (maximum adult dose 0.3-0.5 mL). The dose may be repeated approximately every 5 to 10 minutes if there is persistence or recurrence of symptoms. Endotracheal epinephrine should be considered if intravenous access is not possible during life-threatening reactions.
- Administration of H_1-receptor and H_2-receptor antagonists also is recommended in the initial treatment of anaphylaxis.
  - Administer diphenhydramine 50-75 mg IV or IM.
  - Cimetidine 300 mg IV over 3 to 5 minutes or ranitidine 50 mg IV should be given initially; subsequent doses of H_1-blockers and H_2-blockers can be given orally every 6 hours for 48 hours.
- Corticosteroids are not useful in an acute episode because of their slow onset of action; however, they should be administered in most cases to prevent prolonged or recurrent anaphylaxis. Commonly used agents are hydrocortisone sodium succinate 250-500 mg IV q4-6h in adults (4-8 mg/kg in children) or methylprednisolone 60-125 mg IV in adults (1-2 mg/kg in children).
- Aerosolized $β_2$-agonists (i.e., albuterol 2.5 mg, repeat as needed in 20 minutes) are useful to control bronchospasm.
- Additional useful agents in specific circumstances include atropine for refractory bradycardia, dopamine for refractory hypotension (despite volume expansion), and glucagon in patients taking β-blocking drugs.

CLINICAL PEARL

- A prescription for a prefilled epinephrine syringe (EpiPen) should be given, and the patient should be instructed on the use of this emergency epinephrine kit in case of recurrent anaphylactic episodes.

Anemia, aplastic

Definition: Bone marrow failure resulting from a variety of causes and characterized by stem cell destruction or suppression leading to pancytopenia

DIAGNOSIS

- Diagnostic workup consists primarily of bone marrow aspiration and biopsy and laboratory evaluation (complete blood count and examination of blood film).
- Bone marrow examination generally reveals paucity or absence of erythropoietic and myelopoietic precursor cells; patients with pure red blood cell (RBC) aplasia show only absence of RBC precursors in the marrow.
- Complete blood count reveals pancytopenia. Macrocytosis and toxic granulation of neutrophils also may be present. Isolated cytopenias may occur in the early stages.
- Reticulocyte count reveals reticulocytopenia.
- Additional initial laboratory evaluation should include Ham's test to exclude paroxysmal nocturnal hemoglobinuria and testing for hepatitis C.
- Diagnostic imaging consists of abdominal sonogram or CT scan to evaluate for splenomegaly and CT scan of thymus region if thymoma-associated RBC aplasia is suspected.

ETIOLOGY

- In most patients with acquired aplastic anemia, bone marrow failure results from immunologically mediated, active destruction of blood-forming cells by lymphocytes.
- Common etiologic factors in aplastic anemia include the following:
  - Toxins (e.g., benzene, insecticides)
  - Drugs (e.g., felbamate [Felbatol], cimetidine, busulfan and other myelosuppressive drugs, gold salts, chloramphenicol, sulfonamides, trimethadione, quinacrine, phenylbutazone)
  - Ionizing irradiation
  - Infections (e.g., hepatitis C, HIV)
  - Idiopathic
  - Inherited (Fanconi's anemia)
  - **Other:** immunologic, pregnancy

TREATMENT

- Neutropenic fevers should be treated aggressively with parenteral broad-spectrum antibiotics.

- Platelet and RBC transfusions should be given as needed; however, transfusions should be avoided in patients who are candidates for bone marrow transplantation.

Immunosuppressive therapy is with antithymocyte globulin (ATG) or cyclosporine. ATG is given in combination with prednisone (1-2 mg/kg/day initially) to avoid complications of serum sickness.

- Transplantation of allogeneic marrow or peripheral blood stem cell transplantation from a histocompatible sibling usually cures the underlying bone marrow failure.
- In patients with severe aplastic anemia who are not candidates for allogeneic bone marrow transplantation, use of high-dose cyclophosphamide therapy without bone marrow transplantation is a third treatment option for initial treatment of aplastic anemia.

CLINICAL PEARLS

- ATG with cyclosporine restores hematopoiesis in approximately two thirds of patients; however, recovery of blood cell count is often incomplete. Recurrent pancytopenia requires retreatment. In some patients, myelodysplasia is a late complication of immunosuppressive therapy.
- Response to immunosuppression in aplastic anemia is independent of age, but treatment is associated with increased mortality in older patients.

Anemia, autoimmune hemolytic

Definition: Anemia secondary to premature destruction of red blood cells (RBCs) caused by the binding of autoantibodies or complement or both to RBCs.

DIAGNOSIS

- Evaluation consists primarily of laboratory evaluation to confirm hemolysis and to exclude other causes of anemia.
- Initial laboratory tests include complete blood count (anemia), reticulocyte count (elevated), liver function studies (elevated indirect bilirubin, lactate dehydrogenase), evaluation of peripheral smear, Coombs test (positive direct Coombs test indicates presence of antibodies or complement on the surface of RBCs; positive indirect Coombs test implies presence of anti-RBC antibodies freely circulating in the patient's serum), and haptoglobin level (decreased).
- Tests for autoantibodies IgG (warm) antibody and IgM (cold) antibody are useful.
- Hepatic serology and antinuclear antibody are recommended.

... chest and abdomen to rule out lymphoma also should be considered.

ETIOLOGY

- **Warm antibody mediated:** IgG (often idiopathic or associated with leukemia, lymphoma, thymoma, myeloma, viral infections, and collagen-vascular disease)
- **Cold antibody mediated:** IgM and complement in most cases (often idiopathic, at times associated with infections, lymphoma, or cold agglutinin disease)
- **Drug induced:** three major mechanisms:
  - Antibody directed against Rh complex (e.g., methyldopa)
  - Antibody directed against RBC-drug complex (hapten-induced, e.g., penicillin)
  - Antibody directed against complex formed by drug and plasma proteins; the drug-plasma protein-antibody complex causes destruction of RBCs (innocent bystander, e.g., quinidine)

TREATMENT

- Treat warm antibody autoimmune hemolytic anemia initially with prednisone 1-2 mg/kg/day in divided doses. Corticosteroids are generally ineffective in cold antibody autoimmune hemolytic anemia.
- Splenectomy can be considered in patients responding inadequately to corticosteroids when RBC sequestration studies indicate splenic sequestration.
- Immunosuppressive drugs or immunoglobulins or both are recommended after corticosteroids and splenectomy (unless surgery is contraindicated) have failed to produce an adequate remission.
- Danazol, usually used in conjunction with corticosteroids (may be useful in warm antibody autoimmune hemolytic anemia), is recommended.
- Immunosuppressive drugs (e.g., azathioprine, cyclophosphamide) may be useful in warm antibody autoimmune hemolytic anemia, but are indicated only after corticosteroids and splenectomy (unless surgery is contraindicated) have failed to produce an adequate remission.

CLINICAL PEARL

- Avoid cold exposure in patients with cold antibody autoimmune hemolytic anemia.

Anemia, iron deficiency

Definition: Anemia secondary to inadequate iron supplementation or excessive blood loss

DIAGNOSIS

- Diagnostic workup consists primarily of laboratory evaluation. Most patients with iron deficiency anemia are asymptomatic in the early stages. With progressive anemia, major complaints are fatigue, dizziness, exertional dyspnea, pagophagia (ice eating), and pica. The patient's history also may suggest gastrointestinal blood loss (melena, hematochezia, hemoptysis) or excessive menstrual bleeding.
- Laboratory results vary with the stage of deficiency:
  - Absent iron marrow stores and decreased serum ferritin are the initial abnormalities.
  - Decreased serum iron and increased total iron-binding capacity (TIBC) are the next abnormalities.
  - Hypochromic microcytic anemia is present with significant iron deficiency.
- Peripheral smear in patients with iron deficiency generally reveals microcytic hypochromic red blood cells (RBCs) with a wide area of central pallor, anisocytosis, and poikilocytosis when severe.
- Laboratory abnormalities consistent with iron deficiency are low serum ferritin level, elevated RBC distribution width with values generally >15, low mean corpuscular volume, elevated TIBC, and low serum iron.
- The reticulocyte hemoglobin content may be a good screening test for iron deficiency. It can be measured on an automated hematology analyzer and is a relatively inexpensive and fast way to detect iron deficiency.

ETIOLOGY

- Blood loss from gastrointestinal or menstrual bleeding (genitourinary blood loss less often the cause)
- Dietary iron deficiency (rare in adults)
- Poor iron absorption in patients with gastric or small bowel surgery
- Repeated phlebotomy, recent blood donation
- Increased requirements (e.g., during pregnancy)
- **Other:** traumatic hemolysis (abnormally functioning cardiac valves), idiopathic pulmonary hemosiderosis (iron sequestration in pulmonary macrophages), paroxysmal nocturnal hemoglobinuria (intravascular hemolysis)

- Treatment consists of ferrous sulfate 325 mg PO qd-tid for at least 6 months. Calcium supplements can decrease iron absorption; these two medications should be staggered.
- Parenteral iron therapy is reserved for patients with poor tolerance, noncompliance with oral preparations, or malabsorption.
- Transfusion of packed RBCs is indicated in patients with severe symptomatic anemia (e.g., angina) or life-threatening anemia.

CLINICAL PEARLS
- Dietary iron deficiency occurs often in infants as a result of unsupplemented milk diets. It also commonly is seen in women of childbearing age, as a result of heavy menstrual periods, and during pregnancy (increased demand).
- If the diagnosis of iron deficiency anemia is made, it is mandatory to try to locate the suspected site or etiology of iron loss.

▰ Anemia, macrocytic

Definition: Anemia characterized by macrocytic features of red blood cells (RBCs) (elevated mean corpuscular volume [MCV]). The term *megaloblastic anemias* refers to morphologic abnormalities of cell nuclei caused by various defects in DNA synthesis.

DIAGNOSIS
- **Peripheral blood smear:**
  - Hypersegmented neutrophils (>6 lobes) are present in vitamin B_{12} and folate deficiencies.
- **Laboratory tests:**
  - **Serum vitamin B_{12} level:** A low level indicates vitamin B_{12} deficiency; exceptions are falsely low levels seen in patients with severe folate deficiency or falsely high or normal levels when vitamin B_{12} deficiency coincides with severe liver disease or chronic lymphocytic leukemia.
  - **Serum folate, RBC folate:** Both tests should be ordered because serum folate alone is labile and does not reflect tissue folate levels accurately, whereas RBC folate is a good indicator of tissue stores but may be reduced in severe cobalamin deficiency.
  - Reticulocyte count
  - Thyroid-stimulating hormone, alanine transferase, aspartate transferase
- **Bone marrow examination:** Examination of the bone marrow shows megaloblastic erythroid hyperplasia.

ETIOLOGY

- Folate deficiency
  - Decreased intake (e.g., alcoholism, poor diet)
  - Increased requirements (e.g., hemolysis, pregnancy, dialysis, leukemia, exfoliative dermatitis)
  - Impaired absorption (e.g., sprue, inflammatory bowel disease, ethanol)
  - Drugs (e.g., phenytoin, methotrexate, ethanol, trimethoprim, antituberculous agents)
  - Defective folate interconversion
- Vitamin B₁₂ deficiency
  - Pernicious anemia (antibodies against intrinsic factor and gastric parietal cells)
  - Dietary (e.g., strict lacto-ovovegetarians, food faddists)
  - Malabsorption (e.g., achlorhydria, gastrectomy, ileal resection, Crohn's disease of terminal ileum, pancreatic insufficiency, drugs [omeprazole, metformin, cholestyramine])
  - Chronic alcoholism (multifactorial)
  - *Helicobacter pylori* infection
  - Chronic liver disease (elevated MCV is multifactorial—ineffective erythropoiesis, hemolysis, acute blood loss)
  - Alcoholism (RBC membrane abnormalities)
  - Hypothyroidism (also can cause normochromic, normocytic anemia, or hypochromic, microcytic anemia
  - Elevated reticulocyte count (each increase in the reticulocyte count by 1% increases the MCV by approximately 2 fL)
  - Macrocytic indices (in some patients with aplastic anemia, myelodysplastic syndrome, or sideroblastic anemia)
  - Myelodysplastic syndromes (stem cell disorders characterized by refractory cytopenias, ineffective hematopoiesis, and variable progression to acute myeloid leukemia)
  - Drugs that impair DNA synthesis (e.g., zidovudine, 5-fluorouracil, hydroxyurea, 6-mercaptopurine)

TREATMENT

- **Folate deficiency:** folic acid 1 mg PO qd
- **Vitamin B₁₂ deficiency** Traditional therapy of cobalamin deficiency consists of intramuscular injections of 1000 μg weekly for the first 4 to 6 weeks followed by 1000 μg/mo IM indefinitely.

CLINICAL PEARL

- Oral cobalamin 1000 μg/day is a safe, effective, and inexpensive replacement alternative in most patients after vitamin B₁₂ levels have been normalized, provided that normal cobalamin levels are ensured serum measurements. Oral therapy also can be effective in pernicious anemia because about 1% of an oral dose is absorbed by passive diffusion, a pathway that does not require intrinsic factor.

Anemia, microcytic

Definition: Anemia with a reduced mean corpuscular volume

DIAGNOSIS

- **Peripheral blood smear:**
  - Iron deficiency—microcytic, hypochromic red blood cells (RBCs) with a wide area of central pallor; anisocytosis and poikilocytosis when severe
  - Chronic disease—normocytic or microcytic RBCs
  - Sideroblastic anemia—dimorphic population of cells (hypochromic cells and normochromic, normocytic cells); basophilic stippling also may be present
  - Thalassemia—basophilic stippling, target cells, high RBC count
  - Lead poisoning—basophilic stippling
- **Laboratory studies:**
  - Serum ferritin reflects the quantity of stored iron.
    - A low level is diagnostic of iron deficiency.
    - A normal or elevated level does not rule out iron deficiency because ferritin is an acute-phase reactant and can be increased in the presence of infection, inflammation, or liver disease.
  - A low serum iron and an elevated total iron-binding capacity suggest iron deficiency anemia.
    - Reticulocyte count is elevated with acute blood loss or hemolysis.
  - RBC distribution width >15 is suggestive of iron deficiency.
  - The reticulocyte hemoglobin content also is an excellent screening test for iron deficiency. It can be measured on an automated hematology analyzer and is a relatively inexpensive and fast way to detect iron deficiency.
  - Serum erythropoietin level is useful in the evaluation and treatment of anemia of chronic disease.
- **Bone marrow examination:**
  - Iron deficiency—absent iron stores, absent sideroblasts
  - Chronic disease—normal or increased iron stores, absent or decreased sideroblasts
  - Sideroblastic anemia—normal or increased iron stores, "ringed" sideroblasts present

  • Thalassemia—normal or increased iron stores, normal or increased
    sideroblasts

ETIOLOGY
• Iron deficiency
• Chronic disease
• Sideroblastic anemia (sex-linked)
• Thalassemia
• Lead poisoning

TREATMENT
• **Iron deficiency anemia** ferrous sulfate 325 mg PO qd-tid for at least
  6 months
• **Chronic disease states:** identify and treat underlying disease
• **Sideroblastic anemia:** treat underlying disorder; some primary
  sideroblastic anemias may respond to oral pyridoxine (vitamin B_6)
  100 mg PO tid
• **Thalassemia:** The major points in the management of homozygous
  β-thalassemia are as follows:
    ◦ Periodic transfusions to maintain hemoglobin at approximately
      10 g/dL
    ◦ Chelation therapy with deferoxamine mesylate to achieve negative
      iron balance
    ◦ Splenectomy at age 5 to 10 years
    ◦ Ancillary measures (e.g., folic acid, vitamin C)
• **Lead poisoning:** Children with lead levels of 45 to 69 µg/dL should
  receive chelation therapy using succimer or edetate calcium dis-
  odium. Use of both agents is indicated when blood lead levels are
  >69 µg/dL.

CLINICAL PEARL
• The reticulocyte count should be viewed in relation to the degree of
  anemia; a frequently used correction method is the determination of
  the reticulocyte production index (RPI).
    ◦ RPI = (measured hematocrit [Hct]/normal Hct) × reticulocyte
      count/maturation factor (MF)
    ◦ The MF is 1 if the patient's Hct is 45. Each 10-point decrease in the
      patient's Hct increases the MF by 0.5 (e.g., if the patient's Hct is 35,
      the MF is 1.5).
    ◦ The RPI subdivides anemias into two major classes:
        ▪ RPI >3—proliferative anemia (e.g., hemolysis, hemorrhage,
          response to hematinic agents)
        ▪ RPI <3—hypoproliferative anemia (e.g., marrow failure, iron defi-
          ciency, renal failure, endocrinopathies)

Anemia, normocytic

Definition: Anemia with a normal mean corpuscular volume

DIAGNOSIS

- **Peripheral blood smear:**
  - **Hemolysis:** Findings vary with the cause of the hemolysis.
    - Helmet cells, schistocytes—microangiopathic hemolysis
    - Sickle cells, Howell-Jolly bodies—sickle cell anemia
    - Red blood cell (RBC) fragments in a patient with a mechanical heart valve—traumatic hemolysis
    - Spherocytes—hereditary spherocytosis, autoimmune hemolytic anemias
    - *Spur cells* (irregular borders with thorny projections)—hepatic cirrhosis
  - **Aplastic anemia:** Findings include neutropenia and thrombocytopenia (unless pure RBC aplasia is present).
  - **Myelophthisis:** The peripheral smear shows a leukoerythroblastic picture (normoblasts, granulocyte precursors) caused by premature release from bone marrow.
- **Laboratory results:**
  - **Reticulocyte count:** elevated with RBC destruction (hemolysis), decreased with RBC underproduction (e.g., aplastic anemia, myelophthisis)
  - **Coombs' test**
    - Direct—detects the presence of antibody or complement on the surface of RBCs
    - Indirect—detects the presence of anti-RBC antibodies freely circulating in the patient's serum
  - **Lactate dehydrogenase:** frequently elevated in patients with intravascular or extravascular hemolysis
  - **Haptoglobin:** Haptoglobin is a serum protein that binds hemoglobin (Hb); the Hb-haptoglobin complex is cleared by the liver. Low or absent haptoglobin indicates intravascular hemolysis.
  - **Indirect bilirubin:** increased in intravascular and extravascular hemolysis
  - **Urinary hemosiderin and urinary Hb:** detected in moderate-to-severe intravascular hemolysis
  - **Chromium-51 RBC survival:** expensive and difficult test; should not be done as part of the initial evaluation of hemolytic anemias
  - Additional studies depend on clinical presentation and include blood urea nitrogen, creatinine (to rule out renal failure), and

thyroid screening (TSH). The osmotic fragility test confirms diagnosis of hereditary spherocytosis.

- **Bone marrow examination:**
  - **Aplastic anemia:** scarcity or absence of erythropoietic and myelopoietic precursor cells; patients with pure RBC aplasia show only absence of RBC precursors in the marrow
  - **Myelophthisis:** replacement of normal marrow with fibrosis, granulomas, or tumor cells (e.g., lymphoma, leukemia, metastatic carcinoma)

ETIOLOGY

- Hemolysis
- Aplastic anemia
- Acute hemorrhage (e.g., gastrointestinal, genitourinary), phlebotomy
- Renal failure
- Myelophthisis (marrow replacement by fibrosis, tumor, or granulomatous substance)
- Combined microcytic and macrocytic anemia (e.g., iron and folate deficiency)
- Endocrine disorders (e.g., hypothyroidism, gonadal dysfunction, adrenal insufficiency)
- Chronic disease (e.g., connective tissue disorders, infection, cancer)
- Bone marrow damage (e.g., ionizing radiation, benzene, drugs)
- Lead poisoning

TREATMENT

- Treatment varies with specific cause.

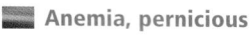

Anemia, pernicious

Definition: Autoimmune disease resulting from antibodies against intrinsic factor and gastric parietal cells

DIAGNOSIS

- The clinical presentation of pernicious anemia varies with the stage. Initially, patients may be asymptomatic. In advanced stages, patients may present with impaired memory, depression, gait disturbances, paresthesias, and complaints of generalized weakness.
- Investigation consists primarily of laboratory evaluation:
  - Complete blood count generally reveals macrocytic anemia and leukopenia with hypersegmented neutrophils.
  - Mean corpuscular volume generally is significantly elevated in advanced stages.
  - Reticulocyte count is low to normal.

severe folate deficiency, when patients are using high doses of ascorbic acid, and when cobalamin levels are measured after nuclear medicine studies (radioactivity interferes with cobalamin RIA measurement).
  - Falsely high normal levels in patients with cobalamin deficiency can occur in severe liver disease or chronic granulocytic leukemia.
- Schilling test is abnormal in part I; part II corrects to normal after administration of intrinsic factor.
- Laboratory tests used for detecting cobalamin deficiency in patients with normal vitamin B_{12} levels include serum and urinary methylmalonic acid level (elevated), total homocysteine level (elevated), and intrinsic factor antibody (positive).
- An increased concentration of plasma methylmalonic acid does not predict clinical manifestations of vitamin B_{12} deficiency and should not be used as the only marker for diagnosis of vitamin B_{12} deficiency.
- Additional laboratory abnormalities include elevated lactate dehydrogenase, direct hyperbilirubinemia, and decreased haptoglobin.
- Endoscopy and biopsy for atrophic gastritis may be performed in selected cases.

ETIOLOGY
- Anti–gastric parietal cell antibodies in >70% of patients, anti–intrinsic factor antibodies in >50% of patients
- Atrophic gastric mucosa

TREATMENT
- Traditional therapy of cobalamin deficiency consists of intramuscular injections of vitamin B_{12} 1000 µg/wk for the first 4 to 6 weeks followed by 1000 µg/mo IM indefinitely. When hematologic parameters have returned to normal range, intranasal cyanocobalamin may be used in place of intramuscular cyanocobalamin. The initial dose of intranasal cyanocobalamin (Nascobal) is one spray (500 µg) in one nostril once per week. Monitor response and increase dose if serum vitamin B_{12} levels decline. Consider return to intramuscular vitamin B_{12} supplementation if decline persists.

CLINICAL PEARLS
- Diagnosis is crucial because failure to treat may result in irreversible neurologic deficits.
- Avoid folic acid supplementation without proper vitamin B_{12} supplementation.
- The absence of anemia or macrocytosis does not exclude the diagnosis of cobalamin deficiency. Anemia is absent in 20% of patients with

cobalamin deficiency, and macrocytosis is absent in >30% of patients at the time of diagnosis. It can be blocked by concurrent iron deficiency or anemia of chronic disease and may be masked by thalassemia trait.

Anemia, sideroblastic

Definition: A blood disorder resulting from defective heme synthesis, classified as hereditary, acquired, and reversible

DIAGNOSIS

- Hypochromic anemia (low mean corpuscular volume, high red blood cell distribution width) is present.
- Peripheral smear shows dimorphic large and small cells revealing Pappenheimer bodies or siderocytes when stained for iron.
- Bone marrow examination shows ringed sideroblasts. These represent iron storage in the mitochondria of erythroblasts.

ETIOLOGY

- Primary hereditary sideroblastic anemia may be inherited as a sex-linked recessive disease.
- Secondary acquired sideroblastic anemia can be caused by alcohol, isoniazid, pyrazinamide, cycloserine, chloramphenicol, and copper deficiency.

TREATMENT

- Patient should avoid alcohol.
- In sideroblastic anemia secondary to isoniazid, pyrazinamide, and cycloserine, use vitamin B$_6$, 50-200 mg/day, and eliminate offending drug.
- Vitamin B$_6$, 50-200 mg/day results in a significant response in 35% of hereditary sideroblastic anemias. The remaining cases require periodic blood transfusions when symptomatic.
- Erythropoietin injections are useful in primary acquired sideroblastic anemia.

CLINICAL PEARLS

- Sideroblastic anemia can be thought of as an iron-loading anemia secondary to defective heme synthesis.
- Organ dysfunction resulting from iron overload requires periodic phlebotomies (indicated when serum iron levels >500 µg/L) and use of desferrioxamine in patients requiring frequent blood transfusions.

Aneurysm, abdominal aorta

Definition: A permanent localized dilation of the abdominal aortic artery to at least 50% compared with the normal diameter (2.3 cm in men, 1.9 cm in women)

DIAGNOSIS
- Abdominal ultrasound is the preferred initial imaging modality. It estimates size within 0.4 cm. Ultrasound is not accurate in estimating proximal extension to renal arteries or involvement of iliac arteries.
- CT and angiography are used preoperatively.
- Almost 75% of abdominal aortic aneurysms are asymptomatic and are discovered on routine examinations (pulsatile epigastric mass) or serendipitously when ordering studies for other complaints.

ETIOLOGY
- Atherosclerotic (degenerative or nonspecific)
- Genetic (e.g., Ehlers-Danlos syndrome)
- Trauma
- Cystic medial necrosis (Marfan syndrome)
- Arteritis, inflammatory
- Mycotic, syphilitic

TREATMENT
- Referral to a vascular surgeon is indicated for aneurysms ≥4 cm, symptomatic patients, and rapidly expanding aneurysms (0.7-1 cm/yr).

CLINICAL PEARLS
- Mortality rate for elective repair of nonruptured aneurysms is 4%.
- Mortality after rupture is >90%.

Angina pectoris

Definition: Angina pectoris is characterized by discomfort that occurs when myocardial oxygen demand exceeds the supply. Myocardial ischemia can be asymptomatic (silent ischemia), particularly in diabetics. The Canadian Cardiovascular Society Classification System divides angina into four classes:

- Class I—Ordinary physical activity does not cause angina, such as walking and climbing stairs. Angina occurs with strenuous, rapid, or prolonged exertion at work or recreation.

- Class II—The individual has slight limitation of ordinary activity. Angina occurs on walking or climbing stairs rapidly; walking uphill; walking or stair climbing after meals, in cold, in wind, or under emotional stress; or only during the few hours after awakening. Angina occurs on walking >2 blocks on level ground and climbing >1 flight of ordinary stairs at a normal pace and in normal conditions.
- Class III—Marked limitations of ordinary physical activity occur. Angina occurs on walking 1 to 2 blocks on level ground and climbing 1 flight of stairs in normal conditions and at a normal pace.
- Class IV—The individual is unable to perform any physical activity without discomfort. Angina may be present at rest.

DIAGNOSIS

- The most important diagnostic factor is the history.
- The physical examination is of little diagnostic help and may be normal in many patients, although the presence of an S_4 gallop suggests ischemic chest pain.
- An ECG taken during the acute episode may show transient T wave inversion or ST-segment depression or elevation, but some patients may have a normal tracing.
- Treadmill exercise tolerance test is useful to identify patients with coronary artery disease who would benefit from cardiac catheterization.
- Echocardiography is indicated in patients with systolic murmur suggesting aortic stenosis, mitral valve prolapse, or hypertrophic cardiomyopathy. Echocardiography combined with treadmill exercise (stress echo) or pharmacologic stress with dobutamine can be used to detect regional wall abnormalities that occur during myocardial ischemia associated with coronary artery disease.
- Coronary angiography remains the gold standard to identify clinically significant coronary artery disease.
- Initial laboratory tests in patients with chronic stable angina should include hemoglobin, fasting glucose, and fasting lipid panel.
- Cardiac isoenzymes (CK-MB every 8 hours × 2) should be obtained to rule out myocardial infarction in patients with unstable angina.
- Cardiac troponins I and T are specific markers of myocardial necrosis and are useful in evaluating patients with acute chest pain.

ETIOLOGY

- **Uncontrollable risk factors for angina:**
  - Advanced age
  - Male sex
  - Genetic predisposition

Risk factors for angina

- Smoking (risk is almost double)
- Hypertension
- Hyperlipidemia
- Impaired glucose tolerance or diabetes mellitus
- Obesity (weight >30% over ideal)
- Hypothyroidism
- Left ventricular hypertrophy
- Sedentary lifestyle
- Oral contraceptive use
- Cocaine use
- Low serum folate levels
- Elevated homocysteine levels
- Elevated levels of highly sensitive C-reactive protein
- Elevated levels of lipoprotein-associated phospholipase A_2
- Elevated fibrinogen levels
- Depression
- Vasculitis
- Low level of red blood cell glutathione peroxidase type 1 activity

TREATMENT

- Implement aggressive modification of preventable risk factors (e.g., weight reduction in obese patients, regular aerobic exercise program, correction of folate deficiency, low-cholesterol and low-sodium diet, cessation of tobacco use).
- Correct possible aggravating factors (e.g., anemia, hypertension, diabetes mellitus, hyperlipidemia, thyrotoxicosis, hypothyroidism).
- The major classes of antiischemic agents are nitrates, β-adrenergic blockers, calcium channel blockers, aspirin, and heparin; they can be used alone or in combination.
  - Aspirin is given as an initial dose of at least 160 mg/day followed by 81-325 mg/day. Aspirin inhibits cyclooxygenase and synthesis of thromboxane A_2 and reduces the risk of adverse cardiovascular events by 33% in patients with unstable angina. Patients intolerant to aspirin can be treated with the antiplatelet agent clopidogrel.
  - Heparin is useful in patients with unstable angina and reduces the frequency of myocardial infarction and refractory angina.
  - Platelet glycoprotein IIb/IIIa receptor antagonists should be administered early in patients with unstable angina, in high-risk patients with positive troponin tests, and in patients undergoing percutaneous revascularization.
- Use lipid-lowering drugs (e.g., statins).
- **Coronary artery bypass graft surgery:** Surgery is recommended for patients with left main coronary disease, for patients with sympto-

matic three-vessel disease, and for patients with left ventricular ejection fraction <40% and critical (>70%) stenosis in all three major coronary arteries. Surgical therapy improves prognosis, particularly in diabetic patients with multivessel disease.

- **Angioplasty and coronary stents:** Percutaneous coronary intervention should be considered for patients with one-vessel or two-vessel disease that does not involve the main left coronary artery and in whom ventricular function is normal or near-normal.

CLINICAL PEARL

Within 12 months of initial diagnosis, 10% to 20% of patients with the diagnosis of stable angina progress to myocardial infarction or unstable angina.

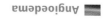

Angioedema

Definition: The cutaneous swelling caused by the release of vasoactive mediators is called *urticaria* and *angioedema*. Urticaria causes edema of the superficial dermis; angioedema involves the deep layers of the dermis and the subcutaneous tissue.

DIAGNOSIS

- Laboratory tests and allergy testing are based on history and physical examination.
- Laboratory tests include complete blood count, erythrocyte sedimentation rate, stool for ova and parasites, serology testing, serum C4 levels, and serum C1 esterase inhibitor (C1 INH) level and activity (if serum C4 level is low).
- Skin testing and radioallergosorbent test are indicated if food allergies are suspected.
- Skin biopsy is indicated in patients with chronic angioedema refractory to corticosteroid treatment.
- Angioedema is characterized by the following: nonpruritic; burning; not well demarcated; involves eyelids, lips, tongue, and extremities; and resolves slowly but can involve the larynx, causing respiratory distress.

ETIOLOGY

- **Acquired (allergic or idiopathic):** usually associated with other diseases, most commonly B-cell lymphoproliferative disorders, but also may result from formation of autoantibodies directed against C1 inhibitor protein. Other causes of angioedema include infections (e.g. herpes simplex, hepatitis B, coxsackie B and B, *Streptococcus*,

...*Asia, Ascaris,* and *Strongyloides*); insect bites and stings; physical factors (e.g., cold, physical exercise, pressure, and vibration); medications (e.g., angiotensin-converting enzyme inhibitors); and connective tissue diseases.
- **Hereditary:** autosomal dominant caused by a deficiency of C1 INH

TREATMENT
- Eliminate offending agent.
- Instruct patient to avoid triggering factors.
- Apply cold compresses to affected areas.
- Acute life-threatening angioedema involving the larynx is treated with the following:
  - Epinephrine 0.3 mg in solution of 1 : 1000 SC
  - Diphenhydramine 50 mg IV or IM
  - Cimetidine 300 mg IV or ranitidine 50 mg IV or IM
  - Methylprednisolone 125 mg IV
- Mainstay therapy in angioedema is H_1 antihistamines (e.g., hydroxyzine, loratadine, fexofenadine).
- H_2 antihistamines (e.g., ranitidine, cimetidine) can be added in severe cases.
- Corticosteroids tapered over several days (e.g., prednisone 60 mg on day 1, decreased by 5 mg every other day until finished) and the tricyclic antidepressant doxepin (25-50 mg qd) are useful in chronic resistant cases.

CLINICAL PEARLS
- Antihistamines achieve symptomatic relief in >80% of patients.
- Chronic angioedema can last for months and even years.

Ankylosing spondylitis

Definition: Chronic inflammatory condition involving the sacroiliac joints and axial skeleton characterized by ankylosis and enthesitis (inflammation at tendon insertions). It is one of a group of several overlapping syndromes, including spondylitis associated with Reiter's syndrome, psoriasis, and inflammatory bowel disease. Patients are typically seronegative for rheumatoid factor, and these disorders now commonly are called *rheumatoid variants* or *seronegative spondyloarthropathies.*

DIAGNOSIS
- The modified New York criteria are often used for diagnosis:
  - Low back pain of >3 months' duration, improved by exercise and not relieved by rest

- Limitation of lumbar spine movement in sagittal and frontal planes
- Decreased chest expansion below normal values for age and sex
- Bilateral sacroiliitis of moderate grade or greater

Back x-rays: Vertebral bodies may become demineralized, and a typical "squaring off" occurs. With progression, calcification of the annulus fibrosus and paravertebral ligaments develops, giving rise to the so-called "bamboo spine" appearance. End result may be a forward-protruding cervical spine and a fixed dorsal kyphosis. Laboratory tests show elevated erythrocyte sedimentation rate and C-reactive protein and negative antinuclear antibody and rheumatoid factor. HLA-B27 antigen is present in >90% of patients.

ETIOLOGY
- Unknown; genetic factors may play a role

TREATMENT
- Exercises primarily to maintain flexibility; general aerobic activity also important
- Postural training
- Patients must be instructed to sit in the erect position and to avoid stooping.
- Sleeping should be in the supine position on a firm mattress; pillows should not be placed under the head or knees.
- Nonsteroidal antiinflammatory drugs for pain control
- New research into the use of disease-modifying antirheumatic drugs (e.g., tumor necrosis factor antagonists such as etanercept) seems promising.

CLINICAL PEARL
Years may pass between the onset of symptoms and ultimate diagnosis because of the frequency of nonspecific low back pain resulting from other disorders.

Anorexia nervosa

Definition: Psychiatric disorder characterized by abnormal eating behavior, severe self-induced weight loss, and a specific psychopathology

DIAGNOSIS
A diagnosis can be made using the following criteria for anorexia nervosa from the *Diagnostic and Statistical Manual of Mental Disorders, Fourth Edition (DSM-IV):*

normal weight for age and height (e.g., weight loss leading to maintenance of BW <85% of that expected or failure to make expected weight gain during a period of growth, leading to BW <85% of that expected)

- Intense fear of gaining weight or becoming fat, even though underweight
- Disturbance in the way in which BW or shape is experienced, undue influence of BW or shape on self-evaluation, or denial of the seriousness of the current low BW
- In postmenarchal women, amenorrhea (i.e., the absence of at least three consecutive menstrual cycles); a woman is considered to have amenorrhea if her periods occur only after hormone (e.g., estrogen) administration
- There are two major types of anorexia nervosa:
  - **Restricting type:** During the current episode of anorexia nervosa, the person has not regularly engaged in binge-eating or purging behavior (i.e., self-induced vomiting or the misuse of laxatives, diuretics, or enemas).
  - **Binge-eating/purging type:** During the current episode of anorexia nervosa, the person has regularly engaged in binge-eating or purging behavior (i.e., self-induced vomiting or the misuse of laxatives, diuretics, or enemas).
- The SCOFF questionnaire is a useful screening tool used in England for eating disorders. It consists of the following five questions:
  - Do you make yourself **S**ick because you feel full?
  - Have you lost **C**ontrol over how much you eat?
  - Have you lost more than **O**ne stone (about 6 kg) recently?
  - Do you believe yourself to be **F**at when others say you are thin?
  - Does **F**ood dominate your life?
- A positive response to two or more questions has a reported sensitivity of 100% for anorexia and bulimia and an overall specificity of 87.5%.
- Baseline ECG should be performed on all patients with anorexia nervosa. Routine monitoring of patients with prolonged Q-T interval is necessary; sudden death in these patients often is caused by ventricular arrhythmias related to Q-T interval prolongation.
- Leukopenia, thrombocytopenia, anemia, reduced erythrocyte sedimentation rate, reduced complement levels, and reduced CD4 and CD8 cells may be present.
- Metabolic alkalosis, hypocalcemia, hypokalemia, hypomagnesemia, hypercholesterolemia, and hypophosphatemia may be present.

- Increased plasma β-carotene levels are useful to distinguish these patients from others on starvation diets.

ETIOLOGY

Etiology is unknown, but probably multifactorial (sociocultural, psychological, familial, and genetic factors).

A history of sexual abuse has been reported in 50% of patients with anorexia nervosa.

Psychological factors: Anorexics often have an incompletely developed personal identity. They struggle to maintain a sense of control over their environment; they usually have a low self-esteem, and they lack the sense that they are valued and loved for themselves.

TREATMENT

- A multidisciplinary approach with psychological, medical, and nutritional support is necessary.
- A goal BW should be set, and the patient should be monitored initially at least once a week in the office setting. The target BW is 100% of ideal BW for teenagers and 90% to 100% for adults.
- Weight gain should be gradual (1-3 lb/wk) to prevent gastric dilation.
- Electrolyte levels should be strictly monitored.
- Mealtime should be a time for social interaction, not confrontation.
- Postprandially, sedentary activities are recommended. The patient's access to a bathroom should be monitored to prevent purging.
- Pharmacologic treatment generally has no role in anorexia nervosa, unless major depression or another psychiatric disorder is present. Selective serotonin reuptake inhibitors can be used to alleviate the depressed mood and moderate obsessive-compulsive behavior in some individuals.

CLINICAL PEARLS

- The long-term prognosis is generally poor and marked by recurrent exacerbations. The percentage of patients with anorexia nervosa who fully recover is modest. Most patients continue to have a distorted body image, disordered eating habits, and psychological difficulties.
- Most patients with anorexia nervosa recover menses within 6 months of reaching 90% of their ideal body weight. Patients with anorexia nervosa can become pregnant despite amenorrhea.
- Mortality rates vary from 5% to 20%. Frequent causes of death are electrolyte abnormalities, starvation, and suicide.
- A prolonged Q-T interval is a marker for risk of sudden death.

Antiphospholipid antibody syndrome (APS)

Definition: APS is characterized by arterial or venous thrombosis or pregnancy loss and the presence of antiphospholipid antibodies. Antiphospholipid antibodies are antibodies directed against either phospholipids or proteins bound to anionic phospholipids. Four types of antiphospholipid antibodies have been characterized:

False-positive serologic tests for syphilis
Lupus anticoagulants
Anticardiolipin antibodies
Anti-β_2 glycoprotein-1 antibodies

APS is referred to as *primary APS* when it occurs alone and as *secondary APS* when it occurs in association with systemic lupus erythematosus, other rheumatic disorders, or certain infections or medications. APS can affect all organ systems and includes venous and arterial thrombosis, recurrent fetal losses, and thrombocytopenia.

DIAGNOSIS
- Diagnostic criteria of APS include at least one of the following clinical criteria and at least one of the following laboratory criteria:
  - **Clinical:**
    - Venous, arterial, or small vessel thrombosis *or*
    - Morbidity with pregnancy (fetal death at >10 weeks' gestation; *or* premature birth at <34 weeks' gestation secondary to eclampsia, preeclampsia, or severe placental insufficiency; *or* three or more unexplained consecutive spontaneous abortions <10 weeks' gestation)
  - **Laboratory:**
    - IgG or IgM anticardiolipin antibody in medium or high titers *or*
    - Lupus anticoagulant activity found on two or more occasions, at least 6 weeks apart

ETIOLOGY
- Etiology is unclear. A binding protein (β_2 glycoprotein I) may be the key immunogen in APS.
- Some APS-positive families exist, and HLA studies have suggested associations with HLA-DR7, HLA-DR4, HLA-Dqw7, and HLA-Drw53.

TREATMENT
- **Positive antiphospholipid antibodies and major thrombotic events or recurrent thrombotic events:** Initiate anticoagulation with heparin, then continue with lifelong warfarin treatment.

- **Positive antiphospholipid antibodies, asymptomatic patient with no previous thrombosis:** Routine prophylaxis is controversial. It is questionable whether acetylsalicylic acid (81 mg) is effective. Women should avoid oral contraceptive pill. Antithrombotic prophylaxis is recommended for major surgery, prolonged immobilization, and pregnancy.
- **Positive antiphospholipid antibodies, pregnant women:** Give acetylsalicylic acid 81 mg at conception and heparin 10,000 IU SC q12h at time of documented viable intrauterine pregnancy.

CLINICAL PEARLS

- One percent to 5% of healthy subjects have anticardiolipin and lupus anticoagulant antibodies.
- Twelve percent to 30% of patients with SLE have anticardiolipin antibodies.
- Fifteen percent to 20% of patients who present with deep venous thrombosis have anticardiolipin antibodies, and 15% to 34% have lupus anticoagulant antibodies.

⚕ Aortic dissection

Definition: Aortic dissection occurs when an intimal tear allows blood to dissect between medial layers of the aorta

DIAGNOSIS

- Clinical presentation includes sudden onset of severe chest pain often described as sharp, tearing, or ripping. Pain in the anterior with ascending aortic dissection or back pain with descending aortic dissection.
- Pulse and blood pressure differentials are common (38%), caused by partial compression of subclavian arteries.
- Most patients present with severe hypertension. Hypotension (25%) can indicate bleeding, cardiac tamponade, or severe aortic regurgitation.
- Chest x-ray may show widened mediastinum (62%).
- Transesophageal echocardiography is the study of choice in unstable patients. Sensitivity is 97% to 100%.
- MRI is the gold standard and gives the best information for surgeons. Sensitivity is 90% to 100%, but length of test and difficult access are not suitable for stable for stable intubated patients.

ETIOLOGY

- Medial degeneration of aorta
- **Risk factors:** hypertension, atherosclerosis, family history of aortic aneurysms, trauma, collagen disorders, bicuspid aortic valve, aortic coarctation, vasculitis, Turner syndrome, cocaine abuse

- Institute hemodynamic monitoring and blood pressure control with intravenous agents.
- Proximal dissections require emergent surgery.
- Distal dissections are treated medically only, unless distal organ involvement or impending rupture occurs. Endovascular stent placement is a new treatment, especially for older high-risk surgical patients.

CLINICAL PEARL
- After surgical repair, patients should be followed with frequent MRI studies because recurrent aneurysm or dissection is common in first 2 years.

Aortic regurgitation

Definition: Retrograde blood flow into the left ventricle from the aorta secondary to incompetent aortic valve

DIAGNOSIS
- **Echocardiography:** coarse diastolic fluttering of the anterior mitral leaflet; left ventricular hypertrophy in patients with chronic aortic regurgitation
- **Cardiac catheterization:** assesses degree of left ventricular dysfunction, confirms the presence of a wide pulse pressure, assesses surgical risk, and determines if there is coexistent coronary artery disease
- **Chest x-ray:**
  - Left ventricular hypertrophy (chronic aortic regurgitation)
  - Aortic dilation
  - Normal cardiac silhouette with pulmonary edema possible in patients with acute aortic regurgitation
- **ECG:** left ventricular hypertrophy
- Clinical presentation varies depending on whether aortic insufficiency is acute or chronic. Chronic aortic insufficiency is well tolerated (except when secondary to infective endocarditis), and patients remain asymptomatic for years. Common manifestations after significant deterioration of left ventricular function are dyspnea on exertion, syncope, chest pain, and congestive heart failure. Acute aortic insufficiency manifests primarily with hypotension secondary to a sudden decrease in cardiac output. A rapid increase in left ventricular diastolic pressure results in a further decrease in coronary blood flow.

- Physical findings in chronic aortic insufficiency include the following:
  - Widened pulse blood pressure (markedly increased systolic blood pressure, decreased diastolic blood pressure) is present.
  - Bounding pulses, head "bobbing" with each systole (de Musset's sign) can be palpated at the wrist or on the femoral arteries (pistol-shot femorals) and is caused by rapid rise and sudden collapse of the arterial pressure during late systolic; capillary pulsations (Quincke's pulse) may occur at the base of the nail beds.
  - A to-and-fro double Duroziez murmur may be heard over femoral arteries with slight compression.
  - Popliteal systolic pressure is increased over brachial systolic pressure 240 mm Hg (Hill's sign).
  - Cardiac auscultation reveals:
    - Displacement of cardiac impulse downward and to the patient's left
    - S_3 heard over the apex
    - Decrescendo, blowing diastolic murmur heard along left sternal border
    - Low-pitched apical diastolic rumble (Austin Flint murmur) caused by contrast of the aortic regurgitant jet with the left ventricular wall
    - Early systolic apical ejection murmur
  - In patients with acute aortic insufficiency, the wide pulse pressure and the large stroke volume are absent. A short blowing diastolic murmur may be the only finding on physical examination.

ETIOLOGY

- Infective endocarditis
- Rheumatic fibrosis
- Trauma with valvular rupture
- Congenital bicuspid aortic valve
- Myxomatous degeneration
- Syphilitic aortitis
- Rheumatic spondylitis
- Systemic lupus erythematosus
- Aortic dissection
- Fenfluramine, dexfenfluramine
- Takayasu's arteritis, granulomatous arteritis

TREATMENT

- **Medical:**
  - Digitalis, diuretics, angiotensin-converting enzyme (ACE) inhibitors, and sodium restriction for congestive heart failure; nitroprusside in patients with acute aortic regurgitation

reducing or delaying the need for aortic valve replacement in asymptomatic patients with severe aortic regurgitation and normal left ventricular function
- Bacterial endocarditis prophylaxis for surgical and dental procedures
- **Surgical:** Reserved for:
  - Symptomatic patients with chronic aortic regurgitation despite optimal medical therapy
  - Patients with acute aortic regurgitation (i.e., infective endocarditis) producing left ventricular failure
  - Evidence of systolic failure:
    - Echocardiographic fractional shortening <25%
    - Echocardiographic and diastolic dimension >55 mm
    - Angiographic ejection fraction <50% or end-systolic volume index >60 mL/m^2
  - Evidence of diastolic failure:
    - Pulmonary pressure >45 mm Hg systolic
    - Left ventricular end-diastolic pressure >15 mm Hg at catheterization
    - Pulmonary hypertension detected on examination
  - In general, the "55 rule" has been used to determine the timing of surgery: Surgery should be performed before ejection fraction is <55% or end-systolic dimension is >55 mm.

CLINICAL PEARL

- Prognosis varies depending on the underlying condition and left ventricular function; aortic regurgitation (except when secondary to infective endocarditis) is generally well tolerated, and patients remain asymptomatic for years.

 # Aortic stenosis (AS)

Definition: Obstruction to systolic left ventricular outflow across the aortic valve

DIAGNOSIS

- **Echocardiography:** thickening of the left ventricular wall; if the patient has valvular calcifications, multiple echos may be seen from within the aortic root, and there is poor separation of the aortic cusps during systole. Gradient across the valve can be estimated, but is less precise than with cardiac catheterization.

- Rough, loud systolic diamond-shaped murmur, best heard at base of heart and transmitted into neck vessels; often associated with a thrill or ejection click; also may be heard well at the apex
- Absence or diminished intensity of sound of aortic valve closure (in severe AS)
- Late, slow-rising carotid upstroke with decreased amplitude
- Strong apical pulse
- Narrowing of pulse pressure in later stages of AS
- Medical history should focus on symptoms and potential complications:
  - Angina
  - Syncope (particularly with exertion)
  - Congestive heart failure (CHF)
  - Gastrointestinal bleeding in patients with associated hemorrhagic telangiectasia (arteriovenous malformation)
- ECG:
  - Left ventricular hypertrophy (found in <80% of patients)
  - ST-T wave changes
  - Atrial fibrillation frequent

ETIOLOGY

- Rheumatic inflammation of aortic valve
- Progressive stenosis of congenital bicuspid valve (found in 1-2% of population)
- Idiopathic calcification of the aortic valve
- Congenital (major cause of AS in patients <30 years old)

TREATMENT

- **Medical:**
  - Diuretics and sodium restriction are needed if CHF is present; digoxin is used only to control rate of atrial fibrillation.
  - Angiotensin-converting enzyme inhibitors are relatively contraindicated.
  - Calcium channel blocker verapamil may be useful only to control rate of atrial fibrillation.
  - Antibiotic prophylaxis is necessary for surgical and dental procedures.
- **Surgical:**
  - Valve replacement is the treatment of choice in symptomatic patients because the 5-year mortality rate after onset of symptoms is extremely high, even with optimal medical therapy; valve replacement is indicated if cardiac catheterization establishes a pressure gradient >50 mm Hg and valve area <1 cm².
  - Balloon aortic valvotomy for adult acquired AS is useful only for

- Symptoms appear when the valve orifice decreases to <1 cm² (normal orifice 3 cm²).
- The stenosis is considered severe when the orifice is <0.5 cm², or the pressure gradient is ≥50 mm Hg.

■ Appendicitis

Definition: Acute inflammation of the appendix

DIAGNOSIS
- Abdominal pain initially may be epigastric or periumbilical in nearly 50% of patients; it subsequently localizes to the right lower quadrant within 12 to 18 hours. Pain can be found in the back or right flank if appendix is retrocecal or in other abdominal locations if there is malrotation of the appendix.
- Pain with right thigh extension (psoas sign) may be present with low-grade fever. Temperature may be >38°C if there is appendiceal perforation.
- Pain with internal rotation of the flexed right thigh (obturator sign) may be present.
- Right lower quadrant pain may occur on palpation of the left lower quadrant (Rovsing's sign). Physical examination may reveal right-sided tenderness in patients with pelvic appendix.
- Point of maximal tenderness is in the right lower quadrant (McBurney's point).
- Nausea, vomiting, tachycardia, and cutaneous hyperesthesias at the level of T12 can be present.
- Complete blood count with differential reveals leukocytosis with a left shift in 90% of patients with appendicitis. Total white blood cell count is generally <20,000/mm³. Higher counts may indicate perforation. Less than 4% have a normal white blood cell count and differential. A low hemoglobin and hematocrit in an older patient should raise suspicion for carcinoma of the cecum.
- Microscopic hematuria and pyuria may occur in <20% of patients.
- Spiral CT of the right lower quadrant of the abdomen has a sensitivity of >90% and an accuracy >94% for acute appendicitis. A distended appendix, periappendiceal inflammation, and a thickened appendiceal wall indicate appendicitis
- Ultrasound has a sensitivity of 75% to 90% for the diagnosis of acute appendicitis. Ultrasound is useful, especially in younger women when

the diagnosis is unclear. Normal ultrasound findings should not deter surgery if the history and physical examination indicate appendicitis.

ETIOLOGY

- Obstruction of the appendiceal lumen with subsequent vascular congestion, inflammation, and edema; common causes of obstruction are:
  - Fecaliths—30% to 35% of cases (most common cause of obstruction in adults)
  - Foreign body—1% (e.g. fruit seeds, pinworms, tapeworms, roundworms, calculi)
  - Inflammation—50% to 60% of cases (submucosal lymphoid hyperplasia [most common etiology in children and teens])
  - Neoplasms—1% (carcinoids, metastatic disease, carcinoma)

TREATMENT

- Urgent appendectomy (laparoscopic or open): correction of fluid and electrolyte imbalance with vigorous intravenous hydration and electrolyte replacement
- Intravenous antibiotic prophylaxis to cover gram-negative bacilli and anaerobes (ampicillin-sulbactam [Unasyn] 3 g IV q6h or piperacillin-tazobactam [Zosyn] 4.5 g IV q8h in adults)

CLINICAL PEARL

- Perforation is common (20%) in adult patients). Indicators of perforation are pain lasting >24 hours, leukocytosis >20,000/mm³, temperature >102°F, palpable abdominal mass, and peritoneal findings.

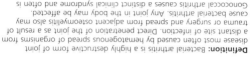

Arthritis, infectious

Definition: Bacterial arthritis is a highly destructive form of joint disease most often caused by hematogenous spread of organisms from a distant site of infection. Direct penetration of the joint as a result of trauma or surgery and spread from adjacent osteomyelitis also may cause bacterial arthritis. Any joint in the body may be affected. Gonococcal arthritis causes a distinct clinical syndrome and often is considered separately.

DIAGNOSIS

- Clinical presentation includes acute onset of a swollen painful joint and fever.
- Physical examination findings include limited range of motion of joint, erythema, and increased warmth around the joint.
- Workup consists of joint aspiration, Gram stain and culture of synovial fluid, blood cultures, complete blood count with differential.

source of infection.

- Synovial fluid leukocyte count usually is elevated (>50,000 cells/mm^3 with a differential count of ≥80% polymorphonuclear cells).
- Imaging studies consist of radiographs of affected joint to rule out osteomyelitis. CT is useful for early diagnosis of infections of the spine, hips, and sternoclavicular and sacroiliac joints. Technetium and gallium scans are positive, but do not allow differentiation of infection from inflammation. Indium-labeled white blood cell scans are less sensitive but more specific.

ETIOLOGY

- Bacteria spread from another locus of infection
- **Most common nongonococcal organisms:** *Staphylococcus aureus*, beta-hemolytic streptococci, and gram-negative bacilli

TREATMENT

- Intravenous antibiotics immediately after joint aspiration and Gram stain of synovial fluid
- **Gram-positive cocci:** nafcillin 2 g IV q4h. If clinical suspicion of methicillin resistant *Staphylococcus aureus*, use vancomycin 1 g IV q12h
- **Gram-negative bacilli:** third-generation cephalosporin or antipseudomonal penicillin plus aminoglycoside
- **Suspected gonococcal infection:** ceftriaxone 1 g IV q24h

CLINICAL PEARLS

- Predisposing factors for infectious arthritis are rheumatoid arthritis, prosthetic joints, advanced age, and immunodeficiency.
- Most commonly affected joints in adults are the knee and hip; the most commonly affected joint in children is the hip.
- In gonococcal infection, typical pattern is a migratory polyarthritis or tenosynovitis and presence of small pustules on the trunk or extremities.

▅▅ Arthritis, juvenile rheumatoid (JRA)

Definition: Arthritis beginning before 16 years of age

DIAGNOSIS

- Clinical presentation is usually one of three types:
  - Systemic or acute febrile JRA (20% of cases)
    - Characterized by extraarticular manifestations, especially spiking fevers and a typical rash that frequently appears in the evening

and may be elicited by gently scratching the skin in susceptible areas (Koebner phenomenon)

- Possible splenomegaly, generalized lymphadenopathy, pericarditis, and myocarditis
- Often minimal articular findings overshadowed by systemic symptoms
- Pauciarticular or oligoarticular JRA (50% of cases)
  - Involves fewer than five joints
  - Usually involves the larger joints, such as the knees, elbows, and ankles
  - Systemic features often minimal
  - Chronic iridocyclitis develops in nearly 30% of cases
  - Accelerated growth of the affected limb from chronic hyperemia possibly resulting in a temporary leg-length discrepancy
- Polyarticular JRA (30% of cases)
  - Involves five or more joints
  - Resembles the adult disease in its symmetric involvement of the small joints of the hands and feet.
  - Cervical spine involvement common and may produce marked loss of motion
  - Early closure of ossification centers of the mandible, often producing a marked receding chin
- Laboratory results include elevated erythrocyte sedimentation, low-grade anemia, and high peripheral white blood cell count. Rheumatoid factor is rarely positive in children. Antinuclear antibody is often positive in children with ocular complications.
- Imaging studies show soft tissue swelling, osteoporosis, bony erosions, and cyst formation. Joint destruction is less frequent than in adults.

ETIOLOGY

- Etiology is unknown.

TREATMENT

- Nonsteroidal antiinflammatory drugs for pain control
- Disease-modifying antirheumatic drugs and biologic response modifiers
- Intraarticular steroids; systemic corticosteroids

CLINICAL PEARLS

- Complete remission occurs in most patients.
- Blindness is the most serious complication of the pauciarticular form; joint deformity is the most serious problem of polyarticular disease.

Arthritis, psoriatic

Definition: An inflammatory spondyloarthritis occurring in patients with psoriasis who usually are seronegative for rheumatoid factor. It is often included in a class of disorders called *rheumatoid variants* or *seronegative spondyloarthropathies*.

DIAGNOSIS

- Clinical presentation includes gradual clinical onset with asymmetric involvement of scattered joints and skin psoriasis.
- Symmetric arthritis similar to rheumatoid arthritis occurs in 15% of patients. Sacroiliitis may occur in a few cases.
- Selective involvement of distal interphalangeal joints (described in "classic cases") occurs in only 5% of patients. When present, it is often accompanied by dystrophic changes in the nails (e.g., pitting, ridging).
- Laboratory studies show slight elevation of erythrocyte sedimentation rate and mild anemia. Positive HLA-B27 antigen often is found in patients with sacroiliitis.
- Imaging studies reveal peripheral joint findings similar to rheumatoid arthritis, but erosive changes in the distal phalangeal tufts characteristic of psoriatic arthritis. Bony osteolysis, periosteal new bone formation, sacroiliitis, and development of vertebral syndesmophytes (osteophytes) are found.

ETIOLOGY

- Etiology is unknown.

TREATMENT

- Nonsteroidal antiinflammatory drugs for pain control
- Splinting, joint protection, physical therapy
- Occasional intraarticular steroid injections
- Disease-modifying antirheumatic drugs rarely required

CLINICAL PEARL

- Early diagnosis may be difficult to establish because the arthritis may develop before skin lesions appear.

Asbestosis

Definition: Slowly progressive diffuse interstitial fibrosis resulting from dose-related inhalation exposure to fibers of asbestos

DIAGNOSIS

- **Chest x-ray:** small, irregular shadows in lower lung zones; thickened pleura; calcified plaques (present under diaphragms and lateral chest wall). CT scan of chest confirms the diagnosis.
- **Pulmonary function testing:** decreased vital capacity, decreased total lung capacity, decreased carbon monoxide gas transfer
- **Arterial blood gases:** hypoxemia, hypercarbia in advanced stages

Physical findings and clinical presentation:
- Insidious onset of shortness of breath with exertion is usually the first sign of asbestosis.
- Dyspnea becomes more severe as the disease advances; with time, progressively less exertion is tolerated.
- Cough is frequent and usually paroxysmal, dry, and nonproductive.
- Scant mucoid sputum may accompany the cough in the later stages of the disease.
- Fine end respiratory crackles (rales, crepitations) are heard more predominantly in the lung bases.
- Digital clubbing, edema, and jugular venous distention may be present.

ETIOLOGY

- Inhalation of asbestos fibers

TREATMENT

- Prompt identification and treatment of respiratory infections
- Supplemental oxygen on an as-needed basis
- Annual influenza vaccination, pneumococcal vaccination

CLINICAL PEARL

- Patients with asbestosis have increased risk for mesotheliomas, lung cancer, and tuberculosis. Reports indicate that the risk of asbestos-induced lung cancer may be overestimated.

Ascariasis

Definition: A parasitic infection caused by the nematode *Ascaris lumbricoides*. Most infected individuals are asymptomatic; however, clinical disease may arise from pulmonary hypersensitivity, intestinal obstruction, and secondary complications.

DIAGNOSIS
- Examine stool sample for *Ascaris* ova
- Expectoration or fecal passage of adult worm may occur.
- Eosinophilia is most prominent early in infection and subsides as adult worm infestation is established in intestines.
- Anti-*Ascaris* IgG4 blood levels by ELISA is a sensitive and specific marker of infection.
- Clinical presentation occurs 9 to 12 days after ingestion of eggs and corresponds to larva migration through the lungs. Nonproductive cough, fever, and substernal chest discomfort may be present. Migration of worms in biliary tree may mimic biliary colic or pancreatitis.
- Chest x-ray may reveal bilateral oval or round infiltrates (Löffler's syndrome).
- Plain films of abdomen and contrast studies may reveal worm masses in loops of bowel.

ETIOLOGY
- Infestation by the nematode *A. lumbricoides*

TREATMENT
- Mebendazole (Vermox) 100 mg tid for 3 days
- Albendazole 400 mg PO as single dose also effective
- Pyrantel pamoate (Antiminth) in pregnant patients
- Piperazine citrate used in cases of intestinal or biliary obstruction

CLINICAL PEARLS
- Transmission is usually hand to mouth, but eggs may be ingested via transported vegetables grown in contaminated soil.
- Within human host, adult worm life span is 1 to 2 years.

Aseptic necrosis

Definition: Disorder characterized by cell death in components of bone

DIAGNOSIS
- MRI is most sensitive imaging modality.
- Bone scan shows early findings of "cold" area; later, increased radionuclide uptake is seen.
- CT scan may reveal central necrosis and area of collapse.
- On plain x-rays, earliest changes include diffuse osteopenia, areas of radiolucency with sclerotic border, and linear sclerosis. Later, subchondral lucency (crescent sign) indicates subchondral fracture. More advanced cases reveal flattening, collapsed bone, and abnormal bone contour. In late disease, osteoarthritic changes are seen.
- Clinical presentation may be asymptomatic; pain in the involved area is exacerbated by movement or weight bearing.

ETIOLOGY
- Impairment of blood supply to the involved bone

TREATMENT
- Decreased weight bearing of affected area
- Core decompression—effectiveness 35% to 95% in early phases
- Bone grafting
- Osteotomies
- Joint replacement

CLINICAL PEARL
- Contralateral joint involvement is common (30-70%).

Aspergillosis

Definition: Several forms of a broad range of illnesses caused by an infection with Aspergillus

DIAGNOSIS
- Clinical presentation varies, but most patients present with cough, fever, dyspnea, and hemoptysis.
- **Allergic bronchopulmonary aspergillosis:**
  - Laboratory test results show peripheral eosinophilia, elevated total serum IgE level, positive Aspergillus serum precipitating antibody (70-100%), positive skin test with Aspergillus antigenic extract

...,and positive sputum cultures for *Aspergillus* (nonspecific).
  * Chest x-ray varies from small patchy, fleeting infiltrates (commonly in upper lobes) to lobar consolidation or cavitation or both. Most patients eventually develop central bronchiectasis.
* **Aspergillomas:**
  * Laboratory tests include sputum culture and serum precipitating antibody.
  * Chest x-ray or CT scan usually shows an intracavity mass partially surrounded by a crescent of air.
* **Invasive aspergillosis:**
  * Definitive diagnosis requires demonstration of tissue invasion as seen on a biopsy specimen or a positive culture from the tissue obtained by an invasive procedure, such as transbronchial biopsy.
  * Chest x-ray and CT scan may reveal cavity formation.

ETIOLOGY
* Infection with the *Aspergillus*. *Aspergillus fumigatus* is the usual cause; *Aspergillus flavus* is the second most important species, particularly in invasive disease of immunosuppressed patients and in lesions beginning in the nose and paranasal sinuses.

TREATMENT
* **Allergic bronchopulmonary aspergillosis:** prednisone 0.5-1 mg/kg PO until chest x-ray has cleared followed by alternate-day therapy at 0.5 mg/kg PO for 3 to 6 months, then graduatlly tapered
* **Aspergillomas:** surgical resection/arterial embolization for patients with severe hemoptysis or life-threatening hemorrhage. For patients at risk for marked hemoptysis with inadequate pulmonary reserve, consider itraconazole 200-400 mg/day PO.
* **Invasive aspergillosis:**
  * Amphotericin B deoxycholate 0.8-1.2 mg/kg IV qd to a total dose of 2-2.5 g; itraconazole 200-400 mg/day PO for 1 year
  * Amphotericin B lipid complex (ABLC) 5 mg/kg in patients intolerant of or refractory to amphotericin B
  * Amphotericin B colloidal dispension (ABCD) 3-6 mg/kg IV qd; stepwise approach in patients who have failed amphotericin B
  * Liposomal amphotericin B (L-AMB) 3-5 mg/kg IV qd; stepwise approach is indicated as empiric therapy for presumed fungal infection in febrile neutropenic patients who are refractory to or intolerant of amphotericin B
  * Itraconazole 200 mg IV bid × 4 doses followed by 200 mg IV qd or 200 mg tid for 4 days, then 200 mg bid PO—first line therapy if not taking P450 inducers

- Voriconazole 6 mg/kg IV bid followed by 6 mg/kg IV for 27 days, then 400 mg/day PO for 24 weeks
- Caspofungin (Cancidas) is the first of a new class of antifungals (echinocandins) approved by the Food and Drug Administration for the treatment of invasive aspergillosis in patients who fail to respond to or are unable to tolerate other antifungal drugs. The recommended dosage is 70 mg the first day and 50 mg daily thereafter given as a single dose intravenously over 1 hour.

Asthma

Definition: The National Asthma Education and Prevention Program (NAEPP) defines asthma as "a chronic inflammatory disorder of the airways in which many cells and cellular elements play a role. In susceptible individuals, this inflammation causes recurrent episodes of wheezing, breathlessness, chest tightness, and coughing, particularly at night and in the early morning. These episodes are usually associated with widespread but variable airflow obstruction that is often reversible either spontaneously or with treatment."

DIAGNOSIS

- Physical examination varies with the stage and severity of asthma and may reveal only increased inspiratory and expiratory phases of respiration.
- The following abnormalities in vital signs indicate severe asthma:
  - Pulsus paradoxus >18 mm Hg
  - Respiratory rate >30 breaths/min
  - Tachycardia with heart rate >120 beats/min
- Useful diagnostic tests for asthma include the following:
  - Pulmonary function studies—during acute severe bronchospasm, forced expiratory volume in 1 second is < 1 L and peak expiratory flow rate is <80 L/min
  - Methacholine challenge test
  - Skin test to assess the role of atopy (when suspected)
- Arterial blood gases can be used in staging the severity of an asthmatic attack:
  - Mild—decreased PaO_2 and $PaCO_2$, increased pH
  - Moderate—decreased PaO_2, normal
  - Severe—marked decreased PaO_2, increased $PaCO_2$, and decreased pH
- Chest x-ray is usually normal, but may show evidence of thoracic hyperinflation (e.g., flattening of the diaphragm, increased volume over the retrosternal air space)

...ows tachycardia, nonspecific ST-T wave changes; it also may show cor pulmonale, right bundle-branch block, right axial deviation, and counterclockwise rotation.

ETIOLOGY

- **Intrinsic asthma:** occurs in patients who have no history of allergies; may be triggered by upper respiratory infections or psychological stress
- **Extrinsic asthma (allergic asthma):** brought on by exposure to allergens (e.g., dust mites, cat allergen, industrial chemicals)
- **Exercise-induced asthma:** seen most frequently in adolescents; manifests with bronchospasm after initiation of exercise and improves with discontinuation of exercise
- **Drug-induced asthma:** often associated with use of nonsteroidal antiinflammatory drugs, β-blockers, sulfites, and certain foods and beverages
- There is a strong association of the *ADAM 33* gene with asthma and bronchial hyperresponsiveness.

TREATMENT

- The Expert Panel of the NAEPP, based on the classification of asthma severity, recommends the following stepwise approach in the pharmacologic management of asthma in adults and children >5 years old:
  - **Step 1 (mild intermittent asthma):** No daily medications are needed.
    - Short-acting inhaled β_2-agonists are used as needed.
  - **Step 2 (mild persistent asthma):** Daily treatment may be needed.
    - Low-dose inhaled corticosteroid can be used.
    - Cromolyn or nedocromil also can be used.
    - Additional considerations for long-term control are the use of the leukotriene receptor antagonist montelukast (Singulair).
    - Quick relief of asthma can be achieved with short-acting inhaled β_2-agonists.
  - Step 3 (moderate persistent asthma): Daily medication is recommended.
    - Low-dose or medium-dose inhaled corticosteroids plus long-acting inhaled β_2-agonist or long-acting oral β_2-agonists can be used. A salmeterol-fluticasone combination for the Discus inhaler (Advair) is now available and simplifies therapy for patients with asthma. It generally should be reserved for patients with at least moderately severe asthma not controlled by an inhaled corticosteroid alone.
    - Short-acting inhaled β-agonists can be used on an as-needed basis for quick relief.

- **Step 4 (severe persistent asthma):**
  - Daily treatment with high-dose inhaled corticosteroids plus long-acting inhaled β-agonists plus long-term systemic corticosteroids (e.g., methylprednisolone, prednisolone, prednisone) can be used.
  - Short-acting β₂-agonists can be used on an as-needed basis for quick relief.

CLINICAL PEARL
- Fifty percent to 80% of children with asthma develop symptoms before 5 years of age.

 Ataxia telangiectasia

Definition: An autosomal recessive disorder of childhood characterized by progressive cerebellar ataxia, choreoathetosis, telangiectasias of the skin and conjunctiva, increased sensitivity to ionizing radiation, and a predisposition to malignancies

DIAGNOSIS
- Children show normal early development until they start to walk, when gait and truncal ataxia become apparent.
- These findings soon are accompanied by polyneuropathy, progressive apraxia of eye movements, choreoathetosis, mild diabetes mellitus, growth failure, and signs of premature aging (graying of the hair).
- Telangiectatic lesions occur in the outer parts of the bulbar conjunctivae, over the ears, on exposed parts of the neck, on the bridge of the nose, and in the flexor creases of the forearms.
- Patients should be evaluated for serum immunoglobulin levels (IgA, IgG, IgE, and IgG subclasses), which are decreased or absent, and α-fetoprotein.
- Karyotype shows high incidence of chromosomal breaks, especially on chromosome 14. Genetic testing for ATM protein and gene is now available.
- CT or MRI shows cerebellar atrophy.
- Fibroblasts can be screened in vitro for x-ray sensitivity and radioresistant DNA synthesis.

ETIOLOGY
- Autosomal recessive, chromosome 11q22-q23. The defective gene product is *ATM*, a protein kinase that is thought to be a regulator of cell cycle checkpoint in response to DNA damage. Virtually every kindred has a distinct mutation.

- Supportive, no effective treatment to date
- Surveillance for infections and neoplasms; consider gamma-globulin injections to supplement immune system
- Minimize radiation because it may induce further chromosomal damage and lead to neoplasms
- Physical and occupational therapy

CLINICAL PEARLS
- Recurrent sinopulmonary infections occur secondary to impaired humoral and cellular immunity in about 70% of children.
- Increased frequency of cancers is noted in approximately 20% of patients, most frequently acute lymphocytic leukemia or lymphoma.

Atelectasis

Definition: Collapse of lung volume

DIAGNOSIS
- Chest x-ray confirms diagnosis.
- CT scan is useful in patients with suspected endobronchial neoplasm or extrinsic bronchial compression.
- Physical examination findings include decreased or absent breath sounds, abnormal chest percussion, diminished chest expansion, tachypnea, and tachycardia.
- Clinical presentation includes cough, dyspnea, decreased vocal fremitus, and vocal resonance.

ETIOLOGY
- Mechanical ventilation with higher fraction of inspired oxygen
- Chronic bronchitis
- Cystic fibrosis
- Endobronchial neoplasms
- Foreign bodies
- Infections (e.g., tuberculosis, histoplasmosis)
- Extrinsic bronchial compression from neoplasms, aneurysms of ascending aorta, enlarged left atrium
- Sarcoidosis
- Silicosis
- Anterior chest wall injury, pneumothorax
- Alveolar injury (e.g., toxic fumes, aspiration of gastric contents)
- Pleural effusion, expanding bullae
- Chest wall deformity (e.g., scoliosis)

- Muscular weaknesses or abnormalities (e.g., neuromuscular disease)
- Mucus plugs from asthma, allergic bronchopulmonary aspergillosis, postoperative state

TREATMENT

- Chest physiotherapy, humidification of inspired air, frequent nasotracheal suctioning
- Positive-pressure breathing (continuous positive airway pressure by facemask, positive end-expiratory pressure for patients on mechanical ventilation)
- Use of mucolytic agents (e.g. acetylcysteine [Mucomyst])
- Recombinant human DNase (dornase alfa) in patients with cystic fibrosis
- Bronchodilator therapy in selected patients

CLINICAL PEARL

Patients should be educated that frequent changes of position are helpful in clearing secretions. Sitting the patient upright in a chair is recommended to increase volume and vital capacity relative to the supine position.

Atrial fibrillation

Definition: Totally chaotic atrial activity caused by simultaneous discharge of multiple atrial foci

DIAGNOSIS

ECG shows the following:

- Irregular nonperiodic waveforms (best seen in V1) reflecting continuous atrial reentry
- Absence of P waves
- Conducted QRS complexes showing no periodicity (Fig. 3)

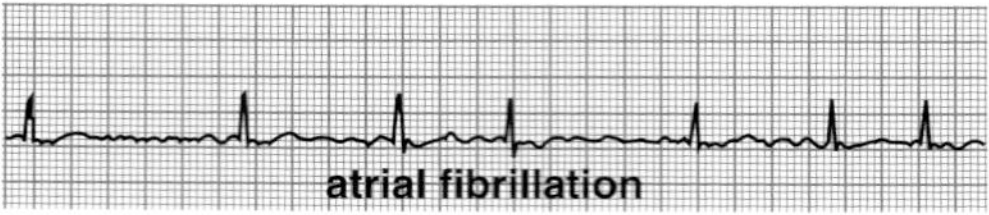

atrial fibrillation

FIGURE 3. Atrial fibrillation with slow ventricular response. (From Goldberger E: Treatment of Cardiac Emergencies, 5th ed. St. Louis, Mosby, 1990.)

ders.

- Holter monitor is useful only in selected patients to evaluate paroxysmal atrial fibrillation.
- Laboratory tests include thyroid-stimulating hormone, free thyroxine, and serum electrolytes.

ETIOLOGY

- Coronary artery disease
- Mitral stenosis, mitral regurgitation, atrial stenosis, atrial regurgitation
- Thyrotoxicosis
- Pulmonary embolism, chronic obstructive pulmonary disease
- Pericarditis
- Myocarditis, cardiomyopathy
- Tachycardia-bradycardia syndrome
- Alcohol abuse
- Myocardial infarction
- Wolff-Parkinson-White syndrome
- Other causes—left atrial myxoma, atrial septal defect, carbon monoxide poisoning, pheochromocytoma, idiopathic, hypoxia, hypokalemia, sepsis, pneumonia

TREATMENT

- **New-onset atrial fiibrillation**
  - If the patient is hemodynamically unstable, perform synchronized cardioversion.
  - If the patient is hemodynamically stable, treatment options include the following:
    - Give diltiazem 0.25 mg/kg given over 2 minutes followed by a second dose of 0.35 mg/kg 15 minutes later if the rate is not slowed. Follow with intravenous infusion 10 mg/hr (range 5-15 mg/hr). Onset of action after intravenous administration is usually within 3 minutes, with peak effect most often occurring within 10 minutes. After the ventricular rate is slowed, the patient can be changed to oral diltiazem 60-90 mg q6h.
    - Give verapamil 2.5-5 mg IV initially, then 5-10 mg IV 10 minutes later if the rate is still not slowed. After the ventricular rate is slowed, the patient can be changed to oral verapamil 80-120 mg q6-8h.
    - Give digoxin 0.5 mg IV loading dose (slow), then 0.25 mg IV 6 hours later. A third dose may be needed after 6 to 8 hours; daily dose varies from 0.125 to 0.25 mg (decrease dosage in patients with renal insufficiency and elderly patients). Digoxin should be avoided in Wolff-Parkinson-White patients with atrial fibrillation.

Procainamide is the preferred pharmacologic agent in these patients.

Esmolol, metoprolol, and atenolol are β-blockers are available in intravenous preparations that can be used in atrial fibrillation.

Other medications useful for converting atrial fibrillation to sinus rhythm are ibutilide, flecainide, propafenone, disopyramide, amiodarone and quinidine.

Intravenous heparin or subcutaneous low-molecular-weight heparin followed by warfarin is indicated.

Long-term anticoagulation with warfarin (adjusted to maintain an international normalized ratio of 2-3) is indicated in all patients with atrial fibrillation and associated cardiovascular disease, including the following:

- Rheumatic valvular disease (mitral stenosis, mitral regurgitation, aortic insufficiency)
- Aortic stenosis
- Prosthetic mitral valve
- History of previous embolism
- Known cardiac thrombus
- Congestive heart failure
- Cardiomyopathy with poor left ventricular function
- Nonrheumatic heart disease (e.g., hypertensive cardiovascular disease, coronary artery disease, atrial septal defect)

Anticoagulation generally is not recommended in young patients with isolated atrial fibrillation (no associated cardiovascular disease)

Aspirin 325 mg/day may be a suitable alternative to warfarin in patients <70 years old with increased risk of bleeding.

CLINICAL PEARLS

- Cardioversion is indicated if the ventricular rate is < 140 beats/min and the patient is symptomatic (particularly in acute myocardial infarction, chest pain, dyspnea, congestive heart failure), or when there is no conversion to normal sinus rhythm after 3 days of pharmacologic therapy.

- Amiodarone therapy should be considered for patients with recent atrial fibrillation and structural heart disease, particularly patients with left ventricular dysfunction. Amiodarone also should be considered for patients with refractory conditions who do not have heart disease, before therapies with irreversible effects, such as atrioventricular nodal ablation, are attempted.

Atrial flutter

Definition: Rapid atrial rate of 280 to 340 beats/min with varying degrees of intraventricular block

DIAGNOSIS

- ECG shows regular, "sawtooth," or F wave pattern, best seen in II, III, and aVF and secondary to atrial depolarization (Fig. 4). Atrioventricular conduction block (2 : 1, 3 : 1, or varying) also is shown.
- Physical examination reveals fast pulse rate (approximately 150 beats/min).
- Clinical presentation includes symptoms of cardiac failure, light-headedness, and angina pectoris.
- Laboratory tests include thyroid function studies and serum electrolytes.

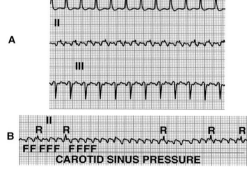

FIGURE 4. Atrial flutter waves (F). **A,** The flutter waves are not apparent in lead I, but are obvious in leads II and III. **B,** Carotid sinus pressure slowed the ventricular rate, but did not change the atrial flutter rate. (From Goldberger E: Treatment of Cardiac Emergencies, 5th ed. St Louis, Mosby, 1990.)

ETIOLOGY
- Atherosclerotic heart disease
- Myocardial infarction
- Thyrotoxicosis
- Pulmonary embolism
- Mitral valve disease
- Cardiac surgery
- Chronic obstructive pulmonary disease

TREATMENT
- Valsalva maneuver or carotid sinus massage usually slows the ventricular rate (increases grade of atrioventricular block) and may make flutter waves more evident.
- Electrical cardioversion is given at low energy levels (20-25 J).
- In the absence of cardioversion, intravenous diltiazem or digitalization may be tried to slow the ventricular rate and convert flutter to fibrillation. Esmolol, verapamil, and adenosine also may be effective.
- Atrial pacing also may terminate atrial flutter.
- Atrial flutter frequently is associated with intermittent atrial fibrillation. It may be prudent to anticoagulate patients with atrial flutter and coexisting medical disorders (e.g., diabetes mellitus, hypertension, cardiac disease) before cardioversion.
- Chronic atrial flutter may respond to amiodarone.
- Radiofrequency ablation to interrupt the atrial flutter also is effective for patients with chronic or recurring atrial flutter.

CLINICAL PEARLS
- Atrial flutter is common during the first week after open heart surgery.
- More than 85% of patients convert to regular sinus rhythm after cardioversion with 25 to 50 J.

Atrial septal defect (ASD)

Definition: Abnormal opening in the atrial septum that allows for blood flow between the atria. There are several forms:

Ostium primum—defect low in the septum
Ostium secundum—occurs mainly in the region of the fossa ovalis
Sinus venous defect—less common form, involves the upper part of the septum

- Echocardiography with saline bubble contrast and Doppler flow studies may show ASD and the presence of shunting. Transesophageal echocardiography is much more sensitive than transthoracic echocardiography in identifying sinus venous defects and is preferred by some clinicians for the initial diagnostic evaluation.
- Cardiac catheterization confirms the diagnosis in patients who are candidates for surgery. It is useful if the patient has some anatomic finding on echocardiography that is not completely clear or has significant elevation of pulmonary artery pressures.
- Physical examination reveals pansystolic murmur best heard at apex secondary to mitral regurgitation (ostium primum defect), widely split S_2, visible and palpable pulmonary artery pulsations, ejection systolic flow murmur, prominent right ventricular impulse, cyanosis, and clubbing (severe cases).
- Exertional dyspnea may be present; however, patients with small defects are generally asymptomatic.

ETIOLOGY
- The etiology is unknown.

TREATMENT
- **Children and infants:** Closure of ASD before age 10 years is indicated if pulmonary: systemic flow ratio is >1.5 : 1.
- **Adults:** ASD closure is indicated in symptomatic patients with shunts >2 : 1.
- Surgery should be avoided in patients with pulmonary hypertension with reversed shunting (Eisenmenger's syndrome) because of increased risk of right heart failure.
- Transcatheter closure is advocated in children when feasible.
- Prophylactic β-blocker therapy to prevent atrial arrhythmias should be considered in adults with ASD.
- Surgical closure is indicated in all patients with ostium primum defect and significant shunting, unless the patient has significant pulmonary vascular disease.

CLINICAL PEARLS
- Surgical mortality varies with the age of the patient and the presence of cardiac failure and systolic pulmonary artery hypertension; mortality ranges from <1% in young patients (<45 years old) to >10% in elderly patients with presence of heart failure and systolic pulmonary hypertension.
- Preoperative atrial fibrillation is a risk factor for immediate postoperative and long-term atrial fibrillation.

Babesiosis

Definition: A tick-transmitted protozoan disease of animals, caused by intraerythrocytic parasites of the genus *Babesia*. Humans are incidentally infected, resulting in a nonspecific febrile illness.

DIAGNOSIS

- Diagnosis made serologically by indirect immunofluorescence assay specific for *Babesia microti*.
  - Titer of ≥1 : 64 indicates seropositivity, whereas a titer of ≥1 : 256 is considered diagnostic of acute infection.
  - Assay is hampered by the inability to distinguish between exposed patients and patients who are actively infected.
  - IgM indirect immunofluorescent-antibody test may be highly sensitive and specific for diagnosis.
  - Babesial DNA by polymerase chain reaction has comparable sensitivity and specificity to microscopic analysis of thin blood smears.
- Giemsa-stained or Wright-stained thick and thin blood films are examined for intraerythrocytic parasites. In its classic, although infrequently seen, form a "tetrad" or "Maltese cross" composed of four daughter cells attached by cytoplasmic strands is observed. More commonly, smaller forms composed of a single chromatin dot are eccentrically located within bluish cytoplasm.
- Other laboratory test results include mild-to-moderate pancytopenia on complete blood count; abnormally elevated serum chemistries, including creatinine, liver function profile, lactate dehydrogenase, and direct and total bilirubin levels; and proteinuria and hemoglobinuria on urinalysis.
- Incubation period is 1 to 4 weeks or 6 to 9 weeks in transfusion-associated disease. There is gradual onset of irregular fever, chills, diaphoresis, headache, myalgia, arthralgia, fatigue, and dark urine.
- On physical examination, petechiae, frank or mild hepatosplenomegaly, and jaundice are found. Infection with *Babesia divergens* produces a more severe illness with a rapid onset of symptoms and increasing parasitemia progressing to massive intravascular hemolysis and renal failure.

TREATMENT

- Therapy is reserved for severely ill patients, especially if asplenic or immunosuppressed.
- Combination of quinine sulfate 650 mg PO tid plus clindamycin 600 mg PO tid (1.2 g parenterally bid) taken for 7 to 10 days is effective, but may not eliminate parasites.

combination of atovaquone 750 mg q12h and azithromycin 500 mg on day 1 and 250 mg/day thereafter for 7 days seems to be as effective as a regimen of clindamycin and quinine with fewer adverse reactions.
- Exchange transfusions in addition to antimicrobial therapy are successful treatment for severe infections in asplenic patients associated with high levels of *B. microti* or *B. divergens* parasitemia.

▰ Balanitis

Definition: Inflammation of the superficial tissues of the penile head

DIAGNOSIS
- Clinical presentation includes itching and tenderness, pain, dysuria, and local edema. Rarely, ulceration and lymph node enlargement may be present. Severe ulcerations can lead to superimposed bacterial infections.

ETIOLOGY
- Poor hygiene, causing erosion of tissue with erythema and promoting growth of *Candida albicans*
- Sexual contact, urinary catheters, and trauma
- Allergic reactions to condoms or medications

TREATMENT
- Clotrimazole 1% cream is applied topically twice daily to affected areas.
- Bacitracin or Neosporin ointment is applied topically four times daily.
- When more severe bacterial superinfection is present, give cephalexin 500 mg PO qid.
- Topical corticosteroids are added four times daily if dermatitis is severe.
- Patient should retract and bathe prepuce several times a day.
- Warm sitz baths ease edema and erythema.
- In uncircumcised patients consider circumcision, especially when symptoms are severe or recurrent.
- Consider biopsy to rule out other diagnoses, such as premalignant or malignant lesions, if lesions are not healing.

Barrett's esophagus

Definition: The squamous lining of the lower esophagus is replaced by columnar epithelium. The condition is associated with an increased risk of esophageal cancer.

DIAGNOSIS

- Symptoms include heartburn, dysphagia for solid food, chest pain, and hematemesis.
- Endoscopy with biopsy is necessary for diagnosis. Diagnosis requires the presence of intestinal metaplasia in columnar epithelium displaced proximal to the gastroesophageal junction.

ETIOLOGY

- Metaplasia is thought to result from reepithelialization of esophageal tissue injured secondary to, and in the background of, chronic gastroesophageal reflux.

TREATMENT

- Proton-pump inhibitors are most effective at relieving symptoms and healing mucosal injury.
- Antireflux surgery may be considered for management of gastroesophageal reflux disease and associated sequelae. Surgical resection is offered for multifocal high-grade dysplasia or carcinoma.

CLINICAL PEARLS

- Only 4% to 10% of patients with reflux symptoms develop Barrett's esophagus.
- Patients with chronic gastroesophageal reflux disease symptoms should be considered for a one-time endoscopy to exclude the presence of Barrett's esophagus. Because many patients with Barrett's esophagus are asymptomatic, some are missed; however, general population screening currently is not recommended.
- Intestinal metaplasia of the gastric cardia is not considered Barrett's esophagus and does not seem to convey the same risk of malignant transformation.

Behçet's disease

Definition: A chronic, relapsing, inflammatory disorder characterized by the presence of recurrent oral aphthous ulcers, genital ulcers, uveitis, and skin lesions

DIAGNOSIS

- The diagnosis of Behçet's disease is a clinical diagnosis. Laboratory tests and x-ray imaging may be helpful in evaluating the complications of Behçet's disease or excluding other diseases in the differential.
- According to the International Study Group for Behçet's disease, the diagnosis of Behçet's disease is established when recurrent oral ulceration is present along with at least two of the following in the absence of other systemic diseases:
  - Recurrent genital ulceration
  - Eye lesions
  - Skin lesions
  - Positive pathergy test

TREATMENT

- **Oral and genital ulcers:**
  - Topical corticosteroids (e.g., triamcinolone acetonide ointment applied three times daily)
  - Tetracycline tablets 250 mg dissolved in 5 mL of water and applied to the ulcer for 2 to 3 minutes
  - Colchicine 0.5-1.5 mg/kg/day PO
  - Thalidomide 100-300 mg PO daily
  - Dapsone 100 mg PO daily
  - Pentoxifylline 300 mg/day PO
  - Azathioprine 1-2.5 mg/kg/day PO
  - Methotrexate 7.5-25 mg/wk PO or IV
- **Ocular lesions:**
  - Anterior uveitis is treated by an ophthalmologist with topical corticosteroids (e.g., betamethasone drops 1-2 drops tid). Topical injection with dexamethasone 1-1.5 mg also has been tried.
  - Infliximab 5 mg/kg single dose
- **Central nervous system (CNS) disease:**
  - Chlorambucil 0.1 mg/kg/day is used in the treatment of posterior uveitis, retinal vasculitis, or CNS disease. Patients not responding to chlorambucil can be given cyclosporine 5-7 mg/kg/day.
  - In CNS vasculitis, cyclophosphamide 2-3 mg/kg/day is used. Prednisone can be used as an alternative.

- **Arthritis:**
  - Nonsteroidal antiinflammatory drugs (e.g., ibuprofen 400-800 mg PO tid or indomethacin 50-75 mg/day PO)
  - Sulfasalazine 1-3 g/day PO is an alternative treatment.
- **Gastrointestinal lesions:**
  - Sulfasalazine 1-3 g/day PO
  - Prednisone 40-60 mg/day PO
- **Vascular lesions:**
  - Prednisone 40-60 mg/day PO
  - Cytotoxic agents as mentioned previously
  - Heparin 5000-20,000 U/day followed by oral warfarin

Bell's palsy

Definition: Idiopathic, isolated, usually unilateral facial weakness in the distribution of the seventh cranial nerve (< 1 % of the facial palsies are bilateral)

DIAGNOSIS

Bell's palsy is a clinical diagnosis. A focused history and neurologic examination confirm the diagnosis:

- Unilateral paralysis of the upper and lower facial muscles (asymmetric eye closure, brow, and smile). Upward rolling of eye on attempted eye closure (*Bell's phenomenon*)
- Ipsilateral loss of taste
- Ipsilateral ear pain, usually 2 to 3 days before presentation
- Hyperacusis
- Increased or decreased unilateral eye tearing
- Subjective (but not objective) ipsilateral facial numbness

Laboratory studies include a fasting blood glucose to evaluate for diabetes and Lyme titer in endemic areas. Consider complete blood count, Venereal Disease Research Laboratory, erythrocyte sedimentation rate, and angiotensin-converting enzyme in selected patients.

Contrast-enhanced MRI to exclude neoplasms is indicated only in patients with atypical features or course.

Chest x-ray may be useful to exclude sarcoidosis or to rule out tuberculosis in selected patients before treating with steroids.

ETIOLOGY

- Most cases are idiopathic.
- The cause is often viral (herpes simplex).

...pes zoster can cause Bell's palsy in association with herpetic blisters affecting the outer ear canal or the area behind the ear (Ramsay Hunt syndrome).
- Bell's palsy also can be a manifestation of Lyme disease.

TREATMENT
- Although the benefits of corticosteroid therapy remain unproven, most practitioners use a brief course of prednisone therapy. Combination therapy with acyclovir and prednisone possibly may be effective in improvement of clinical recovery.
- If used, prednisone therapy should be started within 24 to 48 hours of symptom onset.
- Optimal steroid dose is unknown. Prednisone can be given as one 50-mg tablet qd for 7 days without tapering or can be started at 80 mg and tapered by 5 mg/day until finished. A Medrol Dosepak also may be given.
- Avoid corneal drying by applying skin tape to the upper lid to keep the palpebral fissure narrowed. Lacri-Lube ophthalmic ointment at night and artificial tears during the day also are useful to prevent excessive drying.
- The patient should wear dark glasses when going outside to minimize sun exposure.

CLINICAL PEARLS
- Patients should be monitored for evidence of corneal abrasion and ulceration or hemifacial spasm. Physical therapy, including moist heat and massage, may be beneficial.
- Complete recovery should occur in 71% of patients. Prognosis is improved for patients with clinical improvement within 3 weeks and with less severity of symptoms at onset.

Bite wounds

Definition: A bite wound can be animal or human, accidental or intentional.

DIAGNOSIS
- The appearance of the bite wound varies (e.g., puncture wound, tear, avulsion).
- Cellulitis, lymphangitis, and focal adenopathy may be present in infected bite wounds.
- Patient may experience fever and chills.
- Laboratory tests generally are not necessary. Wound cultures (aerobic and anaerobic) should be performed if there is evidence of sepsis or

the patient is immunocompromised; cultures should be obtained before irrigation of the wound but after superficial cleaning. Consider complete blood count if there has been significant blood loss.

- X-rays are indicated when bony penetration is suspected or if there is suspicion of fracture or significant trauma; x-rays are also useful for detecting presence of foreign bodies (when suspected).

ETIOLOGY

- Most frequent infecting organisms:
  - **Pasteurella:** responsible for most infections within 24 hours of dog (*Pcanis*) and cat (*Pmultocida, Pseptica*) bites
  - *Capnocytophaga canimorsus* (formerly DF2 bacillus): a gram-negative organism responsible for late infection, usually following dog bites
- **Gram-negative organisms (*Pseudomonas, Haemophilus*):** often found in human bites
  - *Streptococcus, Staphylococcus aureus*
  - *Eikenella corrodens* in human bites

Treatment

- Local care comprises débridement, vigorous cleansing, and saline irrigation of the wound and débridement of devitalized tissue.
- High-pressure irrigation cleans the wound and ensures removal of contaminants (e.g., use saline solution with a 30- to 35-mL syringe equipped with a 20-gauge needle or catheter with tip of syringe placed 2-3 cm above the wound).
- Avoid blunt probing of wounds (increased risk of infection).
- Avoid suturing of hand wounds and any wounds that appear infected.
- Puncture wounds should be left open.
- Give antirabies therapy and tetanus immune globulin and toxoid as needed.
- Use empiric antibiotic therapy in high-risk wounds (e.g. cat bite, hand bites, face bites, genital area bites, bites with joint or bone penetration, human bites, immunocompromised host). Give amoxicillin-clavulanate 500-2000 mg bid for 7 days or cefuroxime 250-500 mg bid for 7 days.
- In hospitalized patients, intravenous antibiotics of choice are cefoxitin 1-2 g q6h, ampicillin-sulbactam 1.5-3 g q6h, ticarcillin-clavulanate 3 g q6h, or ceftraxone 1-2 g q24h.
- Prophylactic therapy is warranted for persons bitten by others with HIV and hepatitis B.

- Infection rates are highest for cat bites (30-50%), followed by human bites (15-30%) and dog bites (5%).

Bronchiectasis

Definition: Abnormal dilation and destruction of bronchial walls, which may be congenital or acquired

DIAGNOSIS

- Chest x-ray examination reveals hyperinflation, crowded lung markings, and small cystic spaces at the base of the lungs.
- High-resolution CT of the chest has become the best tool to detect cystic lesions and exclude underlying obstruction from neoplasm. The CT study should be a noncontrast study with the use of a 1- to 1.5-mm window every 1 cm with acquisition time of 1 second. Typical findings on CT include dilation of airway lumen, lack of tapering of an airway toward periphery, ballooned cysts at the end of bronchus, and varicose constrictions along airways.
- Physical examination shows moist crackles at lung bases, halitosis, and skin pallor.
- Clinical presentation includes cough with expectoration of large amount of purulent sputum, fever, night sweats, generalized malaise, weight loss, and hemoptysis.

ETIOLOGY

- Cystic fibrosis
- Lung infections (pneumonia, lung abscess, tuberculosis, fungal infections, viral infections)
- Abnormal host defense (panhypogammaglobulinemia, Kartagener's syndrome, AIDS, chemotherapy)
- Localized airway obstruction (congenital structural defects, foreign bodies, neoplasms)
- Inflammation (inflammatory pneumonitis, granulomatous lung disease, allergic aspergillosis)

TREATMENT

- Postural drainage (reclining prone on a bed with the head down on the side) and chest percussion with use of inflatable vests or mechanical vibrators applied to the chest may enhance removal of respiratory secretions.
- Ensure adequate hydration.
- Provide supplemental oxygen for hypoxemia.

- Antibiotic therapy is based on the results of sputum, Gram stain, and culture and sensitivity in patients with inadequate or inconclusive results, empiric therapy with amoxicillin/clavulanate 500-875 mg q12h, trimethoprim-sulfamethoxazole 800 mg/160 mg q12h, doxycycline 100 mg bid, or cefuroxime 250 mg bid for 10 to 14 days is recommended.
- Bronchodilators are useful in patients with demonstrable airflow obstruction.

CLINICAL PEARL

- Surgical referral for partial lung resection should be considered in patients with localized severe disease unresponsive to medical therapy or in patients with massive hemoptysis.

Budd-Chiari Syndrome (BCS)

Definition: BCS is a rare disease defined by the obstruction of hepatic venous outflow anywhere from the small hepatic veins to the junction of the inferior vena cava and the right atrium. Primary BCS is defined by endoluminal obstruction as seen in thromboses or webs. Secondary BCS occurs when the obstruction is due to nonvascular invasion (malignancy or parasitic masses) or extrinsic compression (tumor, abscess, cysts).

DIAGNOSIS

- **Physical findings:** Variable according to the degree, location, acuity of obstruction, and presence of collateral circulation.
- **Fulminant/acute (uncommon):** severe right upper quadrant abdominal pain, fever, nausea, vomiting, jaundice, hepatomegaly, ascites, marked increase in serum aminotransferases and decrease in coagulation factors, and encephalopathy; early recognition and treatment essential to survival
- **Subacute/chronic (more common):** vague abdominal discomfort, gradual progression to hepatomegaly, portal hypertension with or without cirrhosis, late-onset ascites, lower extremity edema, esophageal varices, splenomegaly, coagulopathy, hepatorenal syndrome, and rarely encephalopathy
- **Asymptomatic:** usually discovered incidentally
- **Imaging studies:**
- Color and pulsed Doppler ultrasound—diagnostic sensitivity of >75%, first-line test
- MRI with gadolinium contrast—better than contrast-enhanced CT, second-line test

gold standard but invasive and mainly indicated to guide percutaneous or surgical intervention, confirm the classic "spiderweb" pattern caused by collateral venous flow, and look for BCS in cases of high clinical suspicion when initial studies are negative

ETIOLOGY
- Myeloproliferative disease
- Hypercoagulable states (can coexist with other causes; 31%)
- Infection
- Malignancy (<5%)
- Other—sarcoid, Behçet's disease, paroxysmal nocturnal hemoglobinuria, abdominal trauma, ulcerative colitis, celiac disease, dacarbazine therapy, idiopathic

TREATMENT
- Angioplasty and stenting, in situ thrombolysis, or removal of inferior vena cava webs to decompress the portal circulation, all combined with anticoagulation—for acute BCS in patients in stable condition
- Transjugular intrahepatic portosystemic stent shunt—may be a decompression option but can be especially hazardous in BCS patients because of the high prevalence of hepatic vein thromboses
- Liver transplant—for fulminant BCS or patients who fail the above-listed therapies
- Lifelong anticoagulation
- Treatment of underlying myeloproliferative or other disorders
- Treatment of liver dysfunction and complications related to portal hypertension

▉ Bulimia nervosa

Definition: A prolonged illness characterized by a specific psychopathology (see next page)

DIAGNOSIS
- The following questions are useful to screen patients for bulimia:
  - "Are you satisfied with your eating habits?"
  - "Do you ever eat in secret?"
  - Answering "no" to the first question or "yes" to the second question has 100% sensitivity and 90% specificity for bulimia. The SCOFF questionnaire also can be used as a screening tool for eating disorders (see "Anorexia Nervosa").

- A diagnosis also can be made using the following *Statistical Manual of Mental Disorders, Fourth Edition (DSM-IV)* diagnostic criteria for bulimia nervosa:
  - Recurrent episodes of binge eating (rapid consumption of a large amount of food in a discrete period of time)
  - A feeling of lack of control over eating behavior during the eating binges
  - Self-induced vomiting, use of laxatives or diuretics, strict dieting or fasting, or rigorous exercise to prevent weight gain
  - A minimum of two binge-eating episodes a week for at least 3 months
  - Persistent overconcern with body shape and weight
- Laboratory evaluation may reveal:
  - Electrolyte abnormalities secondary to vomiting (hypokalemia and metabolic alkalosis) or to diarrhea from laxative abuse (hypokalemia and hyperchloremic metabolic acidosis)
  - Hyponatremia, hypocalcemia, hypomagnesemia (caused by laxative abuse)
  - Elevated cortisol, decreased luteinizing hormone, decreased follicle-stimulating hormone
- Physical examination may reveal:
  - Parotid and salivary gland swelling
  - Scars on the back of the hand and knuckles (Russell's sign) from rubbing against the upper incisors when inducing vomiting
  - Eroded enamel, particularly on the lingual surface of the upper teeth; pyorrhea and other gum disorders possible
  - Petechial hemorrhages of the cornea, soft palate, or face possibly noted after vomiting
  - Loss of gag reflex, well-developed abdominal musculature

ETIOLOGY

- Etiology is unknown, but likely is multifactorial (sociocultural, psychological, familial factors). Bulimia is much more common in Western societies, where there is a strong cultural pressure to be slender. According to the American Psychiatric Association, patients with eating disorders display a broad range of symptoms that occur along a continuum between those of anorexia nervosa and bulimia.

TREATMENT

- Cognitive behavioral therapy is recommended to control abnormal behaviors.
- Use of food diaries, nutritional counseling, and planning meals at least a day in advance is useful to counter abnormal eating behaviors.

- Selective serotonin reuptake inhibitors generally are considered to be the safest medication option in these patients. They are useful in severely depressed patients and in patients who fail to benefit from cognitive behavioral therapy.

CLINICAL PEARL
- Bulimia has a close association with depression, bipolar disorder, obsessive-compulsive disorder, alcoholism, and substance abuse.

▰ Carbon monoxide poisoning

Definition: Carbon monoxide is a colorless, odorless, tasteless, nonirritating gas. When inhaled, it produces toxicity by causing cellular hypoxia.

DIAGNOSIS
- Carboxyhemoglobin level
  - *Note:* Carboxyhemoglobin level >5% in nonsmokers confirms exposure. Heavy smokers may have levels of 10%.
- Direct measurement of arterial oxygen saturation
- Presentation is often nonspecific. Patients with mild to moderately severe poisoning may present with headache, fatigue, dizziness, nausea, dyspnea, confusion, or blurry vision. Patients with severe poisoning may present with arrhythmias, myocardial ischemia, pulmonary edema, lethargy, ataxia, syncope, seizure, coma, or cherry-red skin.
  - *Note:* Pulse oximetry and arterial blood gas may be falsely normal because neither measures oxygen saturation directly. Pulse oximetry is inaccurate because of the similar absorption characteristics of oxyhemoglobin and carboxyhemoglobin. An arterial blood gas is inaccurate because it measures oxygen dissolved in plasma (which is not affected by carbon monoxide), then calculates oxygen saturation.
- Electrolytes, glucose, blood urea nitrogen, creatinine, creatine phosphokinase, arterial blood gas (because lactic acidosis and rhabdomyolysis may develop)
- ECG (rule out ischemia)
- Pregnancy test (fetus at high risk)
- Consider toxicology screen

ETIOLOGY

- Carbon monoxide poisoning occurs when individuals are exposed to smoke from fires; motor vehicle exhaust; or the burning of wood, charcoal, or natural gas for cooking or heating in poorly ventilated areas.

TREATMENT

- Remove from site of carbon monoxide exposure.
- Ensure adequate airway.
- Implement continuous ECG monitoring.
- Administer 100% oxygen by tight-fitting nonrebreather mask or endotracheal tube (this decreases the half-life of carboxyhemoglobin from 4-6 hours to 60-90 minutes).
- Measure carboxyhemoglobin level every 2 to 4 hours.
- Continue oxygen therapy until carboxyhemoglobin level is <10%.
- Hyperbaric oxygen (3 atm) decreases half-life of carbon monoxide to 20 to 30 minutes.
- It is controversial whether there is any beneficial effect of hyperbaric oxygen over regular 100% oxygen.
- A study suggests patients with acute (<24 hours), symptomatic carbon monoxide poisoning treated with three hyperbaric oxygen sessions within 24 hours had lower rates of cognitive sequelae at 6 weeks and 12 hours compared with patients treated with normobaric oxygen.
- Consider hyperbaric oxygen in:
  - Patients with severe intoxication (carboxyhemoglobin >25%, neurologic symptoms or signs, ischemic ECG changes, severe metabolic acidosis, rhabdomyolysis, pulmonary edema, shock)
  - Patients who remain symptomatic after 2 to 4 hours of oxygen at room air
  - Pregnant women with carboxyhemoglobin >15% or signs of fetal distress; lower threshold for treatment suggested given the higher affinity of carbon monoxide for fetal hemoglobin
- Consult local poison control center.
- Consider concomitant poisoning with other toxic/irritant gases that may be present in smoke and thermal injury to the airway.
- Identify source of exposure and determine if poisoning was accidental.

CLINICAL PEARLS

- Survivors of severe poisoning are at 14% to 40% risk for neurologic sequelae ranging from parkinsonism to neuropsychiatric symptoms (personality and memory disorders). Neurologic deficits usually are apparent within 3 weeks of poisoning (but may present months

...y show changes in the white matter and basal ganglia.
- Symptoms of toxicity and prognosis do not correlate well with carboxyhemoglobin levels.

Carcinoid syndrome

Definition: Symptom complex characterized by paroxysmal vasomotor disturbances, diarrhea, and bronchospasm caused by the action of amines and peptides (serotonin, bradykinin, histamine) produced by tumors arising from neuroendocrine cells

DIAGNOSIS
- Cutaneous flushing (75-90%)
  - The patient usually has red-purple flushes starting in the face, then spreading to the neck and upper trunk.
  - The flushing episodes last a few minutes to hours (longer lasting flushes may be associated with bronchial carcinoids).
  - Flushing may be triggered by emotion, alcohol, or foods or may occur spontaneously.
  - Dizziness, tachycardia, and hypotension may be associated with cutaneous flushing.
- Diarrhea (>70%) often associated with abdominal bloating and audible peristaltic rushes
- Intermittent bronchospasm (25%) characterized by severe dyspnea and wheezing
- Facial telangiectasia
- Tricuspid regurgitation from carcinoid heart lesions
- The biochemical marker for carcinoid syndrome is increased 24-hour urinary 5-hydroxyindoleacetic acid, a metabolite of serotonin (5-hydroxytryptamine). False elevations can be seen with ingestion of certain foods (bananas, pineapples, eggplant, avocados, walnuts) and certain medications (acetaminophen, caffeine, guaifenesin, reserpine); patients should be on a restricted diet and should avoid these medications when the test is ordered.
- Chest x-ray is useful to detect bronchial carcinoids.
- CT scan of abdomen or a liver and spleen radionuclide scan is useful to detect liver metastases (palpable in >50% of cases).
- Iodine-123-labeled somatostatin can detect carcinoid endocrine tumors with somatostatin receptors.
- Scanning with radiolabeled octreotide can visualize previously undetected or metastatic lesions.

ETIOLOGY

- The carcinoid syndrome is caused by neoplasms originating from neuroendocrine cells.
- Carcinoid tumors are found principally in the following organs: appendix (40%); small bowel (20%, 15% in the ileum); rectum (15%); bronchi (12%); esophagus, stomach, colon (10%); ovary biliary tract, pancreas (3%).
- Carcinoid tumors do not usually produce the syndrome, unless liver metastases are present or the primary tumor does not involve the gastrointestinal tract.

TREATMENT

- Surgical resection of the tumor can be curative if the tumor is localized or palliative and result in prolonged asymptomatic periods if metastases are present. Surgical manipulation of the tumor can cause severe vasomotor abnormalities and bronchospasm (carcinoid crisis).
- Percutaneous embolization and ligation of the hepatic artery can decrease the bulk of the tumor in the liver and provide palliative treatment of tumors with hepatic metastases.
- **Cytotoxic chemotherapy:** Combination chemotherapy with 5-fluorouracil and streptozotocin can be used in patients with unresectable or recurrent carcinoid tumors; however, it has only limited success.
- **Control of clinical manifestations:**
- Diarrhea usually responds to diphenoxylate with atropine (Lomotil).
- Flushing can be controlled by the combination of H₁-receptor and H₂-receptor antagonists (e.g., diphenhydramine 25-50 mg PO q6h and ranitidine 150 mg bid).
- Somatostatin analogue (SMS 201-995) is effective for flushing and diarrhea in most patients.
- Bronchospasm can be treated with aminophylline or albuterol or both.
- **Nutritional support:** Supplemental niacin therapy may be useful to prevent pellagra because the tumor uses dietary tryptophan for serotonin synthesis, resulting in a nutritional deficiency in some patients.
- Subcutaneous somatostatin analogues (octreotide 150 μg SC tid) have been used successfully for long-term control of symptoms in patients with unresectable neoplasms.

CLINICAL PEARLS

- Echocardiography and monitoring for right-sided congestive heart failure are recommended for patients with unresectable disease because endocardial fibrosis, involving predominantly the endo-

..., ... valves of the right side of the heart, can occur and result in right-sided congestive heart failure.
- Carcinoids of the appendix and rectum have a low malignancy potential and rarely produce the clinical syndrome; metastases also are uncommon if the size of the primary lesion is <2 cm in diameter.

Cardiac tamponade

Definition: Pericardial effusion that significantly impairs diastolic filling of the heart

DIAGNOSIS

- Signs and symptoms include dyspnea, orthopnea, and interscapular pain.
- Physical examination reveals distended neck veins, distant heart sounds, decreased apical impulse, diaphoresis, tachypnea, tachycardia, Ewart's sign (an area of dullness at the angle of the left scapula caused by compression of the lungs by the pericardial effusion), pulsus paradoxus (decrease in systolic blood pressure >10 mm Hg during inspiration), hypotension, and narrowed pulse pressure.
- Chest x-ray shows cardiomegaly (water-bottle configuration of the cardiac silhouette may be seen) with clear lungs; chest x-ray may be normal when acute tamponade occurs rapidly in the absence of prior pericardial effusion.
- ECG reveals decreased amplitude of the QRS complex and variation of the R wave amplitude from beat to beat (electrical alternans). This results from the heart's oscillating in the pericardial sac from beat to beat and frequently occurs with neoplastic effusions.
- Echocardiography detects effusions of 30 mL; a paradoxical wall motion also may be seen.
- Cardiac catheterization reveals equalization of pressures within chambers of the heart, elevation of right atrial pressure with a prominent x but no significant y descent.
- MRI also can be used to diagnose pericardial effusions.

TREATMENT

- Therapy for pericardial tamponade consists of immediate pericardiocentesis preferably by needle paracentesis with the use of echocardiography, fluoroscopy, or CT. In patients with recurrent effusions (e.g., neoplasms), placement of a percutaneous drainage catheter or pericardial window draining in the pleural cavity may be necessary. Aspirated fluid should be sent for analysis (protein, lactate dehydrogenase, cytology, complete blood count, Gram stain, acid-fast bacillus stain) and cultures for acid-fast bacilli, fungi, and bacterial culture and sensitivity.

Cardiomyopathy, dilated (congestive)

Definition: Cardiomyopathies are a group of diseases primarily involving the myocardium and characterized by myocardial dysfunction that is not the result of hypertension, coronary atherosclerosis, valvular dysfunction, or pericardial abnormalities. In dilated cardiomyopathy, the heart is enlarged, and both ventricles are dilated.

DIAGNOSIS

Physical examination may reveal:

- Increased jugular venous pressure
- Small pulse pressure
- Pulmonary rales, hepatomegaly, peripheral edema
- S_3, S_4
- Mitral regurgitation, tricuspid regurgitation (less common)
- Chest x-ray shows cardiac enlargement and possible interstitial pulmonary edema.
- ECG reveals left ventricular hypertrophy with ST-T wave changes, right bundle branch block or left bundle branch block, and arrhythmias (atrial fibrillation, premature ventricular contraction, premature atrial contraction, ventricular tachycardia).
- Echocardiogram reveals low ejection fraction with global akinesia.

ETIOLOGY

- Idiopathic
- Alcoholism (15–40% of all cases in Western countries)
- Collagen vascular disease (systemic lupus erythematosus, rheumatoid arthritis, polyarteritis, dermatomyositis)
- Postmyocarditis
- Peripartum (last trimester of pregnancy or 6 months postpartum)
- Heredofamilial neuromuscular disease
- Toxins (cobalt, lead, phosphorus, carbon monoxide, mercury, doxorubicin, daunorubicin)
- Nutritional (beriberi, selenium deficiency, carnitine deficiency, thiamine deficiency)
- Cocaine, heroin, organic solvents ("glue sniffer's heart")
- Irradiation
- Acromegaly, osteogenesis imperfecta, myxedema, thyrotoxicosis, dia-

- Antiretroviral agents (zidovudine, didanosine, zalcitabine)
- Phenothiazines
- Infections (viral [HIV], rickettsial, mycobacterial, toxoplasmosis, trichinosis, Chagas' disease)
- Hematologic (sickle cell anemia)

TREATMENT
- Treat congestive heart failure (cause of death in 70% of patients) with sodium restriction, diuretics, angiotensin-converting enzyme (ACE) inhibitors, β-blockers, spironolactone, and digitalis.
- Vasodilators (combined with nitrates and ACE inhibitors) are effective agents in all symptomatic patients with left ventricular dysfunction.
- Thromboembolism should be prevented with oral anticoagulants in all patients with atrial fibrillation and in patients with moderate or severe failure.
- Low-dose β-blockade with carvedilol or other β-blockers may improve ventricular function by interrupting the cycle of reflex sympathetic activity and controlling tachycardia.
- Diltiazem and ACE inhibitors also have been reported to have a long-term beneficial effect in idiopathic dilated cardiomyopathy.
- Use antiarrhythmic treatment as appropriate. Empiric pharmacologic suppression of asymptomatic ventricular ectopy does not reduce risk of sudden death or improve long-term survival. In patients with severe left ventricular dysfunction or symptomatic and sustained ventricular tachycardia, the use of an automatic implantable cardioverter-defibrillator should be considered.
- Patients with dilated cardiomyopathy (left ventricular ejection fraction <25%) and associated coronary atherosclerosis (angina, ECG changes, reversible defects on thallium scan) may benefit from surgical revascularization.

CLINICAL PEARL
- Vulnerability to cardiomyopathy among chronic alcohol abusers is partially genetic and is related to the presence of ACE DD genotype.

Cardiomyopathy, hypertrophic (HCM)

Definition: Cardiomyopathies are a group of diseases primarily involving the myocardium and characterized by myocardial dysfunction that is not the result of hypertension, coronary atherosclerosis, valvular dysfunction, or pericardial abnormalities. In HCM, there is marked hypertrophy of the myocardium and disproportionally greater thickening of the intraventricular septum than that of the free wall of the left ventricle (asymmetric septal hypertrophy).

DIAGNOSIS

- Findings on two-dimensional echocardiography include ventricular hypertrophy, ratio of septum thickness to left ventricular wall thickness $\geq 1.3:1$, and increased ejection fraction.
- MRI may be of diagnostic value when echocardiographic studies are technically inadequate. MRI also is useful in identifying segmental left ventricular hypertrophy undetectable by echocardiography.
- Physical examination reveals harsh, systolic, diamond-shaped murmur at the left sternal border or apex that increases with Valsalva maneuver and decreases with squatting.
- Chest x-ray is normal or reveals cardiomegaly.
- ECG is abnormal in 75% to 95% of patients with left ventricular hypertrophy and abnormal Q waves in anterolateral and inferior leads.
- Medical history should be obtained with emphasis in the following manifestations:
  - Dyspnea
  - Syncope (usually seen with exercise)
  - Angina (decreased angina in recumbent position)
  - Palpitations
  - Twenty-four-hour Holter monitor screens for potential lethal arrhythmias (principal cause of syncope or sudden death in obstructive cardiomyopathy).

ETIOLOGY

- Autosomal dominant trait with variable penetrance caused by mutations in any of 1 to 10 genes, each encoding proteins of cardiac sarcomere
- Sporadic occurrence

TREATMENT

- β-Blockers (e.g. propranolol 160-240 mg/day). The beneficial effects of β-blockers on symptoms (principally dyspnea and chest pain) and exercise tolerance seem to be largely a result of a decrease in the passive ventricular filling. By reducing the inotropic response, β-blockers also may lessen myocardial oxygen demand and decrease the outflow gradient during exercise, when sympathetic tone is increased.

- Verapamil also decreases left ventricular outflow obstruction by improving filling and probably reducing myocardial ischemia.
- Intravenous saline infusion in addition to propranolol or verapamil is indicated in patients with congestive heart failure.
- Disopyramide is a useful antiarrhythmic because it is also a negative inotrope.
- Use antibiotic prophylaxis for surgical procedures.
- Avoid use of digitalis, diuretics, nitrates, and vasodilators.
- Encouraging results have been reported on the use of DDD pacing for hemodynamic and symptomatic benefit in patients with drug-resistant HCM.
- Implantable defibrillators are a safe and effective therapy in HCM patients prone to ventricular arrhythmias. Their use is strongly warranted for patients with prior cardiac arrest or sustained spontaneous ventricular tachycardia.
- Surgical treatment (myotomy-myectomy) is reserved for patients who have a large outflow gradient (≥50 mm Hg) and severe symptoms of heart failure that are unresponsive to medical therapy. The risk of sudden death from arrhythmias is not altered by surgery.

CLINICAL PEARLS

- HCM is not a static disease. Some adults may experience subtle regression in wall thickness, whereas others (approximately 5-10%) paradoxically evolve into an end stage resembling dilated cardiomyopathy and characterized by cavity enlargement, left ventricular wall thinning, and diastolic dysfunction.
- Patients with HCM are at increased risk of sudden death, especially if there is onset of symptoms during childhood. Left ventricular outflow at rest is also a strong, independent predictor of severe symptoms of heart failure and of death.

Cardiomyopathy, restrictive

Definition: Cardiomyopathies are a group of diseases primarily involving the myocardium and characterized by myocardial dysfunction that is not the result of hypertension, coronary atherosclerosis, valvular dysfunction, or pericardial abnormalities. Restrictive cardiomyopathies are characterized by decreased ventricular compliance, usually secondary to infiltration of the myocardium.

DIAGNOSIS

- Echocardiogram shows increased wall thickness and thickened cardiac valves (especially in patients with amyloidosis).
- Cardiac catheterization can be used to distinguish restrictive cardiomyopathy from constrictive pericarditis. MRI also may be useful to distinguish restrictive cardiomyopathy from constrictive pericarditis (thickness of the pericardium >5 mm in the latter).
- Chest x-ray shows moderate cardiomegaly and possible evidence of congestive heart failure (CHF) (pulmonary vascular congestion, pleural effusion).
- ECG shows low voltage with ST-T wave changes. Arrhythmias, left axis deviation, and atrial fibrillation also may be present.
- Physical examination reveals edema, ascites, hepatomegaly, distended neck veins, regurgitant murmur, prominent apical impulse, and Kussmaul's sign.
- Patient may complain of fatigue and weakness (secondary to low output).

ETIOLOGY

- Infiltrative and storage disorders (glycogen storage disease, amyloidosis, sarcoidosis, hemochromatosis)
- Scleroderma
- Radiation
- Endocardial fibroelastosis
- Endomyocardial fibrosis
- Idiopathic
- Toxic effects of anthracycline
- Carcinoid heart disease, metastatic cancers
- Diabetic cardiomyopathy
- Eosinophilic cardiomyopathy (Löffler's endocarditis)

TREATMENT

- Cardiomyopathy caused by hemochromatosis may respond to repeated phlebotomies to decrease iron deposition in the heart.
- Sarcoidosis may respond to corticosteroid therapy.

with eosinophilic cardiomyopathy.
- There is no effective therapy for other causes of restrictive cardiomyopathy.

CLINICAL PEARL
- Death usually results from CHF or arrhythmias; therapy should be aimed at controlling CHF by restricting salt, administering diuretics, and treating potentially fatal arrhythmias.

 Carpal tunnel syndrome

Definition: Focal entrapment syndrome involving the median nerve as it passes in the area between the bones of the wrist and the transverse carpal ligament

DIAGNOSIS
- Clinical presentation includes numbness and pain in the distal arm or wrist. It is exacerbated by movement and typically radiates on the palmar surface of the first three digits of the hand. Nocturnal pain is common. Pain may radiate cephalad to the shoulder.
- **Tinel's sign:** Tapping over the median nerve on the flexor surface of the wrist produces a tingling sensation radiating from the wrist to the hand.
- **Phalen's test:** Flexing the wrist 90 degrees for 1 minute causes numbness and dysesthesias in the distribution of the median nerve.
- Diagnosis is confirmed with nerve conduction studies (if necessary and patient is considering surgery).

ETIOLOGY
- Possible causes include rheumatoid tenosynovitis, pregnancy, hypothyroidism, acromegaly, diabetes, mass lesions (lipoma, ganglion, neoplasm), aberrant anatomy, edema, postinjury, repeated trauma, amyloid, and wrist fracture.

TREATMENT
- Have patient minimize wrist movement (e.g., wrist splint, improved positioning of computer keyboard).
- Prescribe nonsteroidal antiinflammatory drugs.
- Corticosteroid wrist injections may be useful in selected patients and result in improvements in 50% to 80% of affected patients, although most of these patients experience recurrence.

- Consider surgical carpal tunnel release if the preceding measures are ineffective. Surgical division of the transverse carpal ligament relieves sensory complaints in >90% of patients.

▇ Cat-scratch disease (CSD)

Definition: A syndrome consisting of gradually enlarging regional lymphadenopathy occurring after contact via scratch with a cat

DIAGNOSIS

- The classic and most common finding is regional lymphadenopathy occurring within 2 weeks of a scratch or contact with a cat.
- Tender, swollen lymph nodes most commonly are found in the head and neck, followed by the axilla and the epitrochlear, inguinal, and femoral areas.
- Erythematous overlying skin shows signs of suppuration from involved lymph nodes.
- On careful examination, evidence of cutaneous inoculation is found in the form of a nonpruritic, slightly tender pustule or papule.
- Three of four of the following criteria are required for diagnosis:
  - History of animal contact in the presence of a scratch, dermal, or eye lesion
  - Culture of lymphatic aspirate that is negative for other causes
  - Positive CSD skin test
  - Biopsied lymph node histology consistent with CSD

ETIOLOGY

- *Major cause: Bartonella (Rochalimaea) henselae*
- **Mode of transmission:** predominantly by direct inoculation through the scratch, bite, or lick of a cat, especially a kitten

TREATMENT

- There is no consensus over therapy because the disease is self-limited in most cases. *Bartonella* is usually sensitive to aminoglyco-sides, tetracycline, erythromycin, and the quinolones.
- When the isolate is proven by culture, the patient should receive antibiotic therapy as directed by the obtained sensitivities.
- Warm compresses can be applied to the affected nodes.

CLINICAL PEARL

- A presentation of CSD, especially in patients with HIV infection or impaired cellular immunity, may be fever of unknown origin.

Cavernous sinus thrombosis

Definition: An uncommon diagnosis usually stemming from infections of the face or paranasal sinuses resulting in thrombosis of the cavernous sinus and inflammation of its surrounding anatomic structures, including cranial nerves III, IV, V (ophthalmic and maxillary branch), and VI and the internal carotid artery

DIAGNOSIS

- Classic findings include:
  - Ptosis
  - Proptosis
  - Chemosis
  - Cranial nerve palsies (III, IV, V, VI)
  - Sixth nerve palsy most common
  - Sensory deficits of the ophthalmic and maxillary branch of the fifth nerve common
- Complete blood count, erythrocyte sedimentation rate, blood cultures, and sinus cultures help establish and identify an infectious primary source.
- Lumbar puncture is necessary to rule out meningitis.
- MRI is the imaging study of choice.

ETIOLOGY

- *Staphylococcus aureus* is the most common infectious microbe (found in 50-60% of cases).
- *Streptococcus* is the second leading cause.
- Gram-negative rods and anaerobes also may cause cavernous sinus thrombosis.
- The most common primary site of infection leading to cavernous sinus thrombosis is sphenoid sinusitis; however, other sites of infection, including the middle ear, orbit, eye, eyelid, and face, can result in the same sequelae.

TREATMENT

- Broad-spectrum intravenous antibiotics are used until a definite pathogen is found.
  - Nafcillin 1.5 g IV q4h
  - Cefotaxime 1.5-2 g IV q4h
  - Metronidazole 15 mg/kg load followed by 7.5 mg/kg IV q6h
- Anticoagulation with heparin is controversial. Retrospective studies show conflicting data. This decision should be made with subspecialty consultation.
- Steroid therapy also is controversial.

Celiac disease

Definition: Chronic disease characterized by malabsorption and diarrhea precipitated by ingestion of food products containing gluten

DIAGNOSIS

- Antigliadin IgA and IgG antibodies are elevated in >90% of patients; however, they are nonspecific. IgA endomysial antibodies are more specific for celiac sprue and are the best screening test for celiac disease except in the case of patients with IgA deficiency. Tissue transglutinase autoantibody by ELISA is a newer serologic test for celiac sprue.
- Biopsy of the small bowel generally is recommended to establish the diagnosis. It reveals absence or shortening of villi, intraepithelial lymphocytes, and crypt lengthening and hyperplasia. Several biopsy specimens should be obtained for proper diagnosis.
- Laboratory evaluation may reveal iron deficiency anemia, folic acid deficiency, vitamin B_{12} deficiency, hypomagnesemia, and hypocalcemia.
- Tests for malabsorption are abnormal. Fecal fat estimation for 72 hours is elevated (>7 g/day); d-xylose testing reveals malabsorption of sugar.

ETIOLOGY

- Celiac sprue results from an inappropriate T cell–mediated immune response against ingested gluten in genetically predisposed people. There is sensitivity to gliadin, a protein fraction of gluten found in wheat, rye, barley, and oats.
- A peptide that resists degradation by proteases in the small bowel has been identified as the potential triggering molecule.

TREATMENT

- Patients should be instructed on a gluten-free diet (avoidance of wheat, rye, and barley). Oats do not damage the mucosa in celiac disease.
- Correct nutritional deficiencies with iron, folic acid, calcium, and vitamin B_{12} as needed.
- Prednisone 20 to 60 mg qd gradually tapered is useful in refractory cases.

CLINICAL PEARLS

- Serial antigliadin or antiendomysial antibody tests can be used to monitor the patient's adherence to a gluten-free diet.

metabolic bone disease or hypocalcemia, especially because gastrointestinal symptoms may be absent or mild. Clinicians also should consider testing children and young adults for celiac disease if unexplained weight loss, abdominal pain or distention, or chronic diarrhea is present.

- The prevalence of celiac disease in patients with dyspepsia is twice that of the general population. Screening for celiac disease should be considered in all patients with persistent dyspepsia.
- Celiac disease is associated with an increased risk for non-Hodgkin's lymphoma, especially of T-cell type and primarily localized in the gut.

 # Cellulitis

Definition: Superficial inflammatory condition of the skin characterized by erythema, warmth, and tenderness of the area involved

DIAGNOSIS

- Physical presentation varies with the causative organism:
  - **Erysipelas:** superficial spreading, warm, erythematous lesion distinguished by its indurated and elevated margin; lymphatic involvement and vesicle formation are common.
  - **Staphylococcal cellulitis:** area involved is erythematous, hot, and swollen; differentiated from erysipelas by nonelevated, poorly demarcated margin; local tenderness and regional adenopathy are common; 85% of cases occur on the legs and feet.
  - ***Haemophilus influenza* cellulitis:** area involved is a blue-red/purple-red color; occurs mainly in children; generally involves the face in children and the neck or upper chest in adults.
  - ***Vibrio vulnificus*** larger hemorrhagic bullae, cellulitis, lymphadenitis, myositis; often found in critically ill patients in septic shock.
- Laboratory evaluation (in severe cases) includes complete blood count with differential, Gram stain and culture (aerobic and anaerobic), blood cultures, and antistreptolysin O titer (in suspected streptococcal disease).

ETIOLOGY

- Group A beta-hemolytic streptococci (may follow a streptococcal infection of the upper respiratory tract)
- Staphylococcal cellulitis
- *H. influenzae*

- **V. vulnificus**—higher incidence in patients with liver disease (75%) and in immunocompromised hosts (e.g. corticosteroid use, diabetes mellitus, renal failure)
- **Erysipelothrix rhusiopathiae**—common in people handling poultry, fish, or meat
- **Aeromonas hydrophila**—generally occurring in contaminated open wound in freshwater
- **Fungi (Cryptococcus neoformans)**—immunocompromised granulopenic patients
- **Gram-negative rods (Serratia, Enterobacter, Proteus, Pseudomonas)**—immunocompromised or granulocytopenic patients

TREATMENT

Erysipelas:
- Nafcillin or oxacillin 2 g IV q4h or cefazolin 1 g IV q8h
- Use erythromycin, cephalosporins, clindamycin, or vancomycin in patients allergic to penicillin.

Staphylococcus cellulitis:
- Dicloxacillin 500 mg PO q6h
- Nafcillin or oxacillin 1-2 g IV q4h
- Dicloxacillin 250-500 mg PO qid
- Cephalosporins (cephalothin, cephalexin, cephradine) also provide adequate antistaphylococcal coverage except for methicillin-resistant *Staphylococcus aureus* (MRSA).
- Use vancomycin in patients allergic to penicillin or cephalosporins and in patients with MRSA.

H. influenzae cellulitis:
- Cefixime 400 mg qd or cefuroxime 500 mg bid is given orally.
- Cefuroxime 1.5 g q8h or ceftriaxone 1.0 g bd is given intravenously.

V. vulnificus:
- Doxycycline 100 mg IV bid with or without a third-generation cephalosporin. Ciprofloxacin is an alternative antibiotic.
- Intravenous support and admission to ICU (mortality rate <50% in septic shock).

- **Erysipelothrix:** penicillin
- **Aeromonas hydrophila:** aminoglycosides or chloramphenicol

CLINICAL PEARLS

- Cellulitis occurs most frequently in diabetics, immunocompromised hosts, and patients with venous and lymphatic compromise.
- Cellulitis frequently is found near skin breaks (trauma, surgical wounds, ulcerations, tinea infections).

Chancroid

Definition: Sexually transmitted disease characterized by painful genital ulceration and inflammatory inguinal adenopathy

DIAGNOSIS

- One to three extremely painful ulcers are present accompanied by tender inguinal lymphadenopathy (especially if fluctuant).
- Inguinal bubo and several ulcers may be present.
- In women, the initial lesion may occur in the fourchette, labia minora, urethra, cervix, or anus. An inflammatory pustule or papule is present that ruptures, leaving a shallow, nonindurated shallow ulceration, usually 1 to 2 cm in diameter with ragged, undermined edges.
- Unilateral lymphadenopathy develops 1 week later in 50% of patients.
- Definitive diagnosis is made by isolation of organism from ulcers by culture or Gram stain. Dark-field microscopy, rapid plasma reagin, herpes simplex virus cultures, *Haemophilus ducreyi* culture, and HIV testing are recommended.

ETIOLOGY

- *H. ducreyi*, a bacillus

TREATMENT

- Azithromycin 1 g PO (single dose) *or*
- Ceftriaxone 250 mg IM (single dose) *or*
- Ciprofloxacin 500 mg PO bid for 3 days *or*
- Erythromycin 500 mg PO qid for 7 days
  - *Note:* Ciprofloxacin is contraindicated in patients who are pregnant, lactating, or <18 years old.
- HIV-infected patients may need more prolonged therapy.

CLINICAL PEARLS

- All sexual partners should be treated with a 10-day course of one of the previous regimens.
- Patients should be reexamined 3 to 7 days after initiation of therapy. Ulcers should improve symptomatically within 3 days and objectively within 7 days after initiation of successful therapy.

Chickenpox

Definition: Viral illness characterized by acute onset of generalized vesicular rash and fever

DIAGNOSIS

- Findings vary with the clinical course. Initial symptoms consist of fever, chills, backache, generalized malaise, and headache.
- Symptoms are generally more severe in adults.
- Initial lesions generally occur on the trunk (centripetal distribution) and occasionally on the face; these lesions consist primarily of 3- to 4-mm red papules with an irregular outline and a clear vesicle on the surface (dew drops on a rose petal appearance).
- Intense pruritus generally accompanies this stage.
- New lesion development generally ceases by day 4 with subsequent crusting by day 6.
- Lesions generally spread to the face and the extremities (centrifugal spread).
- Patients generally present with lesions at different stages at the same time.
- Crusts generally fall off within 5 to 14 days.
- Fever is usually highest during the eruption of the vesicles; temperature generally returns to normal after disappearance of vesicles.
- Signs of potential complications (e.g., bacterial skin infections, neurologic complications, pneumonia, hepatitis) may be present on physical examination.
- Mild constitutional symptoms (e.g. anorexia, myalgias, headaches, restlessness) may be present (most common in adults).
- Excoriations may be present if scratching is prominent.
- Laboratory evaluation is generally not necessary.
- Complete blood count may reveal leukopenia and thrombocytopenia.

ETIOLOGY

- Varicella-zoster virus (human herpesvirus 3) can manifest with either varicella or herpes zoster (i.e., shingles, which is a reactivation of varicella).

TREATMENT

- Use acetaminophen for fever and myalgias; aspirin should be avoided because of the increased risk of Reye's syndrome.
- Oral acyclovir 20 mg/kg qid for 5 days, initiated at the earliest sign (within 24 hours of illness), is useful in healthy, nonpregnant individuals ≥13 years old to decrease the duration and severity of signs and

y systems. Immunocompromised hosts should be treated with acyclovir 500 mg/m^2 or 10 mg/kg IV q8h for 7 to 10 days.
- Varicella-zoster immunoglobulin (VZIG) is effective in preventing chickenpox in susceptible individuals. Dose is 12.5 U/kg IM (maximum of 625 U). Dose may be repeated 3 weeks later if the exposure persists; VZIG must be administered as early as possible after presumed exposure.
- Varicella vaccine is available for children and adults; protection lasts at least 6 years. Patients with HIV or other immunocompromised patients should not receive the live attenuated vaccine.
- Pruritus from chickenpox can be controlled with antihistamines (e.g., hydroxyzine 25 mg q6h) and oral antipruritic lotions (e.g., calamine).
- Oral antibiotics are not routinely indicated and should be used only in patients with secondary infection and infected lesions (most common infective organisms are *Streptococcus* and *Staphylococcus*).

CLINICAL PEARLS
- Infectious period begins 2 days before onset of clinical symptoms and lasts until all lesions have crusted.
- Most patients have lifelong immunity after an attack of chickenpox; protection from chickenpox after varicella vaccine is approximately 6 years.

▆ Cholangitis

Definition: Inflammation or infection (or both) of the hepatic and common bile ducts associated with obstruction of the common bile duct

DIAGNOSIS
- There is acute onset of fever and chills, abdominal pain and tenderness over the right upper quadrant of the abdomen, and jaundice (Charcot's triad).
- Often, dark coloration of the urine results from bilirubinuria.
- Ultrasound allows visualization of the gallbladder and bile ducts to differentiate extrahepatic obstruction from intrahepatic cholestasis. Ultrasound is insensitive but specific for visualization of common duct stones.
- CT scan is less accurate for visualization of gallstones but more sensitive than ultrasound for visualization of the distal part of the common bile duct.
- Endoscopic retrograde cholangiopancreatography (ERCP) is indicated for diagnosis if ultrasound and CT scan are inconclusive. ERCP

confirms obstruction and its level and allows collection of specimens for culture and cytology.

- Laboratory tests usually show the following: elevated white blood cell count with a predominance of polynuclear forms; elevated alkaline phosphatase and bilirubin in chronic obstruction; and elevated transaminases in acute obstruction. Positive blood cultures are present in 50% of cases, typically with enteric gram-negative aerobes (e.g., *Escherichia coli*, *Klebsiella pneumoniae*), enterococci, or anaerobes.

ETIOLOGY

- Obstruction of the common bile duct causing rapid proliferation of bacteria in the biliary tree
- **Most common cause of common bile duct obstruction:** stones, usually migrated from the gallbladder
- **Other causes:** prior biliary tract surgery with secondary stenosis, tumor (usually arising from the pancreas or biliary tree), and parasitic infections from *Ascaris lumbricoides* or *Fasciola hepatica*
- Iatrogenic after contamination of an obstructed biliary tree by ERCP or percutaneous transhepatic cholangiography
- Primary sclerosing cholangitis
- **HIV-associated sclerosing cholangitis:** associated with infection by cytomegalovirus, *Cryptosporidium*, Microsporidia, and *Mycobacterium avium* complex

TREATMENT

- Broad-spectrum antibiotics are directed at gram-negative enteric organisms, anaerobes, and enterococcus. If infection is nosocomial, the patient post-ERCP or the patient is in shock, broader coverage should be strongly considered to include hospital organisms such as *Pseudomonas aeruginosa*, resistant *Staphylococcus aureus*, and others.
- Biliary decompression may be performed in severely ill patients or patients unresponsive to medical therapy within 12 to 24 hours.
- Biliary decompression also may be performed semielectively in patients who respond. Options include ERCP with or without sphincterotomy or placement of a draining stent, percutaneous transhepatic biliary drainage for an acutely ill patient who is a poor surgical candidate, and surgical exploration of the common bile duct.

Cholecystitis

Definition: Acute or chronic inflammation of the gallbladder

DIAGNOSIS

- Workup consists of detailed history and physical examination coupled with laboratory evaluation and imaging studies. No single clinical finding or laboratory test is sufficient to establish or exclude cholecystitis without further testing.
- Ultrasound of the gallbladder is the preferred initial test; it shows the presence of stones and dilated gallbladder with thickened wall and surrounding edema in patients with acute cholecystitis.
- Nuclear imaging (HIDA scan) is useful for diagnosis of cholecystitis; sensitivity and specificity are >90% for acute cholecystis. This test is reliable only when bilirubin is <5 mg/dL. A positive test shows obstruction of the cystic or common hepatic duct; the test does not show the presence of stones.
- Laboratory tests show the following: leukocytosis ($12,000$-$20,000/mm^3$) present in >70% of patients and elevated alkaline phosphatase, alanine aminotransferase, aspartate aminotransferase, and bilirubin. Bilirubin elevation >4 mg/dL is unusual and suggests presence of choledocholithiasis.
- Physical examination reveals pain and tenderness in the right hypochondrium or epigastrium, with pain possibly radiating to the infrascapular region. Palpation of the right upper quadrant elicits marked tenderness and stoppage of inspired breath (Murphy's sign). Examination also may reveal guarding, fever (33%), jaundice (25-50% of patients), and palpable gallbladder.
- Medical history often reveals nausea and vomiting (>70% of patients), fever and chills (>25% of patients), and ingestion of large, fatty meals before onset of pain in the epigastrium and right upper quadrant.

ETIOLOGY

- Gallstones (>95% of cases)
- Ischemic damage to the gallbladder, critically ill patient (acalculous cholecystitis)
- Infectious agents, especially in patients with AIDS (cytomegalovirus, *Cryptosporidium*)
- Strictures of the bile duct
- Neoplasms, primary or metastatic

TREATMENT

- Cholecystectomy (laparoscopic is preferred) is the treatment. Conservative management with intravenous fluids and antibiotics (ampicillin/sulbactam [Unasyn] 3 g IV q6h *or* piperacillin/tazobactam [Zosyn] 4.5 g IV q8h) may be justified in some high-risk patients to convert an emergency procedure into an elective one with a lower mortality.
- Endoscopic retrograde cholangiopancreatography with sphincterectomy and stone extraction can be performed in conjunction with laparoscopic cholecystectomy for patients with choledocholithiasis; approximately 7% to 15% of patients with cholelithiasis also have stones in the common bile duct.
- Intravenous fluids, broad-spectrum antibiotics, and pain management (meperidine as needed) are recommended.

CLINICAL PEARL

- Complication rate is approximately 1% (hemorrhage and bile leak) with laparoscopic cholecystectomy and <0.5% (infection) with open cholecystectomy.

▰ Chronic fatigue syndrome (CFS)

Definition: CFS is characterized by four or more of the following symptoms present concurrently for at least 6 months:

- Impaired memory or concentration
- Sore throat
- Tender cervical or axillary lymph nodes
- Muscle pain
- Multijoint pain
- New headaches
- Unrefreshing sleep
- Postexertion malaise

DIAGNOSIS

- Because CFS is a clinical diagnosis and the symptoms are generally subjective, history and physical examination are essential for excluding other causes of fatigue. A detailed mental status examination is necessary. Abnormalities should be evaluated further with appropriate psychiatric, psychological, or neurologic examination.
- No specific laboratory tests exist for diagnosing CFS. Initial laboratory tests are useful to exclude other conditions that may mimic or may be associated with CFS.

screening laboratory tests, including complete blood count, erythrocyte sedimentation rate, alanine aminotransferase, total protein, albumin, globulin, alkaline phosphatase, calcium, phosphorus, glucose, blood urea nitrogen, creatinine, electrolytes, thyroid-stimulating hormone, and urinalysis, are useful.
- Serologic tests for Epstein-Barr virus, *Candida albicans*, and human herpesvirus 6 and other studies for immune cellular abnormalities are not useful; these tests are expensive and generally not recommended.
- Other tests may be indicated depending on the history and physical examination (e.g., antinuclear antibody and rheumatoid factor in patients presenting with joint complaints or abnormalities on physical examination, Lyme titer in areas where Lyme disease is endemic).
- Imaging studies generally are not recommended unless history and physical examination indicate specific abnormalities (e.g., chest x-ray in any patient suspected to have tuberculosis or sarcoidosis).
- There are no physical findings specific for CFS. The physical examination may be useful to identify fibromyalgia and other rheumatologic conditions that may coexist with CFS.

ETIOLOGY
- The etiology of CFS is unknown.
- Many experts suspect that a viral illness may trigger certain immune responses leading to the various symptoms. Most patients often report the onset of their symptoms with a flu-like illness.
- Initial reports indicated a possible role of Epstein-Barr virus, but subsequent studies disproved this theory.

TREATMENT
- Therapy is generally palliative. The following medications may be helpful:
  - **Antidepressants:** The choice of antidepressant varies with the desired side effects. Patients with difficulty sleeping or fibromyalgia-like symptoms may benefit from low-dose tricyclics (doxepin 10 mg hs or amitriptyline 25 mg qhs). When sedation is not desirable, low-dose selective serotonin reuptake inhibitors (paroxetine 20 mg qd) often help alleviate fatigue and associated symptoms.
  - **Nonsteroidal antiinflammatory drugs** These agents can be used to relieve muscle and joint pain and headaches.

CLINICAL PEARLS
- Moderate-to-complete recovery at 1 year occurs in 22% to 60% of patients.
- Psychiatric referral and treatment are helpful in coping with CFS in most patients.

Chronic obstructive pulmonary disease (COPD)

Definition: A disorder characterized by the presence of airflow limitation that is not fully reversible. COPD encompasses *emphysema*, characterized by loss of lung elasticity and destruction of lung parenchyma with enlargement of air spaces, and *chronic bronchitis*, characterized by obstruction of small airways and productive cough >3 months' duration for >2 successive years.

DIAGNOSIS
- **Physical findings and clinical presentation:**
  - **Blue bloaters (chronic bronchitis):** peripheral cyanosis, productive cough, tachypnea, tachycardia
  - **Pink puffers (emphysema):** dyspnea, pursed-lip breathing with use of accessory muscles for respiration, decreased breath sounds
  - Possible wheezing in patients with chronic bronchitis and emphysema
  - Features of chronic bronchitis and emphysema in many patients with COPD
  - Acute exacerbation of COPD is mainly a clinical diagnosis and generally manifests with worsening dyspnea, increase in sputum purulence, and increase in sputum volume.
- **Workup:**
  - Chest x-ray, pulmonary function testing, arterial blood gases (in patients with acute exacerbation)
- **Laboratory tests:**
  - Complete blood count may reveal leukocytosis with shift to the left during acute exacerbation.
  - Sputum may be purulent with bacterial respiratory tract infections. Sputum staining and cultures usually are reserved for cases that are refractory to antibiotic therapy.
  - Arterial blood gases may show normocapnia and mild-to-moderate hypoxemia.
- **Pulmonary function tests:**
  - Abnormal diffusing capacity, increased total lung capacity or residual volume, and fixed reduction in forced expiratory volume in 1 second are present with emphysema; normal diffusing capacity and reduced forced expiratory volume in 1 second are present with chronic bronchitis. Generally, acute spirometry should not be used to diagnose an exacerbation or assess its severity.

Chest x-ray:
- Hyperinflation with flattened diaphragm, tenting of the diaphragm at the rib, and increased retrosternal chest space
- Decreased vascular markings and bullae in patients with emphysema
- Thickened bronchial markings and enlarged right side of the heart in patients with chronic bronchitis

ETIOLOGY
- Tobacco exposure
- Occupational exposure to pulmonary toxins (e.g., cadmium)
- Atmospheric pollution
- α_1-Antitrypsin deficiency (rare; <1% of COPD patients)

TREATMENT
- Acute exacerbation of COPD can be treated as follows:
  - Give aerosolized β-agonists (e.g., metaproterenol nebulizer solution 5% 0.3 mL or albuterol nebulized 5% solution 2.5-5 mg).
  - Anticholinergic agents have equivalent efficacy to inhaled β-adrenergic agonists. Inhalant solution of ipratropium bromide 0.5 mg can be administered every 4 to 8 hours.
  - Short courses of systemic corticosteroids have been shown to improve spirometric and clinical outcomes. In the hospital, give methylprednisolone 50- to 100-mg bolus IV, then q6-8h; taper as soon as possible. In the outpatient setting, oral prednisone 40 mg/day initially, decreasing the dose by 10 mg every other day, is generally effective.
  - Judicious oxygen administration is recommended (hypercapnia and further respiratory compromise may occur after high-flow oxygen therapy); use of a Venturi-type mask delivering an inspired oxygen fraction of 24% to 28% is preferred to nasal cannula.
  - Noninvasive positive-pressure ventilation delivered by a facial or nasal mask in the treatment of chronic restrictive thoracic disease may obviate the need for intratracheal intubation.
  - Intravenous aminophylline administration is controversial. When used, serum levels should be monitored closely to minimize risks of tachyarrhythmias.
- Antibiotics are indicated in suspected respiratory infection (e.g., increased purulence and volume of phlegm).
  - *Haemophilus influenzae* and *Streptococcus pneumoniae* are frequent causes of acute bronchitis.
  - Oral antibiotics of choice are azithromycin, levofloxacin, amoxicillin/clavulanate, and cefuroxime.

- The use of antibiotics is beneficial in exacerbations of COPD presenting with increased dyspnea and sputum purulence (especially if the patient is febrile).
- Guaifenesin may improve cough symptoms and mucus clearance; however, mucolytic medications are generally ineffective. Their benefits may be greatest in patients with more advanced disease.
- Intubation and mechanical ventilation may be necessary if the above-listed measures fail to provide improvement.

CLINICAL PEARL

- All patients with COPD should receive pneumococcal vaccine and yearly influenza vaccine.

Cirrhosis

Definition: Cirrhosis is defined histologically as the presence of fibrosis and regenerative nodules in the liver.

DIAGNOSIS

- Diagnostic workup is aimed at identifying the most likely cause of cirrhosis.

Laboratory tests:

- **Alcoholic hepatitis and cirrhosis:** There may be mild elevation of alanine aminotransferase (ALT) and aspartate aminotransferase (AST), usually <500 IU; AST > ALT (ratio >2:3).
- **Extrahepatic obstruction:** There may be moderate elevations of ALT and AST to levels <500 IU.
- **Viral, toxic, or ischemic hepatitis:** There are extreme elevations (>500 IU) of ALT and AST.
- Transaminases may be normal despite significant liver disease in patients with jejunoileal bypass operations or hemochromatosis or after methotrexate administration.
- Alkaline phosphatase elevation can occur with extrahepatic obstruction, primary biliary cirrhosis, and primary sclerosing cholangitis.
- Serum lactate dehydrogenase is significantly elevated in metastatic disease of the liver; lesser elevations are seen with hepatitis, cirrhosis, extrahepatic obstruction, and congestive hepatomegaly.
- Serum γ-glutamyl transpeptidase is elevated in alcoholic liver disease and may be elevated with cholestatic disease (primary biliary cirrhosis, primary sclerosing cholangitis).
- Serum bilirubin may be elevated; urinary bilirubin can be present in hepatitis, hepatocellular jaundice, and biliary obstruction.

Serum albumin: Significant liver disease results in hypoalbuminemia.

- **Prothrombin time:** An elevated prothrombin time in patients with liver disease indicates severe liver damage and poor prognosis.
- Presence of hepatitis B surface antigen implies acute or chronic hepatitis B.
- Presence of antimitochondrial antibody suggests primary biliary cirrhosis or chronic hepatitis.
- Elevated serum copper, decreased serum ceruloplasmin, and elevated 24-hour urine may be diagnostic of Wilson's disease.
- Protein immunoelectrophoresis may reveal decreased α_1-globulins (α_1-antitrypsin deficiency), increased IgA (alcoholic cirrhosis), increased IgM (primary biliary cirrhosis), and increased IgG (chronic hepatitis, cryptogenic cirrhosis).
- An elevated serum ferritin and increased transferrin saturation suggest hemochromatosis.
- An elevated blood ammonia suggests hepatocellular dysfunction.
- Antinuclear antibodies may be found in autoimmune hepatitis.
- **Imaging studies:**
  - Ultrasound is the procedure of choice for detection of gallstones and dilation of common bile ducts.
  - CT scan is useful for detecting mass lesions in liver and pancreas, assessing hepatic fat content, identifying idiopathic hemochromatosis, diagnosing Budd-Chiari syndrome, detecting dilation of intrahepatic bile ducts, and detecting varices and splenomegaly.
  - Percutaneous liver biopsy is useful in evaluating hepatic filling defects; diagnosing hepatocellular disease or hepatomegaly; evaluating persistently abnormal liver function tests; and diagnosing hemachromatosis, primary biliary cirrhosis, Wilson's disease, glycogen storage diseases, chronic hepatitis, autoimmune hepatitis, infiltrative diseases, alcoholic liver disease, drug-induced liver disease, and primary or secondary carcinoma.
- **Physical findings:** jaundice, spider angiomata, ecchymosis, gynecomastia in men, small nodular liver, ascites, hemorrhoids, testicular atrophy

ETIOLOGY

- Alcohol abuse
- Secondary biliary cirrhosis, obstruction of the common bile duct (stone, stricture, pancreatitis, neoplasm, sclerosing cholangitis)
- Drugs (e.g., acetaminophen, isoniazid, methotrexate, methyldopa)

- Hepatic congestion (e.g., congestive heart failure, constrictive pericarditis, tricuspid insufficiency, thrombosis of the hepatic vein, obstruction of the vena cava)
- Primary biliary cirrhosis
- Hemochromatosis
- Chronic hepatitis B or C
- Wilson's disease
- α_1-Antitrypsin deficiency
- Infiltrative diseases (amyloidosis, glycogen storage diseases, hemochromatosis)
- Nutritional (jejunoileal bypass)
- **Other causes:** parasitic infections (schistosomiasis), idiopathic portal hypertension, congenital hepatic fibrosis, systemic mastocytosis, autoimmune hepatitis, hepatic steatosis, inflammatory bowel disease

TREATMENT

- Treatment varies with etiology.
- Liver transplantation may be indicated in otherwise healthy patients (<65 years old) with sclerosing cholangitis, chronic hepatitis, cirrhosis, or primary biliary cirrhosis, with prognostic information suggesting <20% chance of survival without transplantation; contraindications to liver transplantation are AIDS, most metastatic malignancies, active substance abuse, uncontrolled sepsis, and uncontrolled cardiac or pulmonary disease.
- Treat complications of portal hypertension (ascites, esophagogastric varices, hepatic encephalopathy, and hepatorenal syndrome).

Cirrhosis, primary biliary

Definition: Chronic progressive disease, most often affecting women, characterized by progressive destruction of the small intrahepatic bile ducts with portal inflammation leading to fibrosis, cirrhosis, liver failure, and need for liver transplantation

DIAGNOSIS

- Clinical presentation varies depending on stage of diagnosis. Fatigue and pruritus are the usual presenting symptoms; however, 48% to 60% of patients may be asymptomatic. Musculoskeletal complaints caused by inflammatory arthropathy occur in 40% to 70% of patients. Hepatomegaly and splenomegaly may be present in more advanced disease.

laboratory studies show the following: antimitochondrial antibodies (found in 95% of patients with primary biliary cirrhosis and are 98% specific), markedly elevated alkaline phosphatase (of hepatic origin), elevated γ-glutamyl transpeptidase, normal or slightly elevated aminotransferases, bilirubin normal early and increases with disease progression (direct and indirect), markedly elevated serum lipids (total cholesterol, low-density lipoprotein, and especially high-density lipoprotein), elevated ceruloplasmin, and eosinophilia.
- Percutaneous liver biopsy is the confirmatory test.

TREATMENT
- Management decisions vary depending on clinical status of patient. Treatment focuses on management of complications (pruritus, metabolic bone diseases, hyperlipidemia) because liver transplantation is the only definitive treatment for this disease.
- Ursodiol, colchicine, and methotrexate have shown encouraging results.
- Ursodiol extends survival and lengthens the time before liver transplantation, normalizes bilirubin, and may mask need for transplantation.
- Colchicine and methotrexate yield less impressive results but are still modestly effective.
- Prednisone, azathioprine, penicillamine, and cyclosporine have limited efficacy and predictable toxicity.

Coccidioidomycosis

Definition: Infectious disease caused by the fungus *Coccidioides immitis*. It is usually asymptomatic and characterized by a primary pulmonary focus with infrequent progression to chronic pulmonary disease and dissemination to other organs.

DIAGNOSIS
- Asymptomatic infections or illness consistent with a nonspecific upper respiratory tract infection occurs in at least 60%. Spontaneous improvement occurs within 2 weeks of illness, with complete recovery usual. Subsequent pulmonary residua in the form of pulmonary nodules and cavities occur in less than 10% of patients with primary infection.
- Symptoms of primary infection—cough, malaise, fever, chills, night sweats, anorexia, weakness, and arthralgias (desert rheumatism)—occur in remaining 40% within 3 weeks of exposure. Skin rashes, such as erythema nodosum and erythema multiforme, may occur. Some

patients, especially if immunocompromised or diabetic, progress to chronic pulmonary disease. Over many years, granulomas rupture, leading to new cavity formation and continued fibrosis, often accompanied by hemoptysis. Disseminated or extrapulmonary disease occurs in approximately 0.5% of acutely infected patients.

- Definitive diagnosis is based on demonstration of the organism by culture from body fluids or tissues. Greatest yield is with pus, sputum, synovial fluid, and soft tissue aspirations, varying with the degree of dissemination.
- Serologic evaluations include latex agglutination and complement fixation. Elevated serum complement-fixing antibody titers $\geq 1:32$ (Smith and Saito) strongly correlate with disseminated disease except with meningitis, where lower titers are seen.
- Other laboratory tests include complete blood count, which may reveal eosinophilia, especially with erythema nodosum. Elevated serum levels of IgE are associated with progressive disease.
- Chest x-ray reveals unilateral infiltrates, hilar adenopathy, or pleural effusion in primary infection.

TREATMENT

- In general, drug therapy is not required for patients with asymptomatic pulmonary disease and most patients with mild symptomatic primary infection.
- In patients with extrapulmonary manifestations involving draining skin, joint, and soft tissue infection, local wound care is provided to avoid possible bacterial superinfection.
- Chemotherapy is indicated under the following circumstances: severe symptomatic primary infection, high serum complement-fixing antibody titers, persistent symptoms (>6 weeks), prostration, progressive pulmonary involvement, pregnancy, infancy, debilitation, concurrent illness (e.g., diabetes, asthma, chronic obstructive pulmonary disease, malignancy), acquired or induced immunosuppression, and racial group with known predisposition for disseminated disease.
- Fluconazole 400 mg/day PO (≤ 1.2 g/day) seems to be the drug of choice for meningeal and deep-seated mycotic infections.
- Itraconazole 400-600 mg/day achieves 90% response rate in bone, joint, soft tissue, lymphatic, and genitourinary infections. Itraconazole may be more efficacious than fluconazole in the treatment of skeletal (bone) infections.
- For pulmonary infections, treatment with either fluconazole or itraconazole (given for 6-12 weeks) seems to be equal in efficacy.
- Amphotericin B is the classic therapy for disseminated extraneural disease; dosage is 1-1.5 mg/kg/day qd for the first week and qid thereafter for a total dose of 1-2.5 g or until clinical and serologic remis-

... Liposomal amphotericin B is probably equally effective, but further studies are needed.
- With meningeal disease, intrathecal amphotericin B is the traditional treatment modality, given alone or preceding the use of oral agents.

▬ Condyloma acuminatum

Definition: Sexually transmitted viral disease of the vulva, vagina, and cervix that is caused by the human papillomavirus

DIAGNOSIS
- Lesions usually are found in genital area, but can be present elsewhere. Lesions usually are in similar positions on both sides of perineum. There are four morphologic types: condylomatous, keratotic, papular, and flat warts.
- Initial lesions are pedunculated, soft papules about 2 to 3 mm in diameter and 10 to 20 mm long. Lesions may occur as a single papule or in clusters.
- Size of lesions varies from pinhead to large cauliflower-like masses. Lesions usually are asymptomatic, but if infected can cause pain, odor, or bleeding.

TREATMENT
- **Keratolytic agents:**
  - Podophyllin is applied directly to lesion weekly and washed off in 6 hours.
  - Trichloroacetic acid (30-80% solution) is applied twice monthly to lesion. It is less painful and irritating to normal tissue than podophyllin.
  - Fluorouracil is applied weekly for 12 weeks and causes necrosis and sloughing of growing tissue. It can be used intravaginally or for vulvar, anal, or urethral lesions.
- **Physical agents:**
  - Cryotherapy can be used weekly for 3 to 6 weeks, with a 62% to 79% success rate. Cryotherapy is not suitable for large warts.
  - Laser therapy is painful and requires anesthesia.
  - Electrocautery and excision are other options.
- **Immunotherapy:**
  - Interferon is injected intralesionally at a dose of 3 million U/m^2 three times weekly for 8 weeks.
  - Imiquimod 5% cream increases wart clearance after 3 months.

CLINICAL PEARLS

- Transmitted disease is spread by skin-to-skin contact. The disease is highly contagious, with 25% to 65% of sexual partners developing it.
- Average incubation time is 2 months (range 1-8 months).

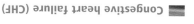

Congestive heart failure (CHF)

Definition: Pathophysiologic state characterized by congestion in the pulmonary or systemic circulation caused by the heart's inability to pump sufficient oxygenated blood to meet the metabolic needs of the tissues

DIAGNOSIS

- The findings on physical examination in patients with CHF vary depending on the severity and whether the failure is right-sided or left-sided.
- Common clinical manifestations are as follows:
  - Dyspnea
  - Orthopnea
  - Paroxysmal nocturnal dyspnea
  - Nocturnal angina
  - Cheyne-Stokes respiration
  - Fatigue, lethargy
- Patients with failure of the left side of the heart have the following abnormalities on physical examination: pulmonary rales, tachypnea, S_3 gallop, cardiac murmurs (atrial stenosis, atrial regurgitation, mitral regurgitation), and paradoxical splitting of S_2.
- Patients with failure of right side of the heart have jugular venous distention, peripheral edema, perioral and peripheral cyanosis, congestive hepatomegaly, ascites, and hepatojugular reflux.
- Laboratory tests include the following:
  - Complete blood count (to rule out anemia, infection), blood urea nitrogen, creatinine, liver enzymes, and thyroid stimulating hormone
  - B-Type natriuretic peptide is a cardiac neurohormone specifically secreted from the ventricles in response to volume expansion and pressure overload. Elevated levels indicate left ventricular dysfunction. Bedside measurement of B-type natriuretic peptide is useful in establishing or excluding the diagnosis of CHF in patients with acute dyspnea.

diomegaly with dilation of the involved heart chamber, and pleural effusions.

- Two-dimensional echocardiography is useful to assess global and regional left ventricular function and to estimate ejection fraction.

ETIOLOGY

- **Left ventricular failure:**
  - Systemic hypertension
  - Valvular heart disease (atrial stenosis, atrial regurgitation, mitral regurgitation)
  - Cardiomyopathy, myocarditis
  - Bacterial endocarditis
  - Myocardial infarction
  - Idiopathic hypertrophic subaortic stenosis (IHSS)
  - Left ventricular failure is differentiated further according to systolic dysfunction (low ejection fraction) and diastolic dysfunction (normal or high ejection fraction), or "stiff ventricle." It is important to make this distinction because treatment is significantly different.
  - Common causes of systolic dysfunction are post-myocardial infarction, cardiomyopathy, and myocarditis.
  - Causes of diastolic dysfunction are hypertensive cardiovascular disease, valvular heart disease (atrial stenosis, atrial regurgitation, mitral regurgitation, IHSS), and restrictive cardiomyopathy.
- **Right ventricular failure:**
  - Valvular heart disease (mitral stenosis)
  - Pulmonary hypertension
  - Bacterial endocarditis (right-sided)
  - Right ventricular infarction
- **Biventricular failure:**
  - Left ventricular failure
  - Cardiomyopathy
  - Myocarditis
  - Arrhythmias
  - Anemia
  - Thyrotoxicosis
  - Arteriovenous fistula
  - Paget's disease
  - Beriberi

TREATMENT

- **Treatment of CHF secondary to systolic dysfunction:**
  - Diuretics
  - Angiotensin-converting enzyme (ACE) inhibitors

- **β-Blockers:** All patients with stable New York Heart Association class II or III heart failure caused by left ventricular systolic dysfunction should receive a β-blocker unless they have a contraindication to its use or are intolerant to it. Effective agents are carvedilol (Coreg) 3.125 mg bid, bisoprolol 1.25 mg qd, or metoprolol 12.5 mg bid initially, titrated upward as tolerated.
  - Angiotensin II receptor blockers are useful in patients unable to tolerate ACE inhibitors.
  - Digitalis is indicated in patients with rapid atrial fibrillation, severe CHF, or ejection fraction <30%.
  - Nesiritide (Natrecor), a recombinant human brain, or B-type, natriuretic peptide, has venous, arterial, and coronary vasodilatory properties that decrease preload and afterload and increase cardiac output without direct inotropic effects.
- **Treatment of CHF secondary to diastolic dysfunction:** Therapeutic options are determined by the cause.
  - **Hypertension:** calcium channel blockers (verapamil), ACE inhibitors, β-blockers, diuretics, angiotensin II receptor blockers
  - **Aortic stenosis:** diuretics, aortic valve replacement in patients with critical stenosis
  - **Aortic insufficiency and mitral regurgitation** ACE inhibitors, diuretics, surgery
  - **IHSS:** β-blockers or verapamil. Restore intravascular volume with intravenous saline solution if necessary in acute pulmonary edema. Septal myotomy and DDD pacing are useful in selected patients.

CLINICAL PEARLS

- Sudden death secondary to ventricular arrhythmias occurs in >40% of patients with heart failure.
- The use of a left ventricular assist device in patients with advanced heart failure can result in a clinically meaningful survival benefit and improve quality of life. It is an acceptable alternative therapy in selected patients who are not candidates for cardiac transplantation.

Conjunctivitis

Definition: Inflammation of the conjunctiva resulting from a variety of causes, including allergies and bacterial, viral, and chlamydial infection

DIAGNOSIS

- Findings are as follows:
  - and chemosis of conjunctivae with discharge

- Vision usually normal
- Cultures are useful if conjunctivitis is not successfully treated with antibiotic medications; initial culture is usually not necessary.

ETIOLOGY
- Bacterial
- Viral
- Chlamydial
- Allergic

TREATMENT
- Warm compresses if infective conjunctivitis
- Cold compresses in irritative or allergic conjunctivitis
- If allergic, nonsteroidal agents, such as diclofenac (Voltaren) ophthalmic solution, and mast cell stabilizers, such as nedocromil (Alocril), olopatadine (Patanol), and ketotifen (Zaditor)
- If infectious, antibiotic drops (e.g., levofloxacin, ofloxacin, ciprofloxacin, tobramycin, gentamicin ophthalmic solution 1-2 drops q2-4h)

CLINICAL PEARL
- *Caution:* Be careful with corticosteroid treatment and avoid unless sure of diagnosis; corticosteroids can exacerbate infections.

▬ Cor pulmonale

Definition: Enlargement of the right ventricle and deterioration of its function secondary to diseases affecting the lungs or pulmonary vasculature that cause pulmonary hypertension; may be acute or chronic

DIAGNOSIS
- Any patient suspected to have cor pulmonale should undergo a workup searching for an underlying pulmonary process resulting in pulmonary hypertension. Workup includes blood tests, chest x-ray, echocardiogram, MRI, and occasionally right-side heart catheterization.
- **Laboratory tests:**
  - Complete blood count may show erythrocytosis secondary to hypoxia
  - Arterial blood gases confirm hypoxemia and acidosis or hypercapnia.
  - Pulmonary function tests are useful.

- **Imaging studies:**
  - Chest x-ray may show evidence of chronic obstructive pulmonary disease (COPD) and pulmonary hypertension (e.g. right atrial, right ventricular, and pulmonary enlargement).
  - ECG may reveal right ventricular hypertrophy, right atrial enlargement (p-pulmonale), right-axis deviation, or incomplete/complete right bundle branch block.
  - Echocardiogram with continuous, pulse, and color Doppler can estimate pulmonary artery pressure. M-mode and two-dimensional echocardiography measures chamber size and wall thickness.
  - Radionuclide ventriculography reveals depressed right ventricular ejection fraction.
  - MRI is a sensitive test to measure right ventricular dimensions and detect hypertrophy.
  - Right-side catheterization measures pulmonary artery pressures and vascular resistance; it also helps determine response to various therapies (e.g. oxygen, calcium blockers, angiotensin-converting enzyme inhibitors).

ETIOLOGY

- Cor pulmonale is caused by pulmonary hypertension. Mechanisms leading to pulmonary hypertension include:
  - Pulmonary vasoconstriction resulting from any condition causing alveolar hypoxia or acidosis or both
  - Lung parenchymal disorders (e.g. emphysema, interstitial lung disease, emboli)
  - Conditions leading to increased blood viscosity (e.g. polycythemia vera, Waldenström's macroglobulinemia)
  - Idiopathic primary pulmonary hypertension
  - Increased pulmonary blood flow (abnormal shunts)

TREATMENT

- The treatment of cor pulmonale is directed at the underlying etiology, while reversing hypoxemia, hypercapnia, and acidosis. Management also is aimed at improving right ventricular contraction and decreasing pulmonary artery vascular resistance.
- Chest physiotherapy is beneficial in patients with COPD and infectious exacerbations.
- Continuous positive airway pressure is used in patients with obstructive sleep apnea.
- Long-term oxygen supplementation has improved survival in hypoxemic patients with COPD.

patients (hematocrit >55%) who have acute decompensation of cor pulmonale. Phlebotomy has been shown to decrease mean pulmonary arery pressure and pulmonary vascular resistance.

Coronary syndromes

Definition: Acute coronary syndromes (ACS) are manifestations of ischemic heart disease and represent a broad clinical spectrum that includes unstable angina (UA)/non-ST elevation myocardial infarction (NSTEMI), and ST elevation myocardial infarction (STEMI).

DIAGNOSIS
- **ECG:**
  - In STEMI, there is the development of the following:
    - Inverted T waves, which indicate an area of ischemia
    - Elevated ST segments, which indicate an area of injury
    - Q waves, which indicate the area of infarction; they usually develop over 12 to 36 hours
  - In UA/NSTEMI, Q waves are absent, but the following indications are present:
    - History and myocardial enzyme elevations compatible with myocardial infarction
    - ECG shows ST segment depression, transient ST segment elevation, or no change followed by T wave inversion.
- **Laboratory tests:**
  - **Serum enzyme studies:** damaged necrotic heart muscle releases cardiac enzymes (CK-MB) into the bloodstream in amounts that correlate with the size of the infarct. Even minor elevations of CK-MB should be considered indicative of acute myocardial infarction.
  - **Cardiac troponin levels:** troponin T (cTnT) and I (cTnI) are highly specific for myocardial injury. Increases in serum levels of cTnT and cTnI may occur relatively early after muscle damage (within 3-12 hours), peak within 24 hours, and be present for several days after myocardial infarction (7 days for cTnI and 10-14 days for cTnT).

ETIOLOGY
- Coronary atherosclerosis
- Coronary artery spasm (Prinzmetal's, cocaine or amphetamine induced)
- Coronary embolism

- Periarteritis and other coronary artery inflammatory diseases
- Dissection into coronary arteries (aneurysmal or iatrogenic)
- Congenital abnormalities of coronary circulation
- Myocardial infarction with normal coronaries (MINC syndrome) (more frequent in younger patients and cocaine addicts)
- Increased blood viscosity (polycythemia vera)
- Hypercoagulable states

TREATMENT

- Any patient with suspected ACS, unless contraindicated, should receive immediately the following: aspirin, nasal oxygen, nitrates, β-adrenergic blocking agents.
- **Adequate analgesia:** Morphine sulfate 2 mg IV q5min as needed can be given for severe pain unrelieved by nitroglycerin.
- **Thrombolytic therapy:** Administer in patients with acute STEMI, if the duration of pain has been <6 hours.
- **Percutaneous coronary intervention:** When available and implemented in a timely fashion (balloon inflation within 180 minutes of onset of pain) by skilled individuals and supported by experienced personnel, percutaneous coronary intervention is preferable to thrombolytic therapy.

Cryptococcosis

Definition: Infection caused by the fungal organism *Cryptococcus neoformans*

DIAGNOSIS

- Culture and India ink stain (60-80% sensitive in culture-proven cases) and examination of the cerebrospinal fluid in all cases when central nervous system involvement is suspected
- Blood and serum cryptococcal antigen assay (>90% sensitivity and specificity)
- Culture and histologic examination of biopsy material
- Chest x-ray to exclude pulmonary involvement
- CT or MRI of the head if focal neurologic involvement is suspected

Clinical presentation: >90% present with meningitis; almost all patients have fever and headache. Meningismus, photophobia, and mental status changes are seen in approximately 25%.

Most common infections outside the central nervous system:
- Lungs (fever, cough, dyspnea)
- Skin (cellulitis, papular eruption)

• Potential involvement of virtually any organ

ETIOLOGY
• Caused by the fungal organism *C. neoformans*
• Transmission almost always in the setting of AIDS or other disorders of cellular immune function (hematologic malignancies, long-term corticosteroid therapy, immunosuppressive therapy after organ transplantation), or pregnancy

TREATMENT
• Therapy is initiated with amphotericin B 0.5 mg/kg/day IV with or without flucytosine.
• After stabilization (usually several weeks), consider fluconazole 200-400 mg PO qd for additional 6 to 8 weeks.
• An alternative is intravenous fluconazole for initial therapy in patients unable to tolerate amphotericin B.
• If increased intracranial pressure is present, consider therapeutic lumbar taps or intraventricular shunt.
• For long-term therapy, fluconazole 200 mg PO qd is highly effective in preventing a relapse in HIV-infected patients.

CLINICAL PEARL
• Cryptococcosis is considered an AIDS-defining infection when it occurs in the absence of other known causes of immunodeficiency. All patients should be advised to having HIV testing.

▬ *Cryptosporidium*

Definition: The intracellular protozoan parasite *Cryptosporidium parvum* is associated with gastrointestinal (GI) disease and diarrhea, especially in AIDS patients or immunocompromised hosts. It also is associated with waterborne outbreak in immunocompetent hosts. Other species, including *C. felis, C. muris,* and *C. meleagridis,* are now described to be pathogens as well.

DIAGNOSIS
• Clinical presentation includes acute GI illness, especially associated with HIV or with travel and waterborne outbreaks. Symptoms usually are limited to the GI tract (diarrhea, severe abdominal pain, impaired digestion, dehydration, nausea, vomiting).
• Stool evaluation is done to look for characteristic oocyst by modified acid-fast stain.
• Serologic testing is investigational.

- The organism may be seen in mucosal surfaces of GI lumen by biopsy.

TREATMENT

- Disease may be self-limited in a normal host; hydration often is required. Antidiarrheal agents (e.g., bismuth subsalicylate [Pepto-Bismol] or loperamide [Kaopectate]) may give symptomatic relief.
- Pharmacologic treatment with antibiotics to date has had a variable and usually poor response. Oocyst excretion reduction has been shown with paromomycin (1 g bid)/azithromycin and nitazoxanide therapy along with decreasing stool frequency. If treatment failure, consider metronidazole or trimethoprim-sulfamethoxazole (Bactrim).
- Nitazoxanide elixir has been approved for the treatment of cryptosporidiosis in children age 1 to 11 years old.
- Biliary cryptosporidiosis can be treated with antiretroviral therapy in the setting of HIV infection.

CLINICAL PEARL

- *Cryptosporidium* may be a significant pathogen causing diarrhea in AIDS.

Cushing's syndrome

Definition: The occurrence of clinical abnormalities associated with glucocorticoid excess secondary to exaggerated adrenal cortisol production or long-term glucocorticoid therapy. Cushing's disease is Cushing's syndrome caused by pituitary adrenocorticotropic hormone (ACTH) excess.

DIAGNOSIS

- **Physical findings and clinical presentation:**
  - Central obesity with rounding of the facies (moon facies); thin extremities
  - Hypertension
  - Hirsutism, menstrual irregularities, hypogonadism
  - Skin fragility, ecchymosis, red-purple abdominal striae, acne, poor wound healing, hair loss, facial plethora, hyperpigmentation (when there is ACTH excess)
  - Psychosis, emotional lability, paranoia
  - Muscle wasting with proximal myopathy
- **Laboratory evaluation:**
  - In patients with a clinical diagnosis of Cushing's syndrome, the initial screening test is the overnight dexamethasone suppression

- • Plasma cortisol level measured 9 hours later (8 A.M.)
  - • Plasma cortisol level <5 µg/100 mL excludes Cushing's syndrome
- Serial measurements (two or three consecutive measurements) of 24-hour urinary free cortisol and creatinine (to ensure adequacy of collection) are undertaken if overnight dexamethasone test suggests Cushing's syndrome. Persistent elevated cortisol excretion (>300 µg/24 hr) indicates Cushing's syndrome.
- The low-dose (2 mg) dexamethasone suppression test is useful to exclude pseudo-Cushing's syndrome if the results of first dexamethasone test are equivocal. Corticotropin-releasing hormone (CRH) stimulation after low-dose dexamethasone administration (dexamethasone-CRH test) also is used to distinguish patients with suspected Cushing's syndrome from patients who have mildly elevated urinary free cortisol level and equivocal findings.
- The high-dose (8 mg) dexamethasone test and measurement of ACTH by RIA are useful to determine the etiology of Cushing's syndrome:
  - ACTH undetectable or decreased and lack of suppression indicates adrenal etiology of Cushing's syndrome
  - ACTH normal or increased and lack of suppression indicates ectopic ACTH production
  - ACTH normal or increased and partial suppression suggests pituitary excess (Cushing's disease)
- A single midnight serum cortisol (normal diurnal variation leads to a nadir around midnight) >7.5 µg/dL has been reported as 96% sensitive and 100% specific for the diagnosis of Cushing's syndrome.
- Other laboratory tests reveal hypokalemia, hypochloremia, metabolic alkalosis, hyperglycemia, hypercholesterolemia, and increased 24-hour urinary free cortisol (>100 µg/24 hr)
- **Diagnostic imaging:**
- CT of adrenal glands is indicated in suspected adrenal Cushing's syndrome.
- MRI of pituitary gland with gadolinium enhancement is indicated in suspected pituitary Cushing's syndrome.

ETIOLOGY
- Iatrogenic from long-term glucocorticoid therapy (common)
- Pituitary ACTH excess (Cushing's disease; 60%)
- Adrenal neoplasms (30%)
- Ectopic ACTH production (neoplasms of lung, pancreas, kidney, thyroid, thymus; 10%)

TREATMENT

- The treatment of Cushing's syndrome varies with its cause:
  - **Pituitary adenoma:** Transsphenoidal microadenomectomy is the therapy of choice in adults. Pituitary irradiation is reserved for patients not cured by transsphenoidal surgery. In children, pituitary irradiation may be considered as initial therapy because 85% of children are cured by radiation. Stereotactic radiotherapy (photon knife or gamma knife) is effective and exposes the surrounding neuronal tissues to less irradiation than conventional radiotherapy. Total bilateral adrenalectomy is reserved for patients not cured by transsphenoidal surgery or pituitary irradiation.
  - **Adrenal neoplasm:**
    - Surgical resection of the affected adrenal
    - Glucocorticoid replacement for approximately 9 to 12 months after the surgery to allow time for the contralateral adrenal to recover from prolonged suppression
  - **Bilateral micronodular or macronodular adrenal hyperplasia:** bilateral total adrenalectomy
  - **Ectopic ACTH:**
    - Surgical resection of ACTH-secreting neoplasm
    - Control of cortisol excess with metyrapone, aminoglutethimide, mifepristone, or ketoconazole
    - Control of the mineralocorticoid effects of cortisol and 11-deoxy-corticosteroid with spironolactone
    - Bilateral adrenalectomy—a rational approach to patients with indolent, unresectable tumors

CLINICAL PEARLS

- In Cushing's syndrome secondary to ectopic ACTH production, many of these tumors secrete a biologically inactive ACTH that does not activate adrenal steroid synthesis. These patients may have only weight loss and weakness.
- Screening for multiple endocrine neoplasia type I should be considered in patients with Cushing's disease.

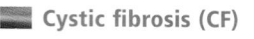

Cystic fibrosis (CF)

Definition: An autosomal recessive disorder characterized by dysfunction of exocrine glands

DIAGNOSIS

- A diagnosis of CF requires a positive quantitative pilocarpine ion-
  sweat test with one or more phenotypic features consistent with

insufficiency) or documented CF in a sibling or first cousin.
- **Laboratory tests:**
  - Pilocarpine iontophoresis ("sweat test") is diagnostic of CF in children if sweat chloride is >60 mmol/L (>80 mmol/L in adults) on two separate tests on consecutive days.
  - DNA testing may be useful to confirm the diagnosis and provide genetic information for family members.
  - Sputum culture and sensitivity and Gram stain are useful because bacterial infections with *Staphylococcus aureus, Pseudomonas, Haemophilus influenzae* are frequent.
  - Low albumin level and increased 72-hour fecal fat excretion are present.
  - Arterial blood gases test for hypoxemia.
  - Pulmonary function test results include decreased total lung capacity, forced vital capacity, and pulmonary diffusing capacity.
- **Imaging studies:**
  - Chest x-ray may reveal focal atelectasis, peribronchial cuffing, bronchiectasis, increased interstitial markings, and hyperinflation.
  - High-resolution chest CT scan shows bronchial wall thickening, cystic lesions, and ring shadows (bronchiectasis).

ETIOLOGY
- Chromosome 7 gene mutation (*CFTR* gene) resulting in abnormalities in chloride transport and water flux across the surface of epithelial cells; the abnormal secretions cause obstruction of glands and ducts in various organs and subsequent damage to exocrine tissue (recurrent pneumonia, atelectasis, bronchiectasis, diabetes mellitus, biliary cirrhosis, cholelithiasis, intestinal obstruction, increased risk of gastrointestinal malignancies)

TREATMENT
- Postural drainage and chest percussion
- Encouragement of regular exercise and proper nutrition
- Antibiotic therapy based on results of Gram stain and culture and sensitivity of sputum (oral ciprofloxacin or floxacillin for *Pseudomonas* and cephalosporins for *S. aureus*, intravenous aminoglycosides plus ceftazidime for life-threatening *Pseudomonas* infections). Macrolides also are active against *Paeruginosa*. Azithromycin maintenance in children with CF may be beneficial.
- Bronchodilators for patients with airflow obstruction
- Long-term pancreatic enzyme replacement
- Alternate-day prednisone 2 mg/kg possibly beneficial in children with CF (decreased hospitalization rate, improved pulmonary function); routine use of corticosteroids not recommended in adults. Among

children with CF who have received alternate-day treatment with prednisone, boys, but not girls, have persistent growth impairment after treatment is discontinued.

- Proper nutrition and vitamin supplementation
- Recombinant human deoxyribonuclease I (DNase, dornase alfa) 2.5 mg qd or bid given by aerosol for patients with viscid sputum. DNase is useful to improve mucociliary clearance by liquefying difficult-to-clear pulmonary secretions. It is, however, very expensive (annual cost to the pharmacist is <$10,000). It most beneficial in patients with forced vital capacity values <50% of predicted. Cost can be decreased by using alternate-day DNase therapy.
- Intermittent administration of inhaled tobramycin has been reported beneficial in CF
- Treatment of glucose intolerance and diabetes mellitus
- Pneumococcal vaccination, yearly influenza vaccination
- Lung transplantation is the only definitive treatment; 3-year survival after transplantation is >50%.

CLINICAL PEARL

- Genetic testing for CF should be offered to adults with a positive family history of CF to couples currently planning a pregnancy, and to couples seeking prenatal care.

Cysticercosis

Definition: An infection with the larval stage of the pork tapeworm (*Taenia solium*). Humans acquire cysticercosis through fecal-oral contamination with *T. solium* eggs from tapeworm carriers. Oncospheres (embryos) in the eggs are liberated by the action of gastric and intestinal fluids and cross the bowel wall, enter the bloodstream, and are carried to muscles and other tissues, including the central nervous system (neurocysticercosis). At small vessels, they establish and encyst as cysticerci, reaching a size of about 1 cm in 2 to 3 months.

DIAGNOSIS

- A comprehensive clinical history must be obtained. Epilepsy caused by intracerebral cysts is the most common manifestation of neurocysticercosis (70-90% of cases). Less common findings are headache, nausea, and vomiting resulting from increased intracranial pressure and altered mental status, including psychosis.
- Inflammation around degenerating cysts can cause focal encephalitis, vasculitis, chronic meningitis, and cranial nerve palsies.

suspected.

- **Imaging studies:** Brain MRI is the most accurate technique to assess the degree of infection, the location, and the evolutionary stage of the parasites. Head CT scan can be substituted if MRI is unavailable or contraindicated.
- **Laboratory tests (serology):** Immunotesting of serum and cerebrospinal fluid (CSF) can be done to look for antibodies. ELISA has a sensitivity and specificity >90% when done in inflammatory CSF.
- CSF examination may show pleocytosis, with lymphocytic or eosinophilic predominance, low glucose, and elevated protein with neurocysticercosis

ETIOLOGY

- Ingestion of the *Taenia solium* cysticerci in infected, undercooked pork

TREATMENT

- **Inactive infection:** Patients with seizures and calcifications alone on neuroimaging studies are not thought to have viable parasites. Cysticidal therapy usually is not undertaken. Anticonvulsants can control seizures. For patients with hydrocephalus, ventriculoperitoneal shunting can resolve symptoms.
- **Active parenchymal infection (most common presentation):** Eradication of cysts is less controversial for active disease. Anticonvulsants should be given to control seizures. Some authors argue that only treatment of seizures, not antiparasitic therapy, is needed.
- **Extraparenchymal neurocysticercosis:** Refer to a neurosurgeon.
  - **Ventricular**—usually presents with obstructive hydrocephalus. The mainstay of therapy is the rapid correction of hydrocephalus.
  - **Subarachnoid**—associated with arachnoiditis. Diversion of CSF and steroid therapy may be needed.
- **Cysticidal therapy:** Praziquantel has been the mainstay of therapy and is effective; albendazole is now being used more frequently, and it may have greater efficacy at a lesser cost than praziquantel.

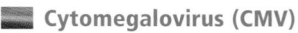

Cytomegalovirus (CMV)

Definition: Infection with CMV, a herpesvirus

DIAGNOSIS
- Demonstration of virus in tissue or serologic testing, including CMV IgM antibodies, rising titers of complement fixation, and indirect fluorescent antibody or anticomplement indirect fluorescent antibody, makes the diagnosis.
- Funduscopy shows necrotic patches with white granular component of retina.
- Culture findings include (viral) human fibroblast from urine, cervical swab, or tissue buffy coat.
- "Owl's eye" inclusion bodies are visible on tissue biopsy sample.

TREATMENT
- Highly active antiretroviral therapy in patients with CD4 count <50/mm^3 for the goal of CD4 >100/ mm^3 for 3 to 6 months
- For compromised hosts with CMV retinitis or pneumonitis:
  - Ganciclovir 5 mg/kg IV bid × 21 days, then 5 mg/kg/day IV or 1 g PO tid or ocular implant
  - Foscarnet 60 mg/kg tid × 3 weeks, then 90 mg/kg/day
  - Cidofovir 5 mg/kg IV, repeat 1 week later, then every 2 weeks IV
  - Fomivirsen (salvage therapy for CMV retinitis) 300 μg injected into vitreous

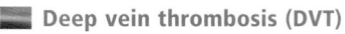

Deep vein thrombosis (DVT)

Definition: The development of thrombi in the deep veins of the extremities or pelvis

DIAGNOSIS
- The clinical diagnosis of DVT is inaccurate. Pain, tenderness, swelling, or color changes are not specific for DVT. Compression ultrasonography is preferred as the initial study to diagnose DVT. An initial negative test should be repeated after 5 days (if the clinical suspicion of DVT persists) to detect propagation of any thrombosis to the proximal veins.
- **Laboratory tests:**
  - Laboratory tests are not specific for DVT. Baseline prothrombin time (international normalized ratio [INR]), partial thromboplastin time, and platelet count should be obtained on all patients before starting anticoagulation.

... ... by ELISA may be useful in the management of suspected DVT. The combination of a normal D dimer study on presentation with a normal compression venous ultrasound is useful to exclude DVT and generally eliminate the need to do repeat ultrasound at 5 to 7 days. Trials indicate that DVT can be ruled out in patients who are clinically unlikely to have DVT and who have a negative D dimer test. Compressive ultrasonography can be omitted safely in such patients.

- Laboratory evaluation of young patients with DVT, patients with recurrent thrombosis without obvious causes, and patients with a family history of thrombosis should include protein S, protein C, fibrinogen, antithrombin III level, lupus anticoagulant, anticardiolipin antibodies, factor V Leiden, factor VIII, factor IX, and plasma homocysteine levels.

- **Imaging studies:**
- Compression ultrasonography generally is preferred as the initial study because it is noninvasive and can be repeated serially (useful to monitor suspected acute DVT); ultrasound has good sensitivity for detecting proximal vein thrombosis (in the popliteal or femoral vein). Its disadvantages are poor visualization of deep iliac and pelvic veins and poor sensitivity in isolated or nonocclusive calf vein thrombi.
- Contrast venography is the gold standard for evaluation of DVT of the lower extremity. It is, however, invasive and painful. Additional disadvantages are the increased risk of phlebitis, new thrombosis, renal failure, and hypersensitivity reaction to contrast media; it also gives poor visualization of the deep femoral vein in the thigh and internal iliac vein and its tributaries.
- Magnetic resonance direct thrombus imaging is an accurate noninvasive test for diagnosis of DVT. Current limitations are cost and lack of widespread availability.

ETIOLOGY

- The etiology is often multifactorial (prolonged stasis, coagulation abnormalities, vessel wall trauma). The following are risk factors for DVT:
  - Prolonged immobilization (≥3 days)
  - Postoperative state
  - Trauma to pelvis and lower extremities
  - Birth control pills, high-dose estrogen therapy. Conjugated equine estrogen, but not esterified estrogen, is associated with increased risk of DVT. Estrogen plus progestin is associated with doubling the risk of venous thrombosis.

- Visceral cancer (lung, pancreas, alimentary tract, genitourinary tract)
- Age >60 years old
- History of thromboembolic disease
- Hematologic disorders (e.g. antithrombin III deficiency; protein C deficiency; protein S deficiency; heparin cofactor II deficiency; sticky platelet syndrome; G20210A prothrombin mutation; lupus anticoagulant; dysfibrinogenemias; anticardiolipin antibody; hyperhomocysteinemia; concurrent homocystinuria; high levels of factors VIII, XI, and factor V Leiden mutation)
- Pregnancy and early puerperium
- Obesity, congestive heart failure
- Surgery, fracture, or injury involving lower leg or pelvis
- Surgery requiring >30 minutes of anesthesia
- Gynecologic surgery (particularly gynecologic cancer surgery)
- Recent travel (within 2 weeks, lasting >4 hours)
- Smoking and abdominal obesity
- Central venous catheter or pacemaker insertion
- Superficial vein thrombosis, varicose veins

TREATMENT

Traditional treatment consists of intravenous unfractionated heparin for 4 to 7 days followed by warfarin therapy. Low-molecular-weight heparin enoxaparin (Lovenox) also is effective for initial management of DVT and allows outpatient treatment. Recommended dose is 1 mg/kg SC q12h and continued for a minimum of 5 days and until a therapeutic INR (2-3) has been achieved with warfarin. Once-daily fondaparinux (Arixtra), a synthetic analogue of heparin, is as effective and safe as twice-daily enoxaparin in the initial treatment of patients with symptomatic DVT. Warfarin therapy should be initiated when appropriate (usually within 72 hours of initiation of heparin). A 5-mg loading dose of warfarin is recommended in inpatients. In the outpatient setting, a warfarin monogram using 10-mg loading doses may be more effective in reaching a therapeutic INR. Low-molecular-weight heparin, when used, should be overlapped with warfarin for at least 5 days and until the INR has exceeded 2 for 2 consecutive days.

Insertion of an inferior vena cava filter to prevent pulmonary embolism is recommended in patients with contraindications to anticoagulation.

Thrombolytic therapy (streptokinase) can be used in rare cases (unless contraindicated) in patients with extensive iliofemoral venous thrombosis and a low risk of bleeding.

- Exclusions from outpatient treatment of DVT include patients with potential high complication risk (e.g., hemoglobin <7 g/dL, platelet count <75,000/mm³, guaic-positive stool, recent cerebrovascular accident or noncutaneous surgery, noncompliance).
- The optimal duration of anticoagulant therapy varies with the cause of DVT and the patient's risk factors:
  - Therapy for 3 to 6 months is generally satisfactory in patients with reversible risk factors (low-risk group).
  - Anticoagulation for at least 6 months is recommended for patients with idiopathic venous thrombosis or medical risk factors for DVT (intermediate-risk group).
  - Indefinite anticoagulation is necessary in patients with DVT associated with active cancer; long-term anticoagulation also is indicated in patients with inherited thrombophilia (e.g., deficiency of protein C or S antibody), antiphospholipid, and recurrent episodes of idiopathic DVT (high-risk group).
  - Measurement of D dimer after withdrawal of oral anticoagulation may be useful to estimate the risk of recurrence. Patients with a first spontaneous DVT and a D dimer level <250 ng/mL after withdrawal of oral anticoagulation have a low risk of DVT recurrence.

Diabetes insipidus (DI)

Definition: Polyuric disorder resulting from insufficient production of antidiuretic hormone (ADH) (pituitary [neurogenic] DI) or unresponsiveness of the renal tubules to ADH (nephrogenic DI)

DIAGNOSIS

- **Clinical presentation:** The following physical findings and clinical manifestations are generally not evident until vasopressin secretory capacity is reduced <20% of normal.
  - Polyuria (urinary volumes 2.5-6 L/day)
  - Polydipsia (predilection for cold or iced drinks)
  - Neurologic manifestations (seizures, headaches, visual field defects)
  - Evidence of volume contractions
- **Laboratory tests:**
  - Decreased urinary specific gravity (≤1.005)
  - Decreased urinary osmolarity (usually <200 mOsm/kg) even in the presence of high serum osmolality

- Hypernatremia, increased plasma osmolarity, hypercalcemia, hypokalemia

Imaging: MRI of the brain if neurogenic diabetes insipidus is confirmed

Workup: The diagnostic workup is aimed at showing that the polyuria is caused by the inability to concentrate urine and determining whether the problem is secondary to decreased ADH or insensitivity to ADH. This is done with the water deprivation test.

ETIOLOGY

- **Neurogenic DI:**
  - Idiopathic
  - Neoplasms of brain or pituitary fossa (craniopharyngiomas, metastatic neoplasms from breast or lung)
  - Postthereapeutic neurosurgical procedures (e.g., hypophysectomy)
  - Head trauma (e.g., basal skull fracture)
  - Granulomatous disorders (sarcoidosis or tuberculosis)
  - Histiocytosis (Hand-Schüller-Christian disease, eosinophilic granuloma)
  - Familial (autosomal dominant)
  - **Other:** intraventricular hemorrhage, aneurysms, meningitis, postencephalitis, multiple sclerosis

- **Nephrogenic DI:**
  - Drugs (lithium, amphotericin B, demeclocycline, methoxyflurane anesthesia)
  - Familial (X-linked)
  - Metabolic (hyperkalemia or hypokalemia)
  - **Other:** sarcoidosis, amyloidosis, pyelonephritis, polycystic disease, sickle cell disease, postobstructive

TREATMENT

- Therapy varies with the degree and type of DI.
- **Neurogenic DI:**
  - Desmopressin acetate 10–40 μg qd intranasally in one to three divided doses or in tablet form 0.05 mg bid. Usual oral dose is 0.1–1.2 mg/day in two to three divided doses. Desmopressin also is available in injectable form given as 2–4 μg/day SC or IV in two divided doses.
  - Vasopressin tannate in oil 2.5–5 U IM q24–72h; this is useful for long-term management because of its long half-life.
  - In mild cases of neurogenic DI, the polyuria may be controlled with hydrochlorothiazide 50 mg or chlorpropamide (Diabinese) 250 mg qd.

- Adequate hydration
- Low-sodium diet and chlorothiazide to induce mild sodium depletion
- Polyuria of DI secondary to lithium can be ameliorated by using amiloride 5 mg PO bid initially, increased to 10 mg bid after 2 weeks

▰ Diabetic ketoacidosis (DKA)

Definition: A life-threatening complication of diabetes mellitus caused by severe insulin deficiency and manifested clinically by severe dehydration and alterations in the sensorium

DIAGNOSIS
- **Physical examination:**
  - Evidence of dehydration (tachycardia, hypotension, dry mucous membranes, sunken eyeballs, poor skin turgor)
  - Clouding of mental status
  - Tachypnea with air hunger (Kussmaul's respiration)
  - Fruity breath odor (caused by acetone)
  - Lipemia retinalis in some patients
  - Possible evidence of precipitating factors (infected wound, pneumonia)
  - Abdominal or costovertebral angle tenderness in some patients
- **Laboratory tests:**
  - Glucose level reveals severe hyperglycemia (serum glucose generally >300 mg/dL).
  - Arterial blood gases reveal acidosis: arterial pH usually <7.3 with PCO_2 <40 mm Hg.
  - Serum electrolytes:
    - Serum bicarbonate is usually <15 mEq/L.
    - Serum potassium may be low, normal, or high. There is always significant total body potassium depletion regardless of the initial potassium level.
    - Serum sodium usually is decreased as a result of hyperglycemia, dehydration, and lipemia. Assume 1.6 mEq/L decrease in extracellular sodium for each 100 mg/dL increase in glucose concentration.
    - Calculate the anion gap (AG):
      - $AG = Na^+ - (Cl^- + HCO_3^-)$

- In DKA, the AG is increased; hyperchloremic metabolic acidosis may be present in unusual circumstances when the glomerular filtration rate and the plasma volume are well maintained.
- Complete blood count with differential, urinalysis, and urine and blood cultures to rule out infectious precipitating factor are performed.
- Serum calcium, magnesium, and phosphorus are measured; the plasma phosphate and magnesium levels may be significantly depressed and should be rechecked within 24 hours because they may decrease further with correction of DKA.
- Blood urea nitrogen and creatinine generally reveal significant dehydration.
- Amylase and liver enzymes should be checked in patients with abdominal pain.
- **Imaging:** Chest x-ray is helpful to rule out an infectious process. The initial chest x-ray may be negative if the patient has significant dehydration. Repeat chest x-ray after 24 hours if pulmonary infection is strongly suspected.

ETIOLOGY

Metabolic decompensation in diabetics usually is precipitated by an infectious process (40% of cases). Poor compliance with insulin therapy and severe medical illness (e.g. cerebrovascular accident, myocardial infarction) are other common causes. Cocaine abuse has been reported as a risk factor for DKA, particularly in patients with multiple admissions.

TREATMENT

- **Fluid replacement (usual deficit is8-8 L):**
- Do not delay fluid replacement until laboratory results have been received.
- The initial fluid replacement should be with 0.9% normal saline until blood pressure and organ perfusion are restored (usually ≥1 L). In patients with severe hypernatremia (serum sodium >160 mEq/L), 0.45% saline infusion can be used. Careful monitoring for fluid overload is necessary in elderly patients and patients with a history of congestive heart failure.
- The rate of fluid replacement varies with the age of the patient and the presence of significant cardiac or renal disease.
- The usual rate of infusion is 500 mL to 1 L over the first hour and 300-500 mL/hr for the next 12 hours.
- Continue infusion at a rate of 200-300 mL/hr, using 0.45% normal saline until the serum glucose level is <300 mg/dL, then change

glycemia, replenish free water, and introduce additional glucose substrate (necessary to suppress lipolysis and ketogenesis).

- **Insulin administration:**
  - The patient should be given an initial loading intravenous bolus of 0.15-0.2 U/kg of regular insulin followed by a constant infusion at 0.1 U/kg/hr (e.g., 25 U of regular insulin in 250 mL of 0.9% saline solution at 70 mL/hr equals 7 U/hr for a 70-kg patient).
  - Monitor serum glucose hourly for the first 2 hours, then monitor q2-4h.
  - The goal is to decrease serum glucose level by 80 mg/dL/hr (after an initial drop because of rehydration); if the serum glucose level is not decreasing at the expected rate, double the rate of insulin infusion.
  - When the serum glucose level approaches 250 mg/dL, decrease the rate of insulin infusion to 2-3 U/hr, and continue this rate until the patient has received adequate fluid replacement, HCO_3^- is close to normal, and ketones have cleared.
  - Approximately 30 to 60 minutes before stopping the intravenous insulin infusion, administer a subcutaneous dose of regular insulin (dose varies with the patient's demonstrated insulin sensitivity); this subcutaneous dose of regular insulin is necessary because of the extremely short half-life of the insulin in the intravenous infusion.
  - When the patient is able to eat, NPH insulin 10-15 U is given in the morning, and regular insulin is administered before each meal and at bedtime by using a sliding scale. In newly diagnosed diabetics, the total daily dose to maintain metabolic control is 0.5-0.8 U/kg/day. Split-dose therapy with regular and NPH insulin may be given, with two thirds of the total daily dose administered in the morning and one third in the evening.
- **Electrolyte replacement:**
  - **Potassium replacement:** The average total potassium loss in DKA is 300 to 500 mEq.
    - The rate of replacement varies with the patient's serum potassium level, degree of acidosis (decreased pH, increased potassium level), and renal function (potassium replacement should be used with caution in patients with renal failure).
    - As a rule of thumb, potassium replacement may be started when there is no ECG evidence of hyperkalemia (tall, narrow, or tent-shaped T waves; decreased or absent P waves; short Q-T intervals; widening of QRS complex).
    - In patients with normal renal function, potassium replacement can be started by adding potassium chloride 20-40 mEq/L to

intravenous hydrating solution if serum potassium is 4 to 5 mEq/L; more can be added if serum potassium level is <4 mEq/L.

- Monitor serum potassium level hourly for the first 2 hours, then monitor q2-4h.
- **Phosphate replacement:** If the serum PO₄ is <1.5 mEq/L, give elemental phosphate 2.5 mg/kg IV over 6 hours. Routine replacement of phosphate (in the absence of laboratory evidence of significant hypophosphatemia) is not indicated. Rapid intravenous phosphate administration can cause hypocalcemia.
- **Magnesium replacement:** Replacement is indicated only in the presence of significant hypomagnesemia or refractory hypokalemia.
- **Bicarbonate therapy:** Routine use of bicarbonate in DKA is contraindicated because it can worsen hypokalemia and intracellular acidosis and cause cerebral edema. Bicarbonate therapy should be used only if the arterial pH is <7. In these patients, 44-88 mEq of sodium bicarbonate can be added to 1 L of 0.45% normal saline q2-4h until pH increases >7.

CLINICAL PEARLS

Although DKA occurs more commonly in type 1 diabetes mellitus, a significant proportion (>20%) occurs in patients with type 2 diabetes mellitus.

Twenty percent of DKA admissions involve newly diagnosed diabetes.

Diffuse interstitial lung disease

Definition: Group of disorders involving the lung interstitium and characterized by inflammation of the alveolar structures and progressive parenchymal fibrosis

DIAGNOSIS

- **Physical examination:**
- The patient generally presents with progressive dyspnea and non-productive cough; other clinical manifestations vary with the underlying disease process.
- Physical examination typically shows end respiratory dry rales (Velcro rales), cyanosis, clubbing, and right-sided heart failure.
- **Imaging:** Chest x-ray may be normal in 10% of patients.
- Ground-glass appearance is often an early finding.
- A coarse reticular pattern is usually a late finding.

must always be ruled out.
- Differential diagnosis of interstitial patterns include the following: pulmonary fibrosis, pulmonary edema, *Pneumocystis carinii* pneumonia, tuberculosis, sarcoidosis, eosinophilic granuloma, pneumoconiosis, and lymphangitic spread of carcinoma.
- **Laboratory tests:**
  - Arterial blood gases provide only limited information; initially, arterial blood gases may be normal, but with progression of the disease, hypoxemia may be present.
  - Antineutrophil cytoplasmic antibody is frequently positive in Wegener's granulomatosis.
  - Anti–glomerular basement membrane (anti-GBM) and anti–pulmonary basement membrane antibody are often present in Goodpasture's syndrome.
  - Pulmonary function testing findings generally are consistent with restrictive disease (decreased vital capacity, total lung capacity, and diffusing capacity).
  - Bronchoscopy with bronchoalveolar lavage is useful in selected patients.
  - Open lung biopsy or transbronchial biopsy is useful to identify the underlying disease process and exclude neoplastic involvement; transbronchial biopsy is less invasive, but provides less tissue for analysis (this factor may be important in patients with irregular pulmonary involvement).

ETIOLOGY
- Occupational and environmental exposure (pneumoconiosis, asbestosis, organic dust, gases, fumes, berylliosis, silicosis)
- Granulomatous lung disease (sarcoidosis, infections [e.g., fungal, mycobacterial])
- Drug-induced (bleomycin, busulfan, methotrexate, chlorambucil, cyclophosphamide, carmustine, gold salts, tetrazolium chloride, amiodarone, tocainide, penicillin, zidovudine, sulfonamide)
- Radiation pneumonitis
- Connective tissue diseases (systemic lupus erythematosus, rheumatoid arthritis, dermatomyositis)
- Idiopathic pulmonary fibrosis (bronchiolitis obliterans, interstitial pneumonitis, diffuse interstitial pneumonitis)
- Infections (viral pneumonia, *P. carinii* pneumonia)
- **Other:** Wegener's granulomatosis, Goodpasture's syndrome, eosinophilic granuloma, lymphangitic carcinomatosis, chronic uremia, chronic gastric aspiration, hypersensitivity pneumonitis, lipoid pneumonia, lymphoma, lymphoid granulomatosis

TREATMENT

- Treat infectious process with appropriate antibiotic therapy.
- Provide supplemental oxygen in patients with significant hypoxemia.
- Give corticosteroids to symptomatic patients with sarcoidosis.
- Immunosuppressive therapy is indicated in selected cases (e.g., cyclophosphamide in patients with Wegener's granulomatosis).
- Treat any complications (e.g., pneumothorax, pulmonary embolism).

CLINICAL PEARLS

- Pulmonary referral for bronchoscopy and bronchoalveolar lavage (selected patients).
- Although open lung biopsy is the gold standard for diagnosis, it may be inappropriate in elderly patients; individual consideration is advisable.
- Consider lung transplantation in selected patients with intractable end-stage interstitial lung disease.

Disseminated intravascular coagulation (DIC)

Definition: Acquired thromboembolic disorder characterized by generalized activation of the clotting mechanism, which results in the intravascular formation of fibrin and ultimately thrombotic occlusion of small and midsize vessels

DIAGNOSIS

- Peripheral blood smear generally shows red blood cell fragments and low platelet count.
- Coagulation factors are consumed at a rate in excess of the capacity of the liver to synthesize them, and platelets are consumed in excess of the capacity of the bone marrow megakaryocytes to release them. Diagnostic characteristics of DIC are increased prothrombin time (PT), partial thromboplastin time (PTT), thrombin time (TT), fibrin split products, and D dimmer and decreased fibrinogen level and thrombocytopenia.
- Coagulopathy secondary to DIC must be differentiated from coagulopathy secondary to liver disease or vitamin K deficiency.
  - Vitamin K deficiency manifests with prolonged PT and normal PTT, TT, platelet, and fibrinogen level; PTT may be elevated in severe cases.
  - Patients with liver disease have abnormal PT and PTT; TT and fibrinogen are usually normal, unless severe disease is present; platelets are usually normal unless splenomegaly is present.

tors V and VIII are low in DIC, but they are normal in liver disease with coagulopathy.

ETIOLOGY
- Infections (gram-negative sepsis, Rocky Mountain spotted fever, malaria, viral or fungal infection)
- Obstetric complications (dead fetus, amniotic fluid embolism, toxemia, abruptio placentae, septic abortion, eclampsia)
- Tissue trauma (burns, hypothermia rewarming)
- Neoplasms (adenocarcinomas [gastrointestinal, prostate, lung, breast], acute promyelocytic leukemia)
- Quinine, cocaine-induced rhabdomyolysis
- Liver failure
- Acute pancreatitis
- Transfusion reactions
- Respiratory distress syndrome
- **Other:** systemic lupus erythematosus, vasculitis, aneurysms, polyarteritis, cavernous hemangiomas

TREATMENT
- Correct and eliminate underlying cause (e.g., antimicrobial therapy for infection).
- Give replacement therapy with fresh frozen plasma and platelets in patients with significant hemorrhage:
  - Fresh frozen plasma 10-15 mL/kg can be given with a goal of normalizing international normalized ratio.
  - Platelet transfusions are given when platelet count is <10,000/mm^3 (or higher if major bleeding is present).
  - Cryoprecipitate 1 U/5 kg is reserved for hypofibrinogen states.
  - Antithrombin III treatment may be considered as a supportive therapeutic option in patients with severe DIC. Its modest results and substantial cost are limiting factors.
- Heparin therapy at a dose lower than that used in venous thrombosis (300-500 U/hr) may be useful in selected cases to increase neutralization of thrombin (e.g., DIC associated with acute promyelocytic leukemia, purpura fulminans, acral ischemia).

CLINICAL PEARL
- The treatment of chronic DIC is controversial. Low-dose subcutaneous heparin or combination antiplatelet agents, such as aspirin and dipyridamole, may be useful.

Diverticular disease

Definitions: *Colonic diverticula* are herniations of mucosa and submucosa through the muscularis. They generally are found along the colon's mesenteric border at the site where the vasa recta penetrates the muscle wall (anatomic weak point).

- *Diverticulosis* is the asymptomatic presence of multiple colonic diverticula.
- *Diverticulitis* is an inflammatory process or localized perforation of diverticulum.

DIAGNOSIS
- **Physical examination:**
  - Physical examination in patients with diverticulosis is generally normal.
  - Painful diverticular disease can present with left lower quadrant pain, often relieved by defecation; location of pain may be anywhere in the lower abdomen because of the redundancy of the sigmoid colon.
  - Diverticulitis can cause muscle spasm, guarding, and rebound tenderness predominantly affecting the left lower quadrant.
- **Laboratory tests:**
  - White blood cell count in diverticulitis reveals leukocytosis with left shift.
  - Microcytic anemia can be present in patients with chronic bleeding from diverticular disease. Mean corpuscular volume may be elevated in acute bleeding secondary to reticulocytosis.
- **Imaging:**
  - Barium enema shows multiple diverticula and muscle spasm ("sawtooth" appearance of the lumen) in patients with painful diverticular disease. Barium enema can be hazardous and should not be performed in the acute stage of diverticulitis because it may produce free perforation.
  - CT scan of the abdomen can be used to diagnose acute diverticulitis; typical findings are thickening of the bowel wall, fistulas, and abscess formation.
  - The following modalities evaluate suspected diverticular bleeding:
    - Arteriography if the bleeding is faster than 1 mL/min (*advantage*—the possible infusion of vasopressin directly into the arteries supplying the bleeding and selective arterial embolization; *disadvantages*—cost and invasive nature)
    - Technetium-99m sulfa colloid

...........um 99mlabeled red blood cells (can detect bleeding
rates 0.12-5 mL/min)

DIFFERENTIAL DIAGNOSIS
- Irritable bowel syndrome
- Inflammatory bowel disease
- Carcinoma of colon
- Endometriosis
- Ischemic colitis
- Infections (pseudomembranous colitis, appendicitis, pyelonephritis, pelvic inflammatory disease)
- Lactose intolerance

TREATMENT
- **Diverticulosis:** increase in dietary fiber intake and regular exercise to improve bowel function in diverticulosis
- **Diverticulitis:**
  - **Mild case:** broad-spectrum oral antibiotics (e.g., ciprofloxin 500 mg bid to cover aerobic component of colonic flora and metronidazole 500 mg q6h for anaerobes) and liquid diet for 7 to 10 days
  - **Severe case:** nothing per mouth and aggressive intravenous antibiotic therapy
    - Ampicillin-sulbactam (Unasyn) 3 g IV q6h *or*
    - Piperacillin-tazobactam (Zosyn) 4.5 g IV q8h *or*
    - Ciprofloxacin 400 mg IV q12h plus metronidazole 500 mg IV q6h *or*
    - Cefoxitin 2 g IV q8h plus metronidazole 500 mg IV q6h
  - **Life-threatening case:** imipenem 500 mg IV q6h *or* meropenem 1 g IV q8h
- Surgical treatment consists of resection of involved areas and reanastomosis (if feasible); otherwise a diverting colostomy with reanastomosis is performed when infection has been controlled; surgery should be considered in patients with the following:
  - Repeated episodes of diverticulitis (two or more)
  - Poor response to appropriate medical therapy (failure of conservative management)
  - Abscess or fistula formation
  - Obstruction
  - Peritonitis
  - Immunocompromised patients; first episode in young patient (<40 years old)
  - Inability to exclude carcinoma (10-20% of patients diagnosed with diverticulosis on clinical grounds subsequently are found to have carcinoma of the colon)

Diverticular hemorrhage:

- Bleeding is painless and stops spontaneously in most patients (60%); it is usually is caused by erosion of a blood vessel by a fecalith present within the diverticular sac.
- Medical therapy consists of blood replacement and correction of volume and any clotting abnormalities.
- Colonoscopic treatment with epinephrine injections, bipolar coagulation, or both may prevent recurrent bleeding and decrease the need for surgery.
- Surgical resection is necessary if bleeding does not stop spontaneously after administration of 4-5 U of packed red blood cells or recurs with severity within a few days; if attempts at localization are unsuccessful, total abdominal colectomy with ileoproctostomy may be indicated (high incidence of rebleeding if segmental resection is performed without adequate localization).

CLINICAL PEARL

- Seventy percent of diverticular bleeding occurs in the right colon.

Dumping syndrome

Definition: Constellation of postprandial symptoms as a result of rapid delivery of stomach contents into the small bowel seen after definitive surgery for peptic ulcer disease

DIAGNOSIS

- **Clinical presentation:** Most patients usually present with early dumping symptoms or a combination of early and late symptoms. Few have late dumping symptoms alone.
- **Early dumping:** Symptoms start within 1 hour after eating food: nausea, vomiting, belching, epigastric fullness, cramping, and diarrhea.
- **Late dumping:** Symptoms occur 1 to 3 hours after eating: diaphoresis, irritability, and difficulty concentrating.
- Typically the diagnosis is made on clinical grounds. In certain clinical settings (e.g., symptoms in patients with no prior history of gastric surgery), a workup, including oral glucose challenge and imaging studies, may be pursued.

ETIOLOGY

- Dumping syndrome occurs almost exclusively in patients having gastric surgery.

rapid shifts of fluid from the intravascular space into the lumen of the bowel.
- An increase in vasoactive substances is thought to play a role in dumping syndrome.
- Late dumping symptoms are thought to be due to reactive hypoglycemia.

TREATMENT
- **Diet modification**
  - Divide calorie intake over six small meals
  - Limit fluid intake with meals (try to avoid 30 minutes before meals)
  - Decrease carbohydrate intake and avoid simple sugars
  - Increase/supplement dietary fibers
  - Avoid milk/milk products
- Acarbose 50 mg PO qd can be tried if dietary modification does not help.
- Octreotide 25-50 µg SC 30 minutes before meals is effective in relieving symptoms of dumping syndrome.
- Surgery is considered in patients with severe symptoms refractory to the above-mentioned dietary and acute general treatment.
- Surgical procedures include reconstruction of the pylorus, converting a Billroth II to a Billroth I anastomosis, and a Roux-en-Y reconstruction.

Echinococcosis

Definition: Chronic infection caused by the larval stage of several animal cestodes (flat worms) of the genus *Echinococcus*. *Echinococcus granulosus* is the cause of cystic hydatid disease; *Echinococcus multilocularis* and *Echinococcus vogeli* are the causes of alveolar and polycystic disease.

DIAGNOSIS
- Antibody assays (ELISA and Western blot) are >90% sensitive and specific for liver cysts, but less accurate for cysts in other sites.
- Ultrasonography and CT are extremely sensitive for the detection of cysts, especially in the liver (Fig. 5); however, both modalities lack specificity and are inadequate to establish the diagnosis of echinococcosis with certainty.
- Histologic examination of cyst or contents obtained by aspiration or resection (if possible) confirms diagnosis.

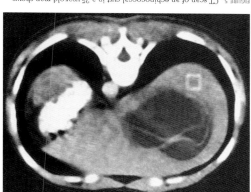

FIGURE 5. CT scan of an echinococcal cyst in a 25-year-old man shows the complex structure of the wall and the interior. (From Goldman L, Bennet JC [eds]: Cecil Textbook of Medicine, 21st ed. Philadelphia, WB Saunders, 2000.)

TREATMENT

- Treatment of choice for echinococcal cysts is surgical resection.
- If resection is not feasible, perform percutaneous drainage with instillation of 95% ethanol to prevent dissemination of viable larvae.
- Surgery is followed by medical therapy with albendazole 400 mg bid for 28 days followed by 14 days of rest for at least three cycles.
- Mebendazole 50-70 mg/kg qd can be used if albendazole is not available.

CLINICAL PEARL

- Long-term follow-up is necessary after surgery or medical therapy because of the high incidence of late relapse. Antibody assays and imaging studies should be repeated every 6 to 12 months for several years after successful surgical or medical therapy.

Ehlers-Danlos syndrome (EDS)

Definition: EDS refers to a group of inherited, clinically variable, and genetically heterogeneous connective tissue disorders characterized by skin hyperextensibility, skin fragility, joint laxity, and joint hyperextensibility.

DIAGNOSIS

- **Classic (EDS I and II):** hyperextensibility (Gorlin's sign—ability to touch tip of tongue to nose); easy scarring and bruising ("cigarette-paper scars"); smooth, velvety skin; subcutaneous spheroids (small, firm cystlike nodules) along shins or forearms
- **Hypermobility (EDS III):** joint hypermobility and some skin hypermobility with or without very smooth skin
- **Vascular (EDS IV):** thin, translucent skin with visible veins; marked bruising; pinched nose; acrogeria; spontaneous rupture of medium and large arteries and hollow organs, especially large intestine and uterus
- **Kyphoscoliosis (EDS VI):** joint hypermobility, progressive scoliosis, ocular fragility and possible globe rupture, mitral valve prolapse and aortic dilation
- **Arthrochalasis (EDS VIIA and VIIB):** prominent joint hypermobility, with subluxations, congenital hip dislocation, skin hyperextensibility, tissue fragility
- **Dermatosparaxis (EDS VIIC):** severe skin fragility with decreased elasticity, bruising, hernias
- **Unclassified type**
  - **EDS V:** classic characteristics
  - **EDS VIII:** classic characteristics and periodontal disease
  - **EDS IX:** classic characteristics
  - **EDS X:** mild classic characteristics, mitral valve prolapse
  - **EDS XI:** joint instability

ETIOLOGY

- Defects of collagen in extracellular matrices of multiple tissues (skin, tendons, blood vessels, and viscera) underlie all forms of EDS. EDS I and II are associated with defects in type V collagen, corresponding to mutations of the *COL5A* genes. EDS IV involves a deficiency in type III collagen, and several studies suggest that mutations of the *COL3A1* gene lead to this deficiency. EDS VIIA and VIIB result from a defect in type I collagen, caused by mutations in the *COL1A1* and *COL1A2* genes.

TREATMENT
- All patients should receive genetic counseling about the mode of inheritance of their EDS and the risk of having children with EDS.
- Management of most skin and joint problems should be conservative and preventive. Joint hypermobility and pain in EDS usually does not require surgical intervention. Physical therapy to strengthen muscles is helpful. Surgical repair and tightening of joint ligaments can be performed, but ligaments frequently do not hold sutures. Surgical intervention should be considered on an individual basis.
- Vascular type requires special surgical care because of increased friability of tissues. Women with EDS type IV should be counseled to avoid pregnancy.
- Patients should be advised to avoid contact sports, and elevated blood pressure should be treated aggressively.

Encephalitis, acute viral

Definition: Acute febrile syndrome with evidence of meningeal involvement and of derangement of the function of the cerebrum, cerebellum, or brainstem; can be caused by a host of viruses, with herpes simplex the most common virus identified

DIAGNOSIS
- The initial clinical presentation includes fever and evidence of meningeal irritation with headache and stiff neck. Later, signs of cortical dysfunction develop, including lethargy, coma, stupor, weakness, seizures, facial weakness, and brainstem findings. The presence of classic herpetic skin lesions suggests herpes encephalitis.
- Lumbar puncture reveals pleocytosis, usually lymphocytic (although neutrophils may be seen early on), elevated cerebrospinal fluid (CSF) protein, and normal or low CSF glucose. In herpes simplex encephalitis, red blood cells and xanthochromia may be present.
- Electroencephalogram changes show periodic high-voltage sharp waves in the temporal regions and slow wave complexes suggestive of herpes encephalitis.
- CT and MRI may reveal edema and hemorrhage in the frontal and temporal lobes.
- Polymerase chain reaction that amplifies DNA from the CSF is useful for herpes simplex encephalitis.

- No specific pharmacologic therapy for most viral pathogens. Acyclovir 30 mg/kg/day IV for 14 days is used for herpes simplex encephalitis.
- Short courses of corticosteroids to control brain edema and prevent herniation
- Supportive care, frequent evaluation, and neurologic examination
- Ventilatory assistance for patients who are moribund or at risk for aspiration
- Avoidance of infusion of hypotonic fluids to minimize the risk of hyponatremia
- Anticonvulsant therapy and follow-up in a critical care setting for patients who develop seizures
- Aggressive care to avoid decubiti, contractures, and deep venous thrombosis for comatose patients

Endocarditis

Definition: Infection of the endocardial surface of the heart, which most commonly involves heart valves. The lesions, known as *vegetations*, are composed of microorganisms, inflammatory cells, fibrin, and platelets. Infective endocarditis can be classified as *acute* or *subacute* based on the tempo and severity of the clinical presentation and progression.

DIAGNOSIS
- **Clinical presentation:**
  - Heart murmur—usually present in subacute bacterial endocarditis, but may be absent in acute bacterial endocarditis and right-sided endocarditis
  - Fever—generally present; may be absent in elderly or immunocompromised patients
  - Flame-shaped retinal hemorrhages with pale centers (*Roth spots*).
  - Painless erythematous papules and macules on the palms of the hands and soles of the feet (*Janeway lesions*) from embolic or immunologic cause
  - Painful erythematous subcutaneous papules (*Osler nodes*) generally found in the fleshy pads of fingers or toes and caused by local vasculitis
  - Petechiae (microemboli)
  - Subungual splinter hemorrhages (microemboli)

Splenomegaly (splenic sequestration) and hepatomegaly (passive congestion)
- **Other:** headaches, backache, arthralgias, confusion

Laboratory tests:
- Blood cultures—positive in 85% to 95% of patients
- Decreased hemoglobin and hematocrit—usually a result of decreased red blood cell production caused by inflammatory state
- Normal, elevated, or decreased white blood cells, usually with shift to left
- **Echocardiography:**
  Useful to show valvular vegetations and to evaluate valvular damage and left ventricular function. A normal echocardiogram does not rule out infective endocarditis; if normal, echocardiogram should be repeated in 1 week.
  Two-dimensional echocardiography is preferred over M mode because of increased sensitivity (can detect 85-95% of vegetations); transesophageal echocardiography further enhances sensitivity and is the preferred diagnostic modality.

ETIOLOGY
- Staphylococci have surpassed streptococci as the most common overall cause of infective endocarditis.
  Staphylococcus aureus—most common organism in right-sided endocarditis in drug addicts and HIV-positive patients
  Staphylococcus epidermidis—most common organism in prosthetic valve endocarditis within months postoperatively
  Streptococci
    Streptococcus viridans—most common organism except for organisms causing right-sided and prosthetic valve endocarditis
    Enterococci (Group D streptococci)—often occur in elderly men with genitourinary disorders
    Streptococcus bovis and other streptococci
  Others: fungi (intravenous drug abusers, immunocompromised patients), gram-negative bacilli, gonococci, pneumococci
  HACEK group (*Haemophilus, Actinobacillus, Cardiobacterium, Eikenella, Kingella*)

TREATMENT
- Antibiotic therapy (after identification of the organism) should be guided by susceptibility testing (minimal inhibitory concentration, minimal bactericidal concentration).
- Initial intravenous antibiotic therapy (before culture results) is aimed at the most likely organism.

but allergic to penicillin, use vancomycin plus rifampin and gentamicin.
- In intravenous drug addicts, use penicillinase-resistant penicillin (oxacillin or nafcillin) plus gentamicin.
- In patients with native valve endocarditis, use the combination of penicillin and gentamicin; a penicillinase-resistant penicillin or vancomycin should be added if acute bacterial endocarditis is present or if *S. aureus* is suspected as one of the possible causative organisms; the combination of vancomycin and gentamicin provides broad empiric coverage while awaiting culture results.

Eosinophilic fasciitis

Definition: A rare inflammatory disease of the skin and subcutaneous tissue that initially is characterized by pain, swelling, and peripheral eosinophilia. This condition starts with erythema and edema on an extremity or on the trunk, and later it may progress to sclerosis of the dermis and subcutaneous fascia and contractures.

DIAGNOSIS
- Initial presentation consists of swelling and pain with or without erythema.
- The extremities usually are symmetrically involved.
- Upper extremities are more commonly affected than lower extremities.
- The face, fingers, and toes tend to be spared.
- The skin may appear deeply rippled with an orange peel texture (peau d'orange).
- Sunken veins may be seen when the extremity is elevated.
- The groove sign marks the borders of different muscle groups.
- Arthritis is found in 40% of cases.
- Chronic complications are carpal tunnel syndrome, which was seen in 23% of patients in one series, and flexion contractures.
- **Laboratory tests:**
  - Peripheral eosinophilia (70%)
  - Elevated erythrocyte sedimentation rate (29%)
  - Hypergammaglobulinemia (35%)
  - Occasionally thrombocytopenia and anemia
- Skin biopsy that penetrates to muscle is optimal for diagnosis.

ETIOLOGY

- The etiology is unclear. A defect in humoral immunity has been hypothesized to cause the disease.
- Elevated polyclonal IgG levels and immune complexes have been associated with the disease.

TREATMENT

- Although there are no controlled trials, oral steroids are effective in most patients, but the duration and extent of symptom reduction vary.
- Methotrexate and cimetidine also have been used.
- Surgery is sometimes required to reduce contractures and maintain function.

CLINICAL PEARL

- Hematologic abnormalities other than eosinophilia are present in 10% of cases, including aplastic anemia, megakaryocytic thrombocytopenia, myeloproliferative disorders, myelodysplastic syndrome, leukemia, lymphoma, and multiple myeloma.

Eosinophilic pneumonia

Definition: A group of disorders characterized by infiltrates on chest radiographs, pulmonary parenchymal eosinophilia, and peripheral blood eosinophilia

DIAGNOSIS AND TREATMENT

- Diagnosis varies depending on the specific cause of the eosinophilic pneumonia and usually involves a combination of chest radiograph, peripheral eosinophil count, and bronchoalveolar lavage (BAL).

Simple pulmonary eosinophilia (Löffler's syndrome)

- Transient infiltrates are present.
- Symptoms range from asymptomatic to dyspnea and dry cough.
- Disease is usually idiopathic.
- Pneumonia may be secondary to parasitic infection or drugs such as nitrofurantoin or penicillin.
- Therapy consists of removing the offending agent.
- If idiopathic and symptoms are severe, give glucocorticoid therapy.

Chronic eosinophilic pneumonia:

- Disease is idiopathic.
- Patient presents with productive cough, dyspnea, malaise, weight loss, night sweats, and fever.
- Progressive peripheral pulmonary infiltrates are present.
- Blood eosinophilia is not always present.

- ~~~ by BAL or lung biopsy.
  - Spontaneous remission occurs in 10% of cases.
  - Treatment with glucocorticoids is rapidly effective.
  - Relapses are common.
- **Acute eosinophilic pneumonia:**
  - Acute onset occurs with cough, dyspnea, fever, tachypnea, and rales.
  - Patients often require mechanical ventilation.
  - Disease tends to affect young patients.
  - Often blood eosinophilia is present.
  - Chest radiographs show alveolar infiltrates.
  - BAL eosinophils are often >20%.
  - Glucocorticoid therapy often leads to rapid improvement.
  - Relapses are rare.
  - Disease may be secondary to drugs or cigarette smoking.

Epididymitis

Definition: Inflammatory reaction of the epididymis caused by either an infectious agent or local trauma

DIAGNOSIS
- Men with epididymitis typically have unilateral testicular pain and tenderness; palpable swelling of the epididymis is usually present.
- The evaluation of men for epididymitis should include the following procedures:
  - Gram-stained smear of urethral exudate or intraurethral swab specimen for *Neisseria gonorrhoeae* and for nongonococcal urethritis (≥5 polymorphonuclear neutrophils per oil immersion field)
  - A culture of urethral exudate or intraurethral swab specimen or nucleic acid amplification test (either on intraurethral swab or first-void urine) for *N. gonorrhoeae*
  - Examination of first-void urine for leukocytes if the urethral Gram stain is negative; culture and Gram stain smear of uncentrifuged urine should be obtained
  - Syphilis serology and HIV counseling and testing

ETIOLOGY
- Among men <35 years old, epididymitis is caused most often by *N. gonorrhoeae* or *Chlamydia trachomatis.*
- Epididymitis is caused by sexually transmitted *Escherichia coli* infection and occurs among homosexual men who are the insertive partners during anal intercourse.

- Non–sexually transmitted epididymitis associated with urinary tract infections caused by gram-negative enteric organisms is more common among men >35 years old and among men who recently have undergone urinary tract instrumentation or surgery.

TREATMENT

- For epididymitis most likely caused by gonococcal or chlamydial infection, use ceftriaxone 250 mg IM in a single dose *plus* doxycycline 100 mg PO bid for 10 days.
- For epididymitis most likely caused by enteric organisms or for patients allergic to cephalosporins or tetracyclines, use ofloxacin 300 mg PO bid for 10 days *or* levofloxacin 500 mg PO qd for 10 days.
- Patients who have epididymitis that is known or suspected to be caused by *N. gonorrhoeae* or *C. trachomatis* should be instructed to refer sex partners for evaluation and treatment.

Erysipelas

Definition: A type of cellulitis caused by infection of the superficial layers of the skin and cutaneous lymphatics. Erysipelas is characterized by redness, induration, and a sharply demarcated, raised border.

DIAGNOSIS

- A distinctive red, warm, tender skin lesion with induration and a sharply defined, advancing, raised border is present.
- The most common sites are the lower extremities or face.
- Systemic signs of infection (fever) are often present.
- Vesicles or bullae may develop.
- After several days, lesions may appear ecchymotic.
- After 7 to 10 days, desquamation of the affected area may occur.

ETIOLOGY

- Usually group A beta-hemolytic streptococci
- Less often group B, C, or G streptococci
- Rarely *Staphylococcus aureus*

TREATMENT

- Typical erysipelas of extremity in nondiabetic patient:
  - Oral—penicillin V 250-500 mg qid
  - Intravenous—penicillin G (aqueous) 1-2 million U q6h
  - *Note:* Use erythromycin or cephalosporin in patients allergic to penicillin.

coverage for *S. aureus*):

- Oral—dicloxacillin 500 mg q6h
- Intravenous—nafcillin or oxacillin 2 g q4h

▆ Erythema multiforme (EM)

Definition: Inflammatory disease believed to be secondary to immune complex formation and subsequent deposition in the skin and mucous membranes

DIAGNOSIS

- Symmetric skin lesions with a classic "target" appearance (caused by the centrifugal spread of red maculopapules to circumference of 1-3 cm with a purpuric, cyanotic, or vesicular center) are present.
- Lesions are most common on the back of the hands and feet and extensor aspect of the forearms and legs. Trunk involvement can occur in severe cases.
- Urticarial papules, vesicles, and bullae also may be present and generally indicate a more severe form of the disease.
- Individual lesions heal in 1 or 2 weeks without scarring.
- Bullae and erosions also may be present in the oral cavity.

DIFFERENTIAL DIAGNOSIS

- Chronic urticaria
- Secondary syphilis
- Pityriasis rosea
- Contact dermatitis
- Pemphigus vulgaris
- Lichen planus
- Serum sickness
- Drug eruption

ETIOLOGY

- Immune complex formation and subsequent deposition in the cutaneous microvasculature may play a role in the pathogenesis of EM.
- Most EM cases follow outbreaks of herpes simplex.
- In >50% of patients, no specific cause is identified.
- EM associated with bupropion use has been reported.

TREATMENT

- Mild cases generally do not require treatment; lesions resolve spontaneously within 1 month.
- Potential drug precipitants should be removed.

- Treatment of associated diseases (e.g., acyclovir for herpes simplex, erythromycin for *Mycoplasma* infection).
- Prednisone 40-80 mg/day for 1 to 3 weeks may be tried in patients with many target lesions; however, the role of systemic steroids is controversial.
- Levamisole, an immunomodulator, may be effective in treatment of patients with chronic or recurrent clinical lesions (dose is 150 mg/day for 3 consecutive days used alone or in combination with prednisone).

CLINICAL PEARL

- The rash of EM generally evolves over 2 weeks and resolves within 1 to 4 weeks without scarring. A severe bullous form can occur (see "Stevens-Johnson syndrome").

Erythema nodosum

Definition: Acute, tender, erythematous, nodular skin eruption resulting from inflammation of subcutaneous fat, often associated with bruising

DIAGNOSIS

- There is an acute onset of tender nodules typically located on the shins and occasionally seen on the thighs and forearms.
- The nodules are usually (1/8) to 1 inch in diameter, but can be 4 inches; they begin as light red lesions, then become darker and often ecchymotic. The nodules heal within 8 weeks without ulceration.
- Associated findings include fever, lymphadenopathy, and arthralgia.
- Laboratory tests include erythrocyte sedimentation rate, throat culture, antistreptolysin O titer, and purified protein derivative.
- Chest x-ray is obtained to look for sarcoidosis and tuberculosis.

ETIOLOGY

- Cell-mediated hypersensitivity reaction is seen more frequently in persons with HLA antigen B8. The lesion results from an exaggerated interaction between an antigen and cell-mediated immune mechanisms leading to granuloma formation; it may be secondary to infections, drugs, sarcoidosis, cancer (usually lymphoma), ankylosing spondylosis, and reactive arthropathies (e.g., associated with inflammatory bowel disease).

TREATMENT

- The disease is self-limited, and treatment is symptomatic:
  - Nonsteroidal antiinflammatory drugs for pain
  - Systemic steroids in severe cases

Definition: A predominantly postural and action tremor that is bilateral and tends to progress slowly over the years in the absence of other neurologic abnormalities

DIAGNOSIS

- Patients complain of tremor that is most bothersome when writing or holding something, such as a newspaper, or trying to drink from a cup. Tremor worsens under emotional duress.
- The tremor measures 4 to 12 Hz and is a bilateral postural and action tremor of the upper extremities. It also may affect the head, voice, trunk, and legs. Typically the tremor is the same amplitude throughout the action, such as bringing a cup to the mouth. No other neurologic abnormalities are apparent on examination. Patients often note improvement with a small amount of alcohol.

ETIOLOGY

- Often an inherited disease, autosomal dominant; sporadic cases without a family history are encountered frequently

TREATMENT

- **First-line agents:**
  - Propranolol—usual starting dose 30 mg; usual therapeutic dose 160-320 mg. Propranolol must be used with caution in patients with asthma, depression, cardiac disease, and diabetes.
  - Primidone—usual starting dose 12.5-25 mg at bedtime; usual therapeutic dose 62.5-75 mg daily. Sedation and nausea when medication is first begun are biggest side effects.
- **Other agents:**
- Neurontin—400 mg at bedtime; usual therapeutic dose 1200-3600 mg
- Topiramate—25 mg at bedtime; may titrate to about 400 mg
- Alprazolam—0.75-2.75 mg

CLINICAL PEARLS

- Essential tremor is the most common of all movement disorders.
- There is no need to treat essential tremor unless it is functionally impairing. Patients need to understand that treatments are only 40% to 70% effective.

Felty's Syndrome (FS)

Definition: The triad of rheumatoid arthritis (RA), splenomegaly, and granulocytopenia. This definition requires some modification based on numerous subsequent reviews of the subject. The hallmark of FS is a persistent, idiopathic granulocytopenia, which is defined as a neutrophil count of <2000/mm³. Splenomegaly is extremely variable in its extent and varies over time. It is an extraarticular manifestation of seropositive RA in which recurrent local and systemic infections are the major source of morbidity and mortality.

DIAGNOSIS

- Rarely, splenomegaly and granulocytopenia are present before RA.
- Articular involvement is usually more severe in patients with FS compared with other patients with RA; however, one third may have relatively inactive synovitis with elevated erythrocyte sedimentation rate (ESR).
- The degree of splenomegaly varies and may be detectable only by imaging studies.
- The degree of splenomegaly has no correlation with the degree of granulocytopenia.
- FS patients have a greater frequency of extraarticular manifestations (e.g. nodules, weight loss, Sjögren's syndrome) than other patients with RA.
- Approximately 25% of patients have refractory leg ulcers, often associated with hyperpigmentation of the anterior tibia.
- Mild hepatomegaly is common (68%).
- Complete blood count with differential shows granulocytopenia, mild-to-moderate anemia, mild thrombocytopenia, and elevated ESR.
- Bone marrow biopsy in most patients shows myeloid hyperplasia with an excess of immature granulocyte precursors ("maturation arrest").
- Other laboratory tests include rheumatoid factor (positive in 98%, usually high titer), antinuclear antibody (positive in 67%), antihistone antibody (positive in 83%), antineutrophil cytoplasmic antibodies (positive in 77%), and HLA-DR4 (positive in 95%).

ETIOLOGY

- The pathogenesis of FS is probably multifactorial, and no clear explanation has been elucidated.
- Proposed mechanisms of the granulocytopenia are as follows:
  - Splenic sequestration and peripheral destruction of granulocytes secondary to immune complexes and antineutrophil antibodies

...[h]ematopoiesis in bone marrow as a result of decreased cytokine production, presence of inhibitors, or humoral and cell-mediated immune suppression
- Excessive margination

TREATMENT
- **Splenectomy:** acutely reverses hematologic abnormalities
  - Ongoing infections may resolve after operation as the granulocyte count rises.
  - 25% to 30% have recurrent granulocytopenia, but the granulocyte count usually remains above the presplenectomy level.
  - Improvement in frequency of recurrent infection varies and is not correlated with hematologic improvement.
  - Splenectomy usually is reserved for patients with profound granulocytopenia (<1000/mm³) and severe recurrent infections.
- **Lithium:**
  - Lithium stimulates granulopoiesis.
  - Little evidence is available of long-term benefit or conclusive reduction in infection rate.
  - Lithium can be used as short-term therapy while awaiting response to other measures.
- **Parenteral testosterone:** The efficacy of testosterone is limited by toxicity, especially in women.
- **Corticosteroids:**
  - Pulse dosing is a potential alternative for short-term elevation of neutrophils.
  - Overwhelming infection is the main barrier to the use of corticosteroids.
- **Antirheumatic drugs:** These are second-line drugs that may improve the granulocytopenia in FS.

CLINICAL PEARL
- Patients with FS have a 20 times increased frequency of infections compared with other RA patients.

Fever of unknown origin (FUO)

Definition: FUO was defined by Petersdorf in 1961 as an illness characterized by temperatures >101°F on several occasions for >3 weeks with no known cause despite extensive workup.

DIAGNOSIS

- Accurate history and careful physical examination are essential.
- Laboratory tests and radiologic examinations depend on historical clues and physical findings.
- A "shotgun" approach—ordering every test for every possibility—is rarely helpful.
- Tests and procedures should be thoughtful, directed toward localizing signs and symptoms.
- **Historical clues:**
  - Fever duration, fever tempo, inciting factors
  - Associated symptoms (rash, myalgia, weight loss, pain)
  - Sick contacts
  - Past medical history (HIV, malignancies, surgeries)
  - Medications
  - Family history (tuberculosis in a relative, malignancies, familial Mediterranean fever)
  - Social history, including daily routine, rural residence versus urban residence, pets and animal contacts, arthropod bites, travel (recent and remote), socioeconomic status, occupation, military service, and sexual history
- **Physical findings:**
  - Head, ears, eyes, and throat—rule out sinusitis, dental abscesses; examine eyes carefully
  - Neck—check adenopathy
  - Lungs—auscultate for rales
  - Heart—listen for murmur
  - Abdomen—check for organomegaly
  - Rectal—examine for prostate tenderness
  - Pelvic—rule out cervical motion tenderness; check for inguinal adenopathy
  - Extremities—look for clubbing, splinter hemorrhages; examine intravenous access site
  - Musculoskeletal—examine for joint effusions
  - Skin—note any rashes, wounds

- Base on historical clues and physical findings: blood cultures, complete blood count, urinalysis, transaminases; purified protein derivative testing is important in most FUO workups.
- Base on leads from history and examination: serum antibody testing, lumbar puncture, thyroid function testing, stool culture and *Clostridium difficil* assay, bone marrow biopsy, skin biopsy, antinuclear antibody; may need to repeat laboratory tests at regular intervals until diagnosis is established.
- **Imaging studies:**
  - Base on historical clues and physical findings: Chest x-ray and abdominal CT scan are important eventually in most workups where diagnosis is elusive.

ETIOLOGY

- **Classic (1 week workup after 2 weeks persistently febrile):** divided into infection, malignancy, collagen vascular, and other etiology; proportion for each depends on age, geography, host and microbial factors, and hospital and health services. Etiology also has changed over time. A partial list of eventual etiologies follows, with the most common diagnoses in *italics:*
  - *Factitious fever, Munchausen syndrome*
  - *Abscess—dental, abdominal, pelvic*
  - *Lymphoma and leukemia*
  - Endocarditis (especially caused by difficult-to-isolate organisms)
  - Biliary tract infection
  - Osteomyelitis
  - Tuberculosis
  - Whipple's disease
  - Psittacosis
  - Fungal—histoplasmosis, cryptomycosis
  - Leishmaniasis
  - Renal cell carcinoma, other solid malignancies
  - Systemic lupus erythematosus
  - Still's disease
  - Hypersensitivity vasculitis
  - Temporal arteritis
  - Drug-induced fever
  - Inflammatory bowel disease
  - Sarcoidosis
  - Granulomatous hepatitis
  - Central fever (rare)

- **Neutropenic (polymorphonuclear neutrophils <500/μL and febrile >3 days):** with blood cultures from onset negative, ruling out *Pseudomonas* and other gram-negative bacteremia and staphylococcal bacteremia from line infection; urinalysis and chest x-ray negative. Possible etiologies are as follows:
  - Perianal infection
  - Occult fungal infection
  - Drug fever
  - Cytomegalovirus infection in posttransplant patients or patients who are on immunosuppressants
- **HIV-associated:** Etiology depends on CD4 count. HIV itself may be the cause. With low CD4 count, *Mycobacterium avium intracellulare* bacteremia or non-Hodgkin's lymphoma may be the cause.
- **Nosocomial (febrile for 3 days in hospital):** urinary tract infection, pneumonia, line-related bacteremia, *C. difficile* diarrhea, or sinusitis secondary to intubation
- **Noninfectious etiology:** deep venous thrombosis, hematoma, drug fever

TREATMENT
- Antibiotics and other treatment are indicated only after definitive or highly probable diagnosis is established, unless patient appears severely ill or septic.

CLINICAL PEARL
- When in doubt, perform another complete history and physical examination.
- Persistence for >2 weeks usually separates a FUO from an insignificant viral illness.

Fibromyalgia

Definition: Poorly defined disorder characterized by multiple trigger points and referred pain

DIAGNOSIS
- The primary condition is often suggested by the following criteria from the American College of Rheumatology:
  - History of widespread pain
  - Pain in 11 of 18 selected tender spots on digital palpation (mainly in the spine, elbows, and knees) (Fig. 6)
- There are no abnormalities in fibromyalgia, but laboratory assessment may be required to rule out other conditions:

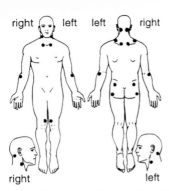

1. Occiput
2. Low cervical
3. Trapezius
4. Supraspinatus
5. Second rib
6. Lateral epicondyle
7. Gluteal
8. Greater trochanter
9. Knees

FIGURE 6. The sites of the 18 tender points of the 1990 American College of Rheumatology criteria for the classification of fibromyalgia. (From Conn R: Current Diagnosis, 9th ed. Philadelphia, WB Saunders, 1997.)

- Complete blood count, erythrocyte sedimentation rate, rheumatoid factor, antinuclear antibody
- Creatine phosphokinase, thyroid-stimulating hormone
- Self-management is possible.
- Patients require an explanation and reassurance.

ETIOLOGY
- Unknown
- Pain magnification may play a role

TREATMENT
- Tricyclic antidepressants for sleep disturbance
- Aerobic and stretching exercise, particularly swimming
- Mild analgesics; avoid long-term narcotic use
- Trigger point injections
- Physical therapy

Folliculitis

Definition: Inflammation of the hair follicle as a result of infection, physical injury, or chemical irritation

DIAGNOSIS

The lesions generally consist of painful yellow pustules surrounded by erythema; a central hair is present in the pustules.

Patients with sycosis barbae may present initially with small follicular papules or pustules that increase in size with continued shaving; deep follicular pustules may occur surrounded by erythema and swelling; the upper lip frequently is involved.

"Hot tub" folliculitis occurs within 1 to 4 days after use of a hot tub with poor chlorination; it is characterized by pustules with surrounding erythema generally affecting the torso, buttocks, and limbs.

Gram stain is useful to identify the infective organisms in infectious folliculitis and to differentiate infectious folliculitis from noninfectious folliculitis.

ETIOLOGY

- *Staphylococcus* infection (e.g. sycosis barbae), *Pseudomonas aeruginosa* (hot tub folliculitis)
- Gram-negative (*Klebsiella, Enterobacter, Proteus*) associated with antibiotic treatment of acne
- Chronic irritation of the hair follicle (use of cocoa butter or coconut oil, chronic irritation from workplace)
- Initial use of systemic corticosteroid therapy (steroid acne), eosinophilic folliculitis (AIDS patients), *Candida albicans* (immuno-compromised patients)
- *Pityrosporum orbiculare*

TREATMENT

- Cleanse affected area with chlorhexidine, and apply saline compresses.
- Apply 2% mupirocin ointment (Bactroban) for bacterial folliculitis affecting a limited area (e.g. sycosis barbae).
- Treat severe cases of *Pseudomonas* folliculitis with ciprofloxacin.
- Treat *Staphylococcus aureus* folliculitis with dicloxacillin 250 mg qid for 10 days.
- Chronic nasal or perineal *S. aureus* carriers with frequent folliculitis can be treated with rifampin 300 mg bid for 5 days.
- Mupirocin (Bactroban ointment 2%) applied to the nares twice daily also is effective for nasal carriers.

- Steroid folliculitis responds to discontinuation of steroids.
- Patients should be instructed in good personal hygiene and avoidance of sharing razors, towels, and washcloths.

Friedreich's ataxia

Definition: The most common neurodegenerative hereditary ataxic disorder, caused by degeneration of dorsal root ganglions, posterior columns, spinocerebellar and corticospinal tracts, and large sensory peripheral neurons

DIAGNOSIS
- Onset is with progressive appendicular and gait ataxia, with absent muscle stretch reflexes in the lower extremities.
- With disease progression (within 5 years), dysarthria, distal loss of position and vibration sense, pyramidal leg weakness, areflexia in all four limbs, and extensor plantar responses occur.
- Common findings include progressive scoliosis, distal atrophy, pes cavus, and cardiomyopathy (symmetric concentric hypertrophic form in most cases).
- Diagnostic criteria include electrophysiologic evidence for a generalized axonal sensory neuropathy.
- ECG shows widespread T wave inversion and evidence of left ventricular hypertrophy in 65% of patients.
- Sural nerve biopsy shows major loss of large myelinated fibers.
- Specific gene testing for the expanded GAA trinucleotide repeat is indicated.

ETIOLOGY
- **Genetic:** Frataxin gene is localized to the centromeric region of chromosome 9q13.
- Normal sequence has 6 to 27 repeats; abnormal sequence has 120 to 1700 GAA repeats.
- Frataxin deficiency leads to impaired mitochondrial iron homeostasis.

TREATMENT
- None established
- An antioxidant, idebenone (short-chain analogue of coenzyme Q_{10}) administered orally 5-10 mg/kg/day with or without vitamin E may improve outcomes in patients with cardiomyopathy without clinical deterioration. This treatment is experimental and research may be reviewed at www.idebenone.org.

- Further research with various antioxidants and iron chelators is ongoing.

CLINICAL PEARLS

- Insulin-requiring diabetes mellitus may occur in 10% of patients, with glucose intolerance occurring in an additional 10% to 20%.
- Loss of ambulation typically occurs within 15 years of symptom onset, and 95% of patients are wheelchair bound by age 45.
- Life expectancy is reduced, particularly if heart disease with or without diabetes mellitus is present. Mean survival from symptom onset is 36 years.

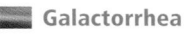 **Galactorrhea**

Definition: Inappropriate lactation (in the absence of pregnancy and postpartum state) secondary to nonphysiologic augmentation of prolactin release

DIAGNOSIS

- Physical examination reveals a milky discharge from nipples usually occurring bilaterally. Visual field defects may be present with prolactinomas. Evidence of acromegaly, Cushing's disease, or hypothyroidism is present when galactorrhea is secondary to these disorders.
- A complete history focuses on menstrual irregularity, infertility, previous pregnancies, duration of galactorrhea, medications, visual complaints, and fatigue.
- **Laboratory tests:**
  - Prolactin level (elevated, usually >200 ng/mL in prolactinoma)
  - Human chorionic gonadotropin level (positive in pregnancy)
  - Thyroid-stimulating hormone (TSH), thyrotropin-releasing hormone (TRH) (both elevated in hypothyroidism)
  - Blood urea nitrogen, creatinine (elevated in renal failure), glucose (elevated in Cushing's syndrome)
  - Urinalysis (hematuria in renal cell carcinoma)
  - Microscopic examination of nipple discharge (scant cellular material, numerous fat globules)
- MRI of brain is performed if prolactin level is elevated, amenorrhea is present, or visual fields defects are detected on physical examination.

- Medications (phenothiazines, metoclopramide, selective serotonin reuptake inhibitors, anxiolytics, buspirone, atenolol, valproic acid, conjugated estrogen and medroxyprogesterone, methyldopa, verapamil, H_2-receptor blockers, octreotide, danazol, tricyclic antidepressants, isoniazid, amphetamine, reserpine, opiates, sumatriptan, rimantidine, oral contraceptive formulations)
- Breast stimulation (prolonged suckling), sexual intercourse
- Pituitary tumors (prolactinomas, craniopharyngiomas
- Chest wall irritation from ill-fitting clothing, herpes zoster, atopic dermatitis, burns
- Hypothyroidism (elevated TSH increases TRH, which increases prolactin)
- Increased stress, major trauma
- Chronic renal failure (decreased prolactin clearance)
- Cushing's disease
- Herbs (e.g., fennel, red clover, anise, red raspberry, marshmallow)
- Cannabis
- Spinal cord surgery or injury, or tumors
- Severe gastroesophageal reflux disease, esophagitis (stimulation of thoracic nerves via cervical and thoracic ganglia)
- Breast surgery
- Idiopathic
- Neonatal
- Lymphomas, Hodgkin's disease, bronchogenic carcinoma, renal adenocarcinomas
- Sarcoidosis and other infiltrative disorders
- Tuberculosis affecting pituitary gland
- Pituitary stalk resection
- Multiple sclerosis
- Empty sella syndrome
- Acromegaly

TREATMENT

- Discontinue potential offending agents.
- Avoid excessive breast stimulation.
- Galactorrhea resulting from prolactinoma can be managed medically, surgically, or with careful surveillance depending on size and growth of tumor, associated symptoms, and prolactin level (see "Prolactinoma").

CLINICAL PEARL

- Neonatal galactorrhea ("witch's milk"), produced by 2% to 5% of neonates, is due to a precipitous drop in maternal estrogen and progesterone after delivery.

Gardner's syndrome

Definition: A variant of familial adenomatous polyposis (FAP), with prominent extraintestinal manifestations. It is an autosomal dominant condition characterized by:

Adenomatous intestinal polyps

Soft tissue tumors

Osteomas

DIAGNOSIS

- In individuals with a family history, diagnosis is confirmed by >100 adenomatous polyps in the colon, >3 pigmented ocular lesions on funduscopic examination, or genetic testing.
- There is phenotypic variability even in families with the same mutation. Soft tissue and bone abnormalities may precede intestinal disease.
- Congenital hypertrophy of the retinal pigment epithelium (often the first sign) is diagnosed by ophthalmologic examination.
- Dental abnormalities include supernumerary teeth and unerupted teeth.
- Soft tissue lesions include epidermoid cysts, sebaceous cysts, fibromas, lipomas, and desmoid tumors.
- Bony abnormalities of skull, mandible, and long bones are present.
- Abdominal mass and occult blood in stool are diagnostic.

ETIOLOGY

- Caused by mutations of the adenomatous polyposis coli (APC) gene on chromosome 5q21. Greater than 300 mutations of the APC gene have been identified. The site of the mutation may explain the extraintestinal lesions that differentiate Gardner's syndrome from other variants of FAP.
- Spontaneous mutations are responsible for 20% to 40% of FAP cases.

TREATMENT

- Colectomy is recommended when polyps are seen on sigmoidoscopy.
- Regular screening of remaining gastrointestinal tract and extraintestinal manifestations must continue after colectomy.

- Polyps occur at a mean age of 16 years.
- Cancer develops in 7% of individuals by age 21 years, 50% by age 39 years, and 90% by age 45 years.

 Gastritis

Definition: Histologically, *gastritis* refers to inflammation in the stomach. Endoscopically, *gastritis* refers to numerous abnormal features, such as erythema, erosions, and subepithelial hemorrhages. Gastritis also can be subdivided into erosive, nonerosive, and specific types of gastritis with distinctive features endoscopically and histologically.

DIAGNOSIS
- Patients with gastritis generally present with nonspecific clinical signs and symptoms (e.g., epigastric pain, abdominal tenderness, bloating, anorexia, nausea [with or without vomiting]). Symptoms may be aggravated by eating.
- Diagnostic workup includes a comprehensive history and endoscopy with biopsy.
- Serologic (IgG antibody to *Helicobacter pylori*) or breath (^{13}C urea) test for *H. pylori* is performed.
- Histologic evaluation of endoscopic biopsy samples is currently the gold standard for accurate diagnosis of *H. pylori* infection.

ETIOLOGY
- Alcohol, nonsteroidal antiinflammatory drugs (NSAIDs), stress (critically ill patients usually on mechanical respiration), hepatic or renal failure, multiorgan failure
- Infection (bacterial, viral)
- Bile reflux, pancreatic enzyme reflux
- Gastric mucosal atrophy, portal hypertension gastropathy
- Irradiation

TREATMENT
- Eradicate infectious agents. Initiate *H. pylori* therapy with
  - Proton-pump inhibitor (PPI) (e.g., omeprazole 20 mg bid or lansoprazole 30 mg bid) *plus* clarithromycin 500 mg bid *and* amoxicillin 1000 mg bid for 7 to 10 days
  - PPI bid *plus* amoxicillin 500 mg bid *plus* metronidazole 500 mg for 7 to 10 days
  - PPI bid *plus* clarithromycin 500 mg bid *and* metronidazole 500 mg bid for 7 days

- Trials indicate that a 1-day quadruple-therapy regimen may be as effective as a 7-day triple-therapy regimen. The 1-day quadruple-theray regimen consists of 2 tablets of 262-mg bismuth subsalicy-late qid, 1 500-mg metronidazole tablet qid, 2 g of amoxicillin suspension qid, and 2 capsules of 30 mg of lansoprazole.
- Prophylaxis and treatment of stress gastritis with sucralfate suspension 1 g PO q4-6h or H$_2$-receptor antagonists
- Misoprostol (Cytotec) in patients on long-term NSAID therapy
- Avoidance of mucosal irritants, such as alcohol and NSAIDs
- Lifestyle modifications with avoidance of tobacco and foods that trigger symptoms

CLINICAL PEARLS

- Patients should not receive PPIs for 2 weeks before undergoing urea breath test for *H. pylori* infection.
- Serum antibody tests are not reliable because of a high rate of false-positive results and the fact that antibodies persist after treatment. The urea breath test is more sensitive and specific; however, it is not readily available.

▬ Gastroesophageal reflux disease (GERD)

Definition: Motility disorder characterized primarily by heartburn and caused by the reflux of gastric contents into the esophagus

DIAGNOSIS

- Clinical signs and symptoms include heartburn, dysphagia, sour taste, regurgitation of gastric contents into the mouth, chronic cough and bronchospasm, chest pain, laryngitis, early satiety, abdominal fullness, bloating with belching, and dental erosions in children.
- Upper gastrointestinal endoscopy is useful to document the type and extent of tissue damage in GERD and to exclude potentially malignant conditions, such as Barrett's esophagus.
- Twenty-four-hour esophageal pH monitoring and Bernstein test are sensitive diagnostic tests; however, they are not practical and generally not done. They are useful in patients with atypical manifestations of GERD, such as chest pain or chronic cough.
- Esophageal manometry is indicated in patients with refractory reflux in whom surgical therapy is planned.
- Upper gastrointestinal series can identify ulcerations and strictures; however, it may miss mucosal abnormalities. Only one third of patients with GERD have radiographic signs of esophagitis.

- Incompetent lower esophageal sphincter (LES)
- Medications that lower LES pressure (calcium channel blockers, β-adrenergic blockers, theophylline, anticholinergics)
- Foods that lower LES pressure (chocolate, yellow onions, peppermint)
- Tobacco abuse, alcohol, coffee
- Pregnancy
- Gastric acid hypersecretion
- Hiatal hernia (controversial)—present in >70% of patients with GERD; however, most patients with hiatal hernia are asymptomatic

TREATMENT
- **Lifestyle modifications**
  - Avoid foods (citrus-based and tomato-based products) and drugs that exacerbate reflux (e.g., caffeine, β-blockers, calcium channel blockers, α-adrenergic agonists, theophylline).
  - Avoid tobacco and alcohol use.
  - Elevate head of bed 4 to 8 inches using blocks.
  - Avoid lying down directly after late or large evening meals.
  - Reduce weight and decrease fat intake.
  - Avoid clothing that is tight around the waist.
- Proton-pump inhibitors (PPIs) (esomeprazole 40 mg qd, omeprazole 20 mg qd, lansoprazole 30 mg qd, rabeprazole 20 mg qd, or pantoprazole 40 mg qd) are safe, tolerated, and effective in most patients.
- H_2-blockers (nizatidine 300 mg at bedtime, famotidine 40 mg at bedtime, ranitidine 300 mg at bedtime, or cimetidine 800 mg at bedtime) can be used but generally are much less effective than PPIs.
- Antacids may be useful for relief of mild symptoms; however, they generally are ineffective in severe cases of reflux.
- Prokinetic agents (metoclopramide) are indicated only when PPIs are not fully effective. They can be used in combination therapy; however, side effects limit their use.
- For refractory cases, surgery with Nissen fundoplication is indicated.
- Endoscopic radiofrequency heating of the gastroesophageal junction (Stretta procedure) is a new treatment modality for GERD patients unresponsive to traditional therapy.

CLINICAL PEARL
- Lifestyle modifications must be followed lifelong because this is generally an irreversible condition.

Giant cell arteritis

Definition: A systemic segmental granulomatous inflammation predominantly involving the arteries of the carotid system in patients >50 years old. Giant cell arteritis (temporal arteritis, cranial arteritis) can involve any large or medium-sized arteries.

DIAGNOSIS

- The presence of any three of the following five items allows the diagnosis of giant cell arteritis with a sensitivity of 94% and a specificity of 91%:
  - Age of disease onset ≥50 years
  - New onset of new type of headache
  - Temporal artery tenderness or decreased pulsation on physical examination
  - Westergren erythrocyte sedimentation rate (ESR) ≥50 mm/hr.
  - Artery biopsy with vasculitis and mononuclear cell infiltrate or granulomatous changes

TREATMENT

- In stable patients without significant ocular involvement, therapy usually is started with prednisone 40–60 mg/day in divided doses, continued for a few weeks until symptoms resolve and ESR returns to normal. If the ESR remains normal, prednisone can be reduced by 5 mg every other week until a dosage of 20 mg/day is reached. Subsequent dosage reductions should be by 2.5 mg/day every 2 to 4 weeks. When the total dosage reaches 5 mg/day, reduction should be by 1 mg every 2 to 4 weeks as tolerated. Usual duration of prednisone treatment is 6 months to 2 years.
- In very ill patients and patients with significant ocular involvement (e.g., visual loss in one eye), rapid aggressive treatment with large doses of intravenous steroids (e.g., methylprednisolone 250 mg IV q6h for 3 days before starting oral prednisone) is indicated to provide optimal protection to the uninvolved eye and to offer improved chance of recovery of the involved eye.
- The addition of methotrexate (10 mg/wk) to prednisone has been reported to be a safe alternative to corticosteroid therapy alone in patients with giant cell arteritis. The combination of methotrexate and prednisone significantly reduces the frequency of first relapses after prednisone alone¹. When initial remission (45% versus 84% with prednisone alone), disease relapses occurred, they were clinically less severe, and prednisone requirements were lower.

Giardiasis

Definition: Intestinal or biliary tract infection (or infection can affect both) caused by the protozoal parasite *Giardia lamblia*

DIAGNOSIS
- In >70% of patients, clinical presentation includes one or more intestinal symptoms (diarrhea, flatulence, cramps, bloating, nausea).
- Stool specimen (three specimens yield 90% sensitivity) or duodenal aspirate for microscopic examination establishes the diagnosis and excludes other pathogens.
- Serum albumin, vitamin B_{12} levels, and stool fat test are performed to exclude malabsorption.

TREATMENT
- Metronidazole 250 mg PO tid for 7 days (metronidazole avoided in pregnancy) *or*
- Paromomycin 25-30 mg/kg/day in three doses for 5 to 10 days

Gilbert's disease

Definition: Autosomal dominant disease characterized by indirect hyperbilirubinemia caused by impaired glucuronyl transferase activity

DIAGNOSIS
- **Laboratory evaluation:** isolated elevation of indirect (unconjugated) bilirubin (rarely >5 mg/dL)

ETIOLOGY
- Probable autosomal dominant disease affecting >5% of U.S. population
- Pathogenesis linked to a reduction in bilirubin UGT-1 gene (*HUG-Br1*) transcription resulting from a mutation in the promoter region

TREATMENT
- Treatment is generally unnecessary. Phenobarbital (if clinical jaundice is present) can decrease rapidly serum indirect bilirubin level.

CLINICAL PEARL
- Fasting for 2 days or significant dehydration may raise the bilirubin level and result in the clinical recognition of jaundice.

Glomerulonephritis, acute

Definition: Immunologically mediated inflammation primarily involving the glomerulus, which can result in damage to the basement membrane, mesangium, or capillary endothelium

DIAGNOSIS

- **Laboratory tests:**
  - Urinalysis (hematuria [dysmorphic erythrocytes and red blood cell casts], proteinuria)
  - Serum creatinine (to estimate glomerular filtration rate), blood urea nitrogen
  - Twenty-four-hour urine for protein excretion and creatinine clearance (to document degree of renal dysfunction and amount of proteinuria). Proteinuria in acute glomerulonephritis typically ranges from 500 mg/day to 3 g/day, but nephrotic-range proteinuria (>3.5 g/day) may be present.
  - Streptococcal tests (Streptozyme), antistreptolysin O (ASO) quantitative titer (highest in 3-5 weeks). ASO titer is not related to severity of renal disease, duration, or prognosis.
  - **Additional useful tests depending on the history:** anti-DNA antibodies (rule out systemic lupus erythematosus), CH_{50} level (if elevated, obtain C_3, C_4 levels), triglycerides, cryoglobulins, hepatitis B and C serologies, antineutrophil cytoplasmic antibody (ANCA), c-ANCA (in suspected cases of Wegener's granulomatosis), p-ANCA (found in pauciimmune [lack of immune deposits], idiopathic, rapidly progressive glomerulonephritis with or without systemic vasculitis), anti-glomerular basement membrane (type α[3] IV collagen) antibodies
  - Hematocrit (decrease in glomerulonephritis), platelet count (thrombocytopenia in cases of lupus nephritis)
  - Anti-glomerular basement membrane antibody (in Goodpasture's syndrome)
  - Blood cultures indicated in all febrile patients
- **Imaging studies:**
  - Chest x-ray useful to rule out pulmonary congestion, Wegener's granulomatosis, and Goodpasture's syndrome
  - Renal ultrasound if glomerular filtration rate is depressed to evaluate renal size and determine extent of fibrosis. A kidney size <9 cm suggests extensive scarring and low likelihood of reversibility
  - Echocardiogram in patients with new cardiac murmurs or positive blood cultures to rule out endocarditis and pericardial effusion

can confirm the diagnosis. Kidney biopsy generally reveals a granular pattern in poststreptococcal glomerulonephritis or a linear pattern in Goodpasture's syndrome; absence of immune deposits suggests vasculitis.

- Immunofluorescence generally reveals C3; negative immunofluorescence suggests Wegener's granulomatosis, idiopathic crescentic glomerulonephritis, or polyarteritis nodosa.
- Angiography or biopsy of other affected organs is indicated if systemic vasculitis is suspected.

ETIOLOGY

- Acute glomerulonephritis may be due to primary renal disease or a systemic disease. Numerous pathogenic processes (e.g., antibody deposition, cell-mediated immune mechanisms, complement activation, hemodynamic alterations) have been implicated in the pathogenesis of glomerular inflammation. Medical disorders generally associated with glomerulonephritis are the following:
  - Post-group A beta-hemolytic *Streptococcus* infection (other infectious etiologies include endocarditis and visceral abscess)
  - Collagen vascular diseases (systemic lupus erythematosus)
  - Vasculitis (Wegener's granulomatosis, polyarteritis nodosa)
  - Idiopathic glomerulonephritis (membranoproliferative, idiopathic, crescentic, IgA nephropathy)
  - Goodpasture's syndrome
  - Other cryoglobulinemia (Henoch-Schönlein purpura)
  - Drug-induced (gold, penicillamine)

TREATMENT

- Instruct patient to avoid salt if edema or hypertension is present.
- Prescribe low protein intake (approximately 0.5 g/kg/day) in patients with renal failure.
- Restrict fluids in patients with significant edema.
- Instruct patient to avoid high-potassium foods.
- Correct electrolyte abnormalities (hypocalcemia, hyperkalemia) and acidosis (if present).
- Treat streptococcal infection with penicillin (or erythromycin in penicillin-allergic patients).
- Give furosemide in patients with significant hypertension or edema or both; alternatively, give hydralazine or nifedipine in patients with hypertension.
- Implement immunosuppressive treatment in patients with heavy proteinuria or rapidly decreasing glomerular filtration rate (high-dose steroids, cyclosporine, cyclophosphamide); corticosteroids generally are not useful in poststreptococcal glomerulonephritis,

- Fish oil (n-3 fatty acids) 12 g/day may prevent or slow down loss of renal function in patients with IgA nephropathy.
- Plasma exchange therapy and immunosuppressive drugs (prednisone and cyclophosphamide) are effective in Goodpasture's syndrome.

CLINICAL PEARL

Prognosis generally is related to histology, with excellent prognosis in patients with minimal change glomerulonephritis and focal segmental proliferative glomerulonephritis; 25% to 30% of patients with mesangial IgA disease and membranous glomerulonephritis generally progress to chronic renal failure; >70% of patients with mesangial capillary glomerulonephritis develop chronic renal failure.

Glossitis

Definition: Inflammation of the tongue that can lead to loss of filiform papillae

DIAGNOSIS

- The appearance of the tongue varies depending on the etiology. Loss of filiform papillae results in a red, smooth-surfaced tongue.
- The tongue may appear pale in patients with significant anemia.
- Pain and swelling of the tongue may be present when glossitis is associated with infections, trauma, or lichen planus.
- Ulcerations may be present in patients with herpetic glossitis, pemphigus, or streptococcal infection.
- Excessive use of mouthwash may result in a "hairy" appearance of the tongue.
- Laboratory evaluation is useful to exclude infectious processes, vitamin deficiencies, and systemic disorders.
  - Complete blood count—decreased hemoglobin and hematocrit, decreased mean corpuscular volume (MCV) (iron deficiency anemia), elevated MCV (vitamin B_{12} deficiency)
  - Vitamin B_{12} level
  - Ten percent potassium hydroxide scrapings in patients with white patches suspicious for candidiasis
  - Biopsy of lesion is indicated only when there is no response to treatment.

ETIOLOGY

- Nutritional deficiencies (vitamin E, riboflavin, niacin, vitamin B_{12}, iron deficiency)
- Infections (viral, candidiasis, tuberculosis, syphilis)
- Trauma (generally caused by poorly fitting dentures)

tongue secondary to toothpaste, medications, alcohol, tobacco, citrus
- Lichen planus, pemphigus vulgaris, erythema multiforme
- Neoplasms

TREATMENT
- Treatment varies with the etiology of the glossitis.
  - Malnutrition with avitaminosis—multivitamins
  - Candidiasis—fluconazole 200 mg on day 1, then 100 mg/day for at least 2 weeks or nystatin 400,000 U suspension qid for 10 days or 200,000 pastilles dissolved slowly in the mouth 4 to 5 times daily for 10 to 14 days
  - Painful oral lesions—rinsing of the mouth with 2% lidocaine viscous, 1-2 tablespoons q4h as needed; triamcinolone 0.1% applied to painful ulcers as needed for symptomatic relief
- Lifestyle changes include elimination of tobacco, alcohol, and other primary irritants.
- Dental evaluation is indicated for correction of ill-fitting dentures.
- Correct associated metabolic abnormalities, such as hyperglycemia from diabetes mellitus.

CLINICAL PEARL
- If the primary cause of glossitis is not identified or cannot be corrected, enteric nutritional replacement therapy should be considered in malnourished patients.

▬ Goodpasture's syndrome

Definition: Triad of glomerulonephritis, pulmonary hemorrhage, and antibody to glomerular basement membrane (GBM) antigens

DIAGNOSIS
- **Clinical presentation:** dyspnea, cough, hemoptysis, skin pallor, fever, arthralgias (may be mild or absent at the time of initial presentation)
- **Laboratory tests:**
  - Urinalysis reveals microscopic hematuria and proteinuria.
  - Circulating serum anti-GBM antibodies are present.
  - Circulating immune complexes, antineutrophils, cytoplasmic antibodies, and cryoglobulins are absent.
  - Elevated blood urea nitrogen and creatinine result from rapidly progressive glomerulonephritis.
  - Immunofluoresence studies of renal biopsy material show linear deposits of anti-GBM antibody, often accompanied by C3 deposition.

- Anemia results from iron deficiency (secondary to blood loss and iron sequestration in the lungs).
- **Chest x-ray:** fluffy alveolar infiltrates, evidence of pulmonary hemorrhage

ETIOLOGY

- Presence of GBM antibody deposition in kidneys and lungs with subsequent pulmonary hemorrhage and glomerulonephritis.

TREATMENT

- Plasma exchange therapy
- Immunosuppressive therapy with prednisone 1 mg/kg/day and cyclophosphamide 2 mg/kg/day
- Dialysis support in patients with renal failure

CLINICAL PEARL

- Goodpasture's syndrome accounts for 5% of all cases of rapidly progressive glomerulonephritis

 Gout

Definition: Disease characterized by deposition of monosodium urate crystals in and about joints, with subsequent acute or chronic arthritis

DIAGNOSIS

- The typical presentation is monoarticular and characterized by sudden severe pain involving the first metatarsophalangeal joint (*podagra*), although the midtarsal and ankle also frequently are affected; any joint may be involved, but acute polyarthritis is uncommon.
- Physical examination reveals a warm, tender, swollen, erythematous joint; fever may be present, particularly if several joints are involved. Extensive soft tissue swelling, heat, and erythema extending to above and below the affected joint are frequently present and may be confused with cellulitis.
- Serum uric acid level may be elevated, but it is often normal during the acute attack, increasing later when the symptoms resolve.
- Aspiration and analysis of synovial fluid from the inflamed joint confirm the diagnosis; examination of the fluid with a polarized light microscope with compensator reveals monosodium urate crystals (needle-shaped, strongly negative birefringent crystals) with synovial fluid leukocytes.

- Give nonsteroidal antiinflammatory drugs (NSAIDs) as follows: indomethacin 50 mg q8h for 3 to 4 days, then gradually tapered off over approximately 1 to 2 weeks (depending on the patient's clinical response). Naproxen, sulindac, and other NSAIDs also are effective; ketorolac (Toradol) 60 mg may be given intramuscularly in patients with nothing-by-mouth status.
- Colchicine can be given orally or intravenously; it is effective, but side effects (diarrhea, abdominal cramps, nausea, vomiting, liver abnormalities) often limit its usefulness. Intravenous administration has been associated with increased risk of bone marrow suppression and renal or hepatic cell damage. Extravasation also can cause tissue necrosis.
- Glucocorticoids (triamcinolone acetonide or adrenocorticotropic hormone [ACTH]) generally are reserved for patients with contraindications to NSAIDs or colchicine or if oral medication is precluded (e.g., postoperatively). Give triamcinolone acetonide 60 mg IM or ACTH 40 UIM or 25 U by slow IV infusion. Intraarticular steroids may be used to treat a single inflamed joint (dexamethasone phosphate 1-6 mg).
- Prednisone 20-40 mg PO daily can be used short-term in patients refractory or intolerant to NSAIDs or colchicine or responding poorly to these agents.

CLINICAL PEARLS

- Uricosuric agents (e.g., probenecid) or xanthine oxidase inhibitors (allopurinol) are used in patients with frequent recurrent attacks. Hypouricemic therapy should not be started for at least 2 weeks after the acute attack has resolved because it may prolong the acute attack and can precipitate new attacks by rapidly lowering the serum uric acid level.
- Colchicine 0.6 mg PO bid is indicated for acute gout prophylaxis before starting hypouricemic therapy. It generally is discontinued 6 to 8 weeks after normalization of serum urate levels. Long-term colchicine therapy (0.6 mg qd or bid) may be necessary in patients with frequent gout attacks despite the use of uricosuric agents. It also can be used as an alternative to uricosuric agents.

Granuloma inguinale

Definition: Infection caused by a gram-negative bacterium, *Calymmatobacterium granulomatis*. It may be sexually transmitted, possibly by anal intercourse. It also can be spread through close, chronic nonsexual contact.

DIAGNOSIS

- The lesion erodes to a granulomatous, heaped ulcer and progresses slowly.
- An indurated nodule, usually painless, is the primary lesion.
- Pathogenic features are as follows:
  - Intracytoplasmic location
  - Large infected mononuclear cell containing many Donovan bodies. Wright stain shows Donovan bodies (intracellular bacteria) and organisms in vacuoles within macrophages.

TREATMENT

- **Recommended regimens:**
  - Doxycycline 100 mg PO bid × 3 weeks minimum
  - Trimethoprim-sulfamethoxazole, one double-strength tablet PO bid × 3 weeks minimum
- **Alternative regimens:**
  - Ciprofloxacin 750 mg PO bid × 3 weeks
  - Erythromycin base 500 mg PO qid × 3 weeks
  - Azithromycin 1 g /wk PO × 3 weeks
  - Gentamicin 1 mg/kg IV q8h if no improvement within the first few days of therapy

Graves' disease

Definition: A hypermetabolic state characterized by thyrotoxicosis, diffuse goiter, and infiltrative ophthalmopathy.

DIAGNOSIS

- **Physical examination:**
  - Tachycardia, palpitations, tremor, hyperreflexia
  - Goiter, exophthalmos (50% of patients), lid retraction, lid lag
  - Nervousness, weight loss, heat intolerance, atrial fibrillation
  - Increased sweating, brittle nails, clubbing of fingers
  - Nervousness, weight loss, heat intolerance, atrial fibrillation

anterolateral aspects of the skin, but can be found at other sites (especially after trauma)
- **Laboratory tests:**
  - Increased free thyroxine (T_4) and free triiodothyronine (T_3)
  - Decreased thyroid-stimulating hormone (TSH)
  - Presence of thyroid autoantibodies (useful in selected patients to differentiate Graves' disease from toxic nodular goiter)
- Twenty-four-hour radioactive iodine (RAI) uptake shows increased homogeneous uptake.
- CT or MRI of the orbits is useful if there is uncertainty about the cause of ophthalmopathy.

ETIOLOGY
- **Autoimmune etiology:** The activity of the thyroid gland is stimulated by the action of T cells, which induce specific B cells to synthesize antibodies against TSH receptors in the follicular cell membrane.

TREATMENT
- Antithyroid drugs (ATDs) (e.g., methimazole [Tapazole]) to inhibit thyroid hormone synthesis or peripheral conversion of T_4 to T_3
- **RAI:** treatment of choice for patients >21 years old and younger patients who have not achieved remission after 1 year of ATD therapy. RAI is contraindicated during pregnancy and lactation.
- **Surgery:** near-total thyroidectomy rarely performed. Indications for surgery are obstructing goiters despite RAI and ATD therapy, patients who refuse RAI and cannot be managed adequately with ATDs, and pregnant women inadequately managed with ATDs.
- **Adjunctive therapy:** propranolol 20-40 mg q6h to alleviate the β-adrenergic symptoms of hyperthyroidism (tachycardia, tremor). Propranolol is contraindicated in patients with congestive heart failure and bronchospasm.
- **Graves' ophthalmopathy:** methylcellulose eye drops to protect against excessive dryness, sunglasses to decrease photophobia, systemic high-dose corticosteroids for severe exophthalmos. Worsening of ophthalmopathy after RAI therapy is often transient and can be prevented by the administration of prednisone.

CLINICAL PEARL
- Elderly patients can have an atypical presentation of Graves' disease (apathetic hyperthyroidism).

Guillain-Barré syndrome

Definition: Acute inflammatory demyelinating polyradiculopathy predominantly affecting motor function

DIAGNOSIS

- **Clinical presentation:**
  - There is rapid progression of acute symmetric progressive weakness, usually greater distally than proximally and worse in the legs than the arms.
  - The patient often reports difficulty in ambulating, getting up from a chair, or climbing stairs.
  - The ascending paralysis affects motor nerves more than sensory nerves. Sensory loss (predominantly deep position and vibration senses) is variable but usually mild.
  - In some patients, initial manifestations may involve the cranial musculature or the upper extremities (e.g., tingling of the hands).
  - Generally, weakness reaches its maximum within 14 days.

- **Physical examination:**
  - Symmetric weakness, initially involving proximal muscles and sub-sequently proximal and distal muscles
  - Depressed or absent reflexes bilaterally early in the disease
  - Minimal-to-moderate glove-and-stocking anesthesia
  - Ataxia and pain in a segmental distribution—may occur in some patients (caused by involvement of posterior nerve roots)
  - Autonomic abnormalities (bradycardia or tachycardia, hypotension or hypertension)
  - Respiratory insufficiency (caused by weakness of intercostal muscles)
  - Facial paresis, difficulty swallowing (secondary to cranial nerve involvement)

- **Lumbar puncture:** Typical findings include elevated cerebrospinal fluid protein (especially IgG) and presence of a few mononuclear leukocytes, usually <10 cells/μL (albuminocytologic dissociation).

- **Electromyography:** Electromyography reveals slowed conduction velocities; prolonged motor, sensory, and F wave latencies also are present.

ETIOLOGY

Two thirds of all patients give a history of respiratory or gastrointesti-nal illness (e.g., *Campylobacter jejuni*) within 30 days of onset of neurologic symptoms.

- Monitor respiratory function closely (frequent [every hour initially] bedside measurements of forced vital capacity and negative inspiratory force to assess pulmonary muscle strength) because respiratory failure is the major potential problem in Guillain-Barré syndrome.
- Infusion of intravenous immunoglobulins (0.4 mg/kg/day for 5 days) has replaced plasmapheresis as the therapy of choice at many centers.
- Early therapeutic plasma exchange (plasmapheresis) started within 7 days of onset of symptoms is beneficial in preventing paralytic complications in patients with rapidly progressive disease. It is contraindicated in patients with cardiovascular disease (recent myocardial infarction, unstable angina), active sepsis, and autonomic dysfunction.
- Mechanical ventilation may be needed if forced expiratory volume is <12 to 15 mL/kg, vital capacity is rapidly decreasing or is <1000 mL, and PaO_2 is <70 mm Hg, or if the patient is having significant difficulty clearing secretions and is aspirating. Approximately 10% to 20% of patients require ventilatory support. When performing endotracheal intubation, avoid use of paralyzing agents (e.g., succinylcholine) because of increased risk of life-threatening hyperkalemia.

Hand-foot-mouth (HFM) disease

Definition: A viral illness characterized by superficial lesions of the oral mucosa and of the skin of the extremities. HFM disease is transmitted primarily by the fecal-oral route and is highly contagious. Although children are predominantly affected, adults also are at risk. HFM disease is usually self-limited and benign.

DIAGNOSIS
- **Symptoms:**
  - After a 4- to 6-day incubation period, patients may complain of odynophagia, sore throat, malaise, and fever (38.3-40°C).
  - The characteristic oral lesions appear 1 to 2 days later.
  - In 75% of cases, skin lesions on the extremities accompany the oral manifestations.
  - Eleven percent of adults have cutaneous findings.
  - Lesions appear over 1 or 2 days.
- **Physical findings:**
  - Oral lesions (usually 5-10) commonly are found on the tongue buccal mucosa, gingivae, and hard palate.

Oral lesions initially start as 1- to 3-mm erythematous macules and evolve into gray vesicles on an erythematous base.

Vesicles frequently are broken by the time of presentation and appear as superficial gray ulcers with surrounding erythema.

Skin lesions of the hands and feet start as linear erythematous papules (3-10 mm in diameter) that evolve into gray vesicles that may be mildly painful. These vesicles are usually intact at presentation and remain so until they desquamate within 2 weeks. Involvement of the buttocks and perineum is present in 31% of cases.

ETIOLOGY

Coxsackievirus group A, type 16, was the first and is the most common viral agent isolated. Coxsackieviruses A5, A7, A9, A10, B1, B2, B3, and B5 and enterovirus 71 also have been implicated.

TREATMENT

Palliative therapy is given for this usually self-limited disease.

One small, uncontrolled case series reported a decrease in duration of symptoms in response to acyclovir.

CLINICAL PEARL

Spontaneous abortion may occur if the infection occurs early in pregnancy.

Heart block, second degree

Definition: Blockage of some (but not all) impulses from the atria to the ventricles. There are two types of second-degree atrioventricular (AV) block:

- **Mobitz type I (Wenckebach):**
  - There is a progressive prolongation of the P-R interval before an impulse is completely blocked; the cycle repeats periodically.
  - Cycle with dropped beat is less than two times the previous cycle.
  - Site of block is usually AV node (proximal to the bundle of His).

- **Mobitz type II:**
  - There is a sudden interruption of AV conduction without prior prolongation of the P-R interval.
  - Site of block is infranodal.

DIAGNOSIS

- **ECG:**
  - Gradual prolongation of P-R interval leading to a blocked beat (Fig. 7) and shortened P-R interval after dropped beat in Mobitz I

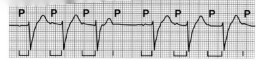

FIGURE 7. Mobitz I second-degree atrioventricular block (Wenckebach). (From Goldberger E: Treatment of Cardiac Emergencies, 5th ed. St Louis, Mosby, 1990.)

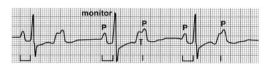

FIGURE 8. Mobitz II second-degree atrioventricular block. Every alternate P wave is blocked. (From Goldberger E: Treatment of Cardiac Emergencies, 5th ed. St Louis, Mosby, 1990.)

- Fixed duration of P-R interval and sudden appearance of blocked beats in Mobitz II (Fig. 8)

ETIOLOGY
- **Mobitz type I:**
  - Vagal stimulation
  - Degenerative changes in the AV conduction system
  - Ischemia at the AV nodes (particularly in inferior wall myocardial infarction [MI])
  - Drugs (digitalis, quinidine, procainamide, adenosine, calcium channel blockers, β-blockers)
  - Cardiomyopathies
  - Aortic regurgitation
  - Lyme carditis
- **Mobitz type II:**
  - Degenerative changes in the His-Purkinje system
  - Acute anterior wall MI
  - Calcific aortic stenosis

TREATMENT
- **Mobitz type I:**
  - Treatment generally is not necessary. This type of block is usually transient.
  - If symptomatic (e.g., dizziness), atropine 1 mg (may repeat once after 5 minutes) may be tried to increase AV conduction; if no response, insert temporary pacemaker.
  - If block is secondary to drugs (e.g., digitalis), discontinue the drug.
  - If associated with anterior wall MI and wide QRS escape rhythm, consider insertion of temporary pacemaker.
  - Significant AV block post-MI may be caused by adenosine produced by the ischemic myocardium. These arrhythmias (which may be resistant to conventional therapy, such as atropine) may respond to theophylline (adenosine antagonist).
- **Mobitz type II:** Pacemaker insertion is needed because this type of block is usually permanent and often progresses to complete AV block.

CLINICAL PEARL
- Patients with Mobitz type I should be followed routinely for potential development of high-grade AV block.

Heart block, third degree

Definition: Complete blockage of all atrioventricular (AV) conduction. The atria and ventricles have separate, independent rhythms.

DIAGNOSIS
- **ECG:**
- P waves constantly change their relationship to the QRS complexes (Fig. 9).
- Ventricular rate is usually <50 beats/min (may be higher in congenital forms).
- Ventricular rate is generally lower than the atrial rate.
- QRS complex is wide.

ETIOLOGY
- Degenerative changes in His-Purkinje system
- Acute anterior wall myocardial infarction
- Calcific aortic stenosis
- Cardiomyopathy
- Trauma
- Cardiovascular surgery

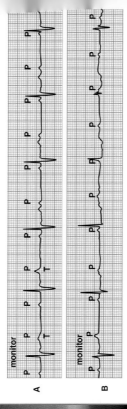

FIGURE 9. Third-degree atrioventricular block. **A**, Atrial rate of 75 beats/min. Ventricles are beating independently at a slow rate of approximately 40 beats/min. **B**, A few hours later in the same patient, variations in the shape of QRS complex from beat to beat. (From Goldberger E: Treatment of Cardiac Emergencies, 5th ed. St Louis, Mosby, 1990.)

TREATMENT
- Immediate pacemaker insertion, unless the patient has congenital third-degree AV block and is completely asymptomatic

CLINICAL PEARL
- Patients may present with dizziness, palpitations, Stokes-Adams syncopal attacks, congestive heart failure, or angina.

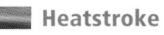 **Heatstroke**

Definition: A life-threatening heat illness characterized by extreme hyperthermia, dehydration, and neurologic manifestations (core temperature >40°C [104°F])

DIAGNOSIS
- **Clinical presentation:**
  - Neurologic manifestations (seizures, tremor, hemiplegia, coma, psychosis, and other bizarre behavior)
  - Evidence of dehydration (poor skin turgor, sunken eyeballs)
  - Tachycardia, hyperventilation
  - Skin hot, red, and flushed
  - Sweating often (not always) absent, particularly in elderly patients
- **Laboratory tests:** Draw initial laboratory studies, including electrolytes, complete blood count, blood urea nitrogen (BUN), creatinine, aspartate aminotransferase (AST), alanine aminotransferase (ALT), creatine phosphokinase (CPK), lactate dehydrogenase (LDH), glucose, international normalized ratio, partial thromboplastin time, platelet count, Ca^{2+}, lactic acid, and arterial blood gases. Laboratory abnormalities may include the following:
  - Elevated BUN, creatinine, hematocrit
  - Hyponatremia or hypernatremia, hyperkalemia or hypokalemia
  - Elevated LDH, AST, ALT, CPK, bilirubin
  - Lactic acidosis, respiratory alkalosis (secondary to hyperventilation)
  - Myoglobinuria, hypofibrinogenemia, fibrinolysis, hypocalcemia

TREATMENT
- Remove the patient's clothes, and place the patient in a cool, well-ventilated room.
- If the patient is unconscious, position patient on his or her side, and clear the airway. Protect airway and augment oxygenation (e.g., nasal oxygen at 4 L/min to keep oxygen saturation >90%).

...y 8 minutes. Measurement of the patient's core temperature with a rectal probe is recommended. The goal is to reduce the body temperature to 39°C (102.2°F) in 30 to 60 minutes.

- Spray the patient with a cool mist and use fans to enhance airflow over the body (rapid evaporation method).
- Immersion of the patient in ice water, stomach lavage with iced saline solution, intravenous administration of cooled fluids, and inhalation of cold air are advisable only when the means for rapid evaporation are not available. Immersion in tepid water (15°C [59°F]) is preferred over ice water immersion to minimize risk of shivering.
- Use of ice packs on axillae, neck, and groin is controversial because they increase peripheral vasoconstriction and may induce shivering.
- Antipyretics are ineffective because the hypothalamic set-point during heatstroke is normal despite the increased body temperature.
- Intubate a comatose patient, insert a Foley catheter, and start nasal oxygen. Continuous ECG monitoring is recommended.
- Insert at least two large-bore intravenous lines and begin intravenous hydration with normal saline or Ringer's lactate.
- Treat complications as follows:
  - Hypotension—vigorous hydration with normal saline or Ringer's lactate
  - Convulsions—diazepam 5-10 mg IV (slowly)
  - Shivering—chlorpromazine 10-50 mg IV
  - Acidosis—use bicarbonate judiciously (only in severe acidosis)
- Observe for evidence of rhabdomyolysis or hepatic, renal, or cardiac failure, and treat accordingly.

▰ Hemochromatosis

Definition: Autosomal recessive disorder characterized by increased accumulation of iron in various organs (adrenals, liver, pancreas, heart, testes, kidneys, pituitary) and eventual dysfunction of these organs if not treated appropriately

DIAGNOSIS
- **Laboratory tests:**
  - Transferrin saturation is the best screening test. Values >45% are an indication for further testing. Plasma ferritin also is a good indicator of total body iron stores but may be elevated in many other conditions (inflammation, malignancy).
  - Measurement of hepatic iron index (hepatic iron concentration ÷ age) in liver biopsy specimen can confirm diagnosis.

- **Imaging:** CT or MRI of the liver is useful to exclude other etiologies and in some cases may show iron overload in the liver
- **Clinical presentation:** Examination may be normal; patients with advanced disease may present with the following:
  - Increased skin pigmentation
  - Hepatomegaly, splenomegaly, hepatic tenderness, testicular atrophy
  - Loss of body hair, peripheral edema, gynecomastia, ascites
  - Amenorrhea (25% of women)
  - Loss of libido (50% of men)

ETIOLOGY

- Arthropathy
  - Joint pain (44%)
  - Fatigue (45%)
- Autosomal recessive disease linked to the region of the short arm of chromosome 6 encoding HLA-A*3. The gene *HFE*, which contains two missense mutations (C 282Y and H 63D), has been identified.

TREATMENT

- Weekly phlebotomies of 1 or 2 U of blood (each containing approximately 250 mg of iron) should be continued for several months until depletion of iron stores is achieved (ferritin level <50 ng/mL, and transferrin saturation <30%). Subsequent phlebotomies can be performed on an as-needed basis to maintain transferrin saturation <50% and ferritin level <100 ng/mL.
- Deferoxamine (iron chelating agent) generally is reserved for patients with severe hemochromatosis with diffuse organ involvement (e.g., liver disease, heart disease) and when phlebotomy is not possible. It is administered in a dose of 0.5-1 g IM qd or 20 mg SC over a 12 to 24 hours with a constant infusion pump.

CLINICAL PEARLS

- Genetic testing (*HFE* genotyping for the C 282Y and H 63D mutations) may be useful in selected patients with liver disease and suspected iron overload (e.g., patients with transferrin saturation >40%). Genetic testing should not be performed as part of initial routine evaluation for hereditary hemochromatosis. When a patient has been identified, first-degree relatives of the index patient should be screened.
- Established cirrhosis, hypogonadism, destructive arthritis, and insulin-dependent diabetes mellitus secondary to hemochromatosis cannot be reversed with repeated phlebotomy, but progress of these disorders can be slowed.

Hemophilia

Definition: Hereditary bleeding disorder caused by low factor VIII coagulant activity (hemophilia A) or low levels of factor IX coagulant activity (hemophilia B)

DIAGNOSIS

- Partial thromboplastin time (PTT) is prolonged.
- Reduced factor VIII:C level distinguishes hemophilia A from other causes of prolonged PTT.
- Factor VIII antigen, prothrombin time, fibrinogen level, and bleeding time are normal.
- Factor IX coagulant activity levels are reduced in patients with hemophilia B.
- Coagulation factor activity measurement is useful to correlate with disease severity. Normal range is 50 to 150 U/dL; 5 to 20 U/dL indicates mild disease, 2 to 5 U/dL indicates moderate disease, and <2 U/dL indicates severe disease with spontaneous bleeding episodes.

ETIOLOGY

- **Hemophilia A:** low factor VIII coagulant (VIII:C) activity; can be classified as mild if factor VIII:C levels are >5%; moderate, levels are 1% to 5%; and severe, levels are <1%
- **Hemophilia B:** low levels of factor IX coagulant activity
- Both disorders are congenital.
- Spontaneous acquisition of factor VIII inhibitors (acquired hemophilia) is rare.

TREATMENT

- **Hemophilia A:**
  - Reversal and prevention of acute bleeding in hemophilia A and B are based on adequate replacement of deficient or missing factor protein.
  - The choice of the product for replacement therapy is guided by availability, capacity, concerns, and cost. Recombinant factors cost two to three times as much as plasma-derived factors, and the limited capacity to produce recombinant factors often results in periods of shortage. In the United States, 60% of patients with severe hemophilia use recombinant products.
  - Factor VIII concentrates are effective in controlling spontaneous and traumatic hemorrhage in severe hemophilia. The new recombinant factor VIII is stable without added human serum albumin (decreased risk of transmission of infectious agents).

- A new recombinant activated factor VII is useful to stop spontaneous hemorrhages and prevent excessive bleeding during surgery
in 75% of patients with inhibitors. Recommended dosage is 90
μg/kg body weight every 2 to 3 hours for treatment of life-threatening hemorrhage. It is, however, expensive ($1/μg).
- Desmopressin acetate 0.3 μg/kg 2h (causes release of factor
VIII:C) may be used in preparation for minor surgical procedures
in patients with mild hemophilia.
- Aminocaproic acid (Amicar) 4 g PO q4h can be given for persistent bleeding that is unresponsive to factor VIII concentrate or
desmopressin.

Hemophilia B:
- Infuse factor IX concentrates. Factor IX concentrates contain other
proteins that may increase the risk of thrombosis with recurrent
use. Factor IX concentrates must be used only when clearly indicated.
- Daily administration of oral cyclophosphamide and prednisone
without empiric factor VIII therapy is an effective and well-tolerated
treatment for acquired hemophilia.

CLINICAL PEARLS
- Despite the advent of virally safe blood products and blood treatment
programs, nearly 70% of hemophiliacs are HIV-seropositive. Survival is
of normal expectancy in HIV-negative patients with mild disease.
- Intracranial bleeds are the second most common cause of death in
hemophiliacs after AIDS. They are fatal in 30% of patients, occur in
10% of patients, and are generally secondary to trauma.

Henoch-Schönlein purpura (HSP)

Definition: Systemic small vessel vasculitis characterized by palpable
purpura in dependent areas (buttocks, legs), gastrointestinal bleeding
and other symptoms, arthralgias, arthritis, and renal involvement

DIAGNOSIS
- Diagnosis of HSP is made on clinical grounds. Skin manifestations are
most common. Palpable purpura is seen in 70% of adult patients and
is less pronounced in children, in whom gastrointestinal complaints
are more common. Skin biopsy specimen shows leukocytoclastic
vasculitis.
- There is palpable purpura of dependent areas, especially lower
extremities, and areas subjected to pressure, such as the belt line.

- Gastrointestinal symptoms are seen in approximately one third of patients. Common findings are nausea, vomiting, diarrhea, cramping, abdominal pain, hematochezia, and melena.
- Anecdotally, HSP may follow upper respiratory infection.
- Renal involvement is seen in 80% of older children, usually within the first month of illness; <5% of cases progress to end-stage renal failure.
- Laboratory abnormalities are not specific for HSP. Leukocytosis and eosinophilia may be seen. IgA levels are elevated in approximately 50% of patients. Glomerulonephritis may be present and result in microscopic hematuria, proteinuria, and red blood cell casts.

ETIOLOGY

- The presumptive etiology is exposure to a trigger antigen that causes antibody formation. Antigen-antibody (immune) complex deposition then occurs in arteriole and capillary walls of skin, renal mesangium, and gastrointestinal tract. IgA deposition is most common. Postulated antigen triggers include drugs, foods, immunization, and upper respiratory and other viral illnesses. Serologic and pathologic evidence exists, suggesting an association between parvovirus B19 and HSP. This association may explain observed cases of HSP that do not respond to corticosteroids or other immunosuppressive therapy.

TREATMENT

- Prednisone 1 mg/kg PO is given if renal or severe gastrointestinal disease is present, although benefits are not clear.
- Corticosteroids and azathioprine may be beneficial if rapidly progressive glomerulonephritis is present. Pulse methylprednisolone therapy also has been proposed in patients with glomerulonephritis, mesenteric vasculitis, or pulmonary involvement.
- Nonsteroidal antiinflammatory drugs are given for arthritis and arthralgias.

▬ Heparin-induced thrombocytopenia (HIT)

Definition: Immunologic drug reaction caused by platelet-activating IgG antibodies that recognize complexes of platelet factor 4 and heparin. It is associated with venous or arterial thrombosis.

DIAGNOSIS

- HIT usually develops within 5 to 8 days after heparin exposure. It may develop earlier (within 2 days) in patients with previous exposure. It

also may occur 3 weeks after exposure to heparin secondary to high titers of platelet-activating IgG induced by heparin (delayed-onset HIT).
- The diagnosis should be differentiated from early, benign, transient thrombocytopenia that can occur with heparin therapy. Factors favoring immune thrombocytopenia are as follows:
  - Platelet count is decreased to <100,000/mm^3 or >50% of baseline value.
  - Falling platelet count generally occurs after 5 days of heparin therapy or earlier if the patient had recent exposure to heparin.
  - Diagnosis can be confirmed with platelet serotonin release assay or ELISA for heparin-PF4 complex.

TREATMENT
- Treatment is empiric and consists of the following:
  - Discontinue heparin.
  - If warfarin had been started few days before HIT, it should be discontinued because it has been reported to cause limb gangrene in this setting.
  - Use other anticoagulant agents. The three agents currently approved for HIT are:
    - Danaparoid, a heparanoid compound—approved for prophylaxis against venous thromboembolism in high-risk patients with HIT
    - Lipirudin, a hirudin derivative—approved for HIT with thrombosis. This is a short-acting agent administered intravenously. Therapy is monitored with partial thromboplastin time (PTT). Excretion is renal; dosage reduction is necessary in renal insufficiency.
    - Argatroban, a direct thrombin inhibitor—approved for HIT with thrombosis. This is a short-acting agent administered intravenously. Therapy is monitored with PTT. It is metabolized by the liver; dosage reduction is necessary in liver disease.

■ Hepatic encephalopathy

Definition: Abnormal mental status occurring in patients with severe impairment of liver function and consequent accumulation of toxic products not metabolized by the liver

DIAGNOSIS
- **Classification** Hepatic encephalopathy can be classified in stages or grades 1 to 4:
  - **Grades 1 and 2:** mild obtundation

...p...is deep coma, with or without decere-
brate posturing
- **Physical examination:** The physical examination in hepatic encephalopathy varies with the stage and may reveal the following abnormalities:
  - **Skin:** jaundice, palmar erythema, spider angiomata, ecchymosis, dilated superficial periumbilical veins (caput medusae) in patients with cirrhosis
  - **Eyes:** scleral icterus, Kayser-Fleischer rings (Wilson's disease)
  - **Breath:** fetor hepaticus
  - **Chest:** gynecomastia in men with chronic liver disease
  - **Abdomen:** ascites, small nodular liver (cirrhosis), tender hepatomegaly (congestive hepatomegaly)
  - **Rectal examination:** hemorrhoids (portal hypertension), guaiac-positive stool (alcoholic gastritis, bleeding esophageal varices, peptic ulcer disease, bleeding hemorrhoids)
  - **Genitalia:** testicular atrophy in men with chronic liver disease
  - **Extremities:** pedal edema from hypoalbuminemia
  - **Neurologic:** flapping tremor (asterixis), obtundation, coma with or without decerebrate posturing
- **Laboratory tests:**
  - Alanine aminotransferase, aspartate aminotransferase, bilirubin, alkaline phosphatase, glucose, calcium, electrolytes, blood urea nitrogen, creatinine, albumin
  - Complete blood count, platelet count, prothrombin time, partial thromboplastin time
  - Serum and urine toxicology screen in suspected medication or illegal drug use
  - Blood and urine cultures, urinalysis
  - Venous ammonia level
  - Arterial blood gases

ETIOLOGY
- Precipitating factors in patients with underlying cirrhosis (upper gastrointestinal bleeding, hypokalemia, hypomagnesemia, analgesic and sedative drugs, sepsis, alkalosis, increased dietary protein)
- Acute fulminant viral hepatitis
- Drugs and toxins (e.g., isoniazid, acetaminophen, diclofenac, statins, methyldopa, loratadine, propylthiouracil, lisinopril, labetalol, halothane, carbon tetrachloride, erythromycin, nitrofurantoin, troglitazone)
- Reye's syndrome
- Shock or sepsis (or both)
- Fatty liver of pregnancy

- Metastatic carcinoma, hepatocellular carcinoma
- **Other:** autoimmune hepatitis, ischemic venocclusive disease, sclerosing cholangitis, heatstroke, amebic abscesses

TREATMENT

- Identification and treatment of precipitating factors
- Restriction of protein intake (30–40 g/day) to reduce toxic protein metabolites
- Reduction of colonic ammonia production:

  Lactulose 30 mL of 50% solution qid initially; dose subsequently is adjusted depending on clinical response. Ornithine aspartate 9 g tid also is effective.

  Neomycin 1 g PO q4-6h or given as a 1% retention enema solution (1 g in 100 mL of isotonic saline solution); neomycin should be used with caution in patients with renal insufficiency Metronidazole 250 mg qid may be as effective as neomycin and is not nephrotoxic; however, long-term use can be associated with neurotoxicity Rifaximin 1200 mg/day is a viable alternative to metronidazole

  A combination of lactulose and neomycin can be used when either agent is ineffective alone.
- **Treatment of cerebral edema:** Cerebral edema often is present in patients with acute liver failure, and it accounts for nearly 50% of deaths. Monitoring intracranial pressure by epidural, intraparenchymal, or subdural transducers and treatment of cerebral edema with mannitol 100–200 mL of 20% solution (0.3–0.4 g/kg of body weight) given by rapid intravenous infusion are helpful in selected patients (e.g., potential transplantation patients); dexamethasone and hyperventilation (useful in head injury) are of little value in treating cerebral edema from liver failure.

CLINICAL PEARLS

- The early stages of hepatic encephalopathy can be managed in the outpatient setting, whereas stages 3 or 4 require hospital admission.
- Patients not responding to supportive therapy should be evaluated for liver transplantation.

Definition: Acute infection of the liver parenchymal cells caused by a virus

DIAGNOSIS

- Acute hepatitis A is diagnosed by detection of IgM antibodies to hepatitis A virus in patient's serum (usually detectable within 1 week of clinically apparent jaundice).
- Acute hepatitis B is diagnosed by the following:
  - Detection of hepatitis B surface antigen (HBsAg) *or*
  - IgM anti-HBc (marker of acute hepatitis B) (Fig. 10)

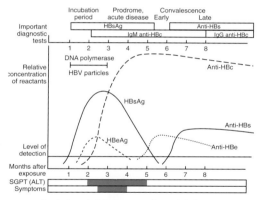

FIGURE 10. Serologic and clinical patterns observed during acute hepatitis B virus (HBV) infection. Patients who do not resolve the HBV infection (chronic carrier state) show persistence of hepatitis B surface antigen (HbsAg) and do not have an elevation of anti-HBs. HBeAg, hepatitis Be antigen; SGPT (ALT), serum glutamic pyruvic transaminase (alanine aminotransferase). (From Hollinger FB, Dienstag JL. In Murray PR, et al [eds]: Manual of Clinical Micriobiology, 6th ed. Washington, DC, American Society of Microbiology, 1995.)

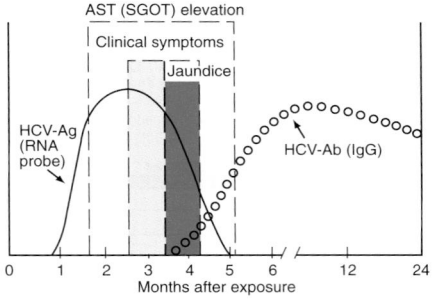

FIGURE 11. Hepatitis C virus antigen (HCV-Ag) and antibody (HCV-Ab). SGOT (AST), serum glutamic oxaloacetic acid (aspartate aminotransferase). (From Ravel R: Clinical Laboratory Medicine, 6th ed. St Louis, Mosby, 1995.)

- Hepatitis C is diagnosed by the following:
  - Hepatitis C enzyme immunoassay for detecting antibody against HCV (anti-HCV) often is used as a screening test for HCV. It is not detectable until about 12 weeks after exposure. It indicates present or past infection, but does not differentiate between acute, chronic, or resolved infection. Because it may miss acute infection and early interferon therapy may decrease risk of progression to chronic hepatitis, it should not be the diagnostic test for patients suspected of having acute HCV hepatitis.
  - The recombinant immunoblot assay for hepatitis C can be performed to confirm the diagnosis in low-risk patients.
  - Most clinicians prefer the test for HCV RNA, which detects the presence of the virus in serum 1 to 2 weeks after exposure (Fig. 11). It is the best initial test in patients who are immunocompromised, have risk factors for infection, or may have acute infection.

reverse transcriptase polymerase chain reaction amplification of HCV RNA by in-house or commercial assays can be used to differentiate between patients who have ongoing infection and patients who have cleared the virus from the circulation. It also is useful to monitor patients receiving antiviral therapy.
  - Testing for HCV genotype is recommended for patients undergoing drug therapy for hepatitis C.
- Hepatitis D is diagnosed by the presence of delta antigen or antibody to delta antigen (anti-HDV) in the patient's serum; it can cause either acute or chronic hepatitis. Acute hepatitis D can occur in two forms:
  - **Coinfection:** simultaneous acute infection with hepatitis B and hepatitis D viruses; diagnosis is confirmed by the presence of anti-HDV and IgM anti-HBc
  - **Superinfection:** occurrence of acute delta infection in a chronic HBV carrier; diagnosis is made by presence of anti-HDV and HBsAg in the serum; IgM anti-HBc is absent
  - Chronic hepatitis D is diagnosed by the presence in the serum of sustained high titers of anti-HDV and HBsAg; liver biopsy confirms the diagnosis by showing HDV antigen in liver tissue.
- Hepatitis E is diagnosed by detection of anti-hepatitis E virus in the serum.
- Diagnosis of hepatitis G virus infection currently depends on the use of polymerase chain reaction to detect viral RNA in serum or other infected fluids or tissues.

TREATMENT
- Patients need to avoid strenuous activity and ingestion of excessive amounts of hepatotoxic agents (e.g., ethanol, acetaminophen); patients should be instructed on possible infectivity to others.
- Correct any metabolic abnormalities (e.g., dextrose solutions for hypoglycemia; vitamin K 10-15 mg SC or PO qd × 3 days if international normalized ratio elevated).
- Pruritus can be treated with hydroxyzine 25-50 mg PO/IM q6h. Cholestyramine 4 g bid may be added in severe cases, but is generally not well tolerated.
- A balanced high-carbohydrate diet is recommended.
- Acute HCV infection should be treated with pegylated interferon alfa, INF alfa, or ribavirin to reduce the risk of chronic hepatitis.
- Hospitalization is rarely indicated except for severe volume depletion, encephalopathy, or intractable vomiting.

CLINICAL PEARL
- Anti-HBc is particularly useful as a serologic marker of acute hepatitis B during the "core antibody window" period when HBsAg and anti-HBs may be negative.

Hepatitis, autoimmune

Definition: A chronic inflammatory condition of the liver, characterized by the presence of circulating autoantibodies. Three types have been described:

- Type 1 or "classic" autoimmune hepatitis is the most predominant form in the United States and is positive for either antinuclear antibodies (ANA) or anti–smooth muscle antibodies (ASMA). There is a bimodal age distribution: Teenagers and adults 50 to 70 years old are most commonly affected.
- Type 2 is rare in the United States and primarily affects young children. Type 2 is characterized by the presence of antibodies to liver/kidney microsomes (anti-LKM).
- Type 3 is characterized by antibodies to soluble liver antigen or liver-pancreas antigen (anti-SLA/LP). A bimodal age distribution also is associated with type 3.

DIAGNOSIS

- Clinical presentation varies from asymptomatic elevations of liver enzymes to advanced cirrhosis.
  - Symptoms may include fatigue, anorexia, nausea, abdominal pain, pruritus, and arthralgia.
  - Jaundice may be present.
  - Hepatomegaly/splenomegaly may be present.
  - Autoimmune findings include arthritis, xerostomia, keratoconjunctivitis, cutaneous vasculitis, and erythema nodosum.
  - For patients presenting with advanced disease, ascites, edema, abnormal bleeding, and jaundice are present.
- **Laboratory tests:**
  - Aminotransferases generally elevated; may fluctuate
  - Bilirubin and alkaline phosphatase moderately elevated or normal
  - Hypergammaglobulinemia usually present
  - Circulating autoantibodies often present
    - Rheumatoid factor
    - ANA—present in two thirds of patients. Typical pattern is homogeneous or speckled. Titer does not correlate with stage, activity, or prognosis.
    - ASMA—present in 87% of patients. Titer does not correlate with course or prognosis.
    - Anti-LKM—typically found in patients who are ANA negative and ASMA negative. It is found in <1/25 of patients in the United States. Anti-LKM is present in children and 20% of adults in ⎯⎯⎯ ⎯⎯⎯ ⎯⎯⎯ present in patients with drug-induced hepatitis.

present in 10% to 30% of patients. The presence of anti-SLA/LP is associated with a higher rate of relapse after corticosteroid therapy. Several studies suggest that patients with anti-SLA/LP have a more severe course.

- Hypoalbuminemia and prolonged prothrombin time with advanced disease
- Liver biopsy reveals interface hepatitis, which consists of a lymphoplasmacytic inflammatroy infiltrate that extends from the portal tract into the lobule.
- **Imaging studies:** Ultrasound of liver and biliary tree is performed to rule out obstruction or hepatic mass.

ETIOLOGY

- Exact etiology is unknown; liver histology shows cell-mediated immune attack against hepatocytes.
- Presence of a variety of autoantibodies suggests an autoimmune mechanism.
- There is a strong genetic predisposition.

TREATMENT

- **Initial treatment:**
  - Prednisone 60 mg/day PO or combination treatment with prednisone 30 mg/day PO plus azathiaprine 50 mg/day PO
  - Combination therapy allows for lower prednisone doses and fewer steroid side effects.
  - Goal of therapy is remission (normalization of gamma globulin and bilirubin, reduction of animotransferases to less than two times the upper limit of normal).
- **Indications for treatment:**
  - Serum aminotransferase >10 times the upper limit of normal
  - Serum aminotransferase more than five times the upper limit of normal, with serum gamma globulin level twice the upper limit of normal
  - Young age
  - Histologic features of bridging necrosis or multiacinar necrosis
- **Evaluation of treatment response:**
  - Goal is normalization of serum transaminase levels.
  - Patients who normalize transaminase levels may continue to have ongoing active hepatitis involving inflammation and fibrosis; 5% to 10% of patients with normal transaminase levels progress to cirrhosis.
  - Histologic improvement may lag behind clinical and laboratory improvement by 6 months.
  - Repeat liver biopsy should be considered after normalization of transaminase levels.

CLINICAL PEARLS
- Persistent interface hepatitis is associated with 90% risk of relapse.
- Complete normalization on biopsy specimen is associated with 15% to 20% risk of relapse.
- 65% of patients achieve remission by 18 months; 80% achieve remission by 3 years.
- Approximately 10% of patients fail to improve with therapy.
- Patients with decompensated cirrhosis usually do not benefit from corticosteroid therapy and should be considered for liver transplantation.

Hepatorenal syndrome (HRS)

Definition: A condition of intense renal vasoconstriction resulting from loss of renal autoregulation occurring as a complication of severe liver disease. There are two types of HRS:

- Type 1—progressive impairment in renal function as defined by a doubling of initial serum creatinine >2.5 mg/dL in <2 weeks
- Type 2—stable or slowly progressive impairment of renal function not meeting the above-mentioned criteria

DIAGNOSIS
Criteria for HRS are:
- Serum creatinine concentration >1.5 mg/dL or 24 hours creatinine clearance <40 mL/min
- Absence of shock, ongoing infection, and fluid loss and no current treatment with nephrotoxic drugs
- Absence of sustained improvement in renal function (decrease in serum creatinine to ≤1 mg/dL) after discontinuation of diuretics and a trial of plasma expansion
- Absence of proteinuria (<500 mg/day) or hematuria (<50 red blood cells/high-power field)
- Absence of ultrasound evidence of obstructive uropathy or parenchymal renal disease
- Urinary sodium concentration <10 mmol/L

ETIOLOGY
- HRS may occur after significant reduction of effective blood volume (e.g., phlebotomy, gastrointestinal bleeding, diuretics) or in the absence of any precipitating factors.

- Volume challenge (to increase mean arterial pressure) followed by large-volume paracentesis (to increase cardiac output and decrease renal venous pressure) is recommended to distinguish HRS from pre-renal azotemia in patients with a fractional excretion of sodium <1%. In patients with prerenal azotemia, the increase in renal perfusion pressure and renal blood flow results in prompt diuresis; the volume challenge can be accomplished by giving a solution of 100 g of albumin in 500 mL of isotonic saline.
- Vasopressin analogues may improve renal perfusion by reversing splanchnic vasodilation, which is the hallmark of HRS. Intravenous norepinephrine combined with albumin and furosemide also may be effective.
- Treat HRS with vasoconstrictors for 5 to 15 days in an attempt to reduce serum creatinine to <1.5 mg/dL with one of the following drugs or drug combinations:
  - Norepinephrine 0.5-3 mg/hr IV
  - Midodrine 7.5 mg PO tid, increased to 12.5 mg tid if needed, in combination with octretide 100 µg SC tid, increased to tid as needed
  - Terlipressin 0.2-2 mg IV q4-12h)
  - Concomitant administration of albumin 1 g/kg IV on day 1, followed by 20-40 g daily

CLINICAL PEARL
- Liver transplantation may be indicated in otherwise healthy patients (age preferably <65 years old) with sclerosing cholangitis, chronic hepatitis with cirrhosis, or primary biliary cirrhosis; contraindications to liver transplantation are AIDS, most metastatic malignancies, active substance abuse, uncontrolled sepsis, and uncontrolled cardiac or pulmonary disease.

▰ Herpes simplex, genital

Definition: A viral infection caused by the herpes simplex virus (HSV); HSV-1 is associated primarily with oral infections, whereas HSV-2 causes mainly genital infections. Each type can infect any site, however.

DIAGNOSIS
- **Primary infection:**
  - Symptoms occur 3 to 7 days after contact (respiratory droplets, direct contact).
  - Constitutional symptoms include low-grade fever, headache and myalgias, regional lymphadenopathy, and localized pain.

- Pain, burning, itching, and tingling last several hours.
- Grouped vesicles usually with surrounding erythema appear and generally ulcerate or crust within 48 hours.
- The vesicles are uniform in size (differentiating it from herpes zoster vesicles, which vary in size).
- During the acute eruption, the patient is uncomfortable; involvement of lips and inside of mouth may make it unpleasant for the patient to eat; urinary retention may complicate involvement of the genital area.
- Lesions generally last 2 to 6 weeks and heal without scarring.
- **Recurrent infection:**
  - Recurrent infection generally is caused by alteration in the immune system; fatigue, stress, menses, local skin trauma, and exposure to sunlight are contributing factors.
  - The prodromal symptoms (fatigue, burning and tingling of the affected area) last 12 to 24 hours.
  - A cluster of lesions generally evolves within 24 hours from macules to papules and then vesicles surrounded by erythema; the vesicles coalesce and subsequently rupture within 4 days, revealing erosions covered by crusts.
  - The crusts generally are shed within 7 to 10 days, revealing a pink surface.
  - The most frequent location of the lesions is on the vermilion border of the lips (HSV-1), the penile shaft or glans penis and the labia (HSV-2), buttocks (seen more frequently in women), fingertips (herpetic whitlow), and trunk (may be confused with herpes zoster).
- **Laboratory tests:**
  - Direct immunofluorescent antibody slide tests provide a rapid diagnosis.
  - Viral culture is the most definitive method for diagnosis; results generally are available in 1 or 2 days; the lesions should be sampled during the vesicular or early ulcerative stage; cervical samples should be taken from the endocervix with a swab.
  - Tzanck smear is a readily available test; it shows multinucleated giant cells. It is not a sensitive test, however.
  - Pap smear detects HSV-infected cells in cervical tissue from women without symptoms.
  - Serologic tests for HSV are for IgG and IgM serum antibodies. Antibodies to HSV occur in 50% to 90% of adults. Routine tests do not discriminate between antibodies that are HSV-1 and HSV-2; the presence of IgM or a fourfold or greater rise in IgG titers indicates

weeks after the acute specimen is drawn).

TREATMENT

- Acyclovir ointment or cream (Zovirax) applied using finger-cot or rubber glove every 3 to 6 hours (six times daily) for 7 days may be useful for the first clinical episode of genital herpes. Severe primary genital infections may be treated with intravenous acyclovir 5 mg/kg infused at a constant rate over 1 hour q8h for 7 days in patients with normal renal function or oral acyclovir 200 mg five times daily for 7 to 10 days. Topical acyclovir 5% cream also can be used for herpes labialis; when started at the prodrome or papule stage, it decreases the duration of an episode by about {1/2} day.
- Valacyclovir caplets (Valtrex) also can be used for the initial episode of genital herpes (1 g bid for 10 days).
- Valacyclovir 2 g PO q12h for 1 day begun with the first symptoms of herpes labialis can modestly shorten its duration.
- Penciclovir 1% cream (Denavir) can be used for recurrent herpes labialis on the lips and face. It should be applied every 2 hours while awake for 4 days. Treatment should be started at the earliest sign or symptom. Its use decreases healing time of orolabial herpes by about 1 day.
- Docosanol 10% cream (Abreva), a long-chain saturated alcohol, inhibits fusion between the plasma membrane and the viral envelope, blocking viral entry and subsequent replication. It is available over the counter, and when applied at the first sign of recurrence of herpes labialis, it may shorten the duration of the episode by about 12 hours.
- Recurrent episodes of genital herpes can be treated with acyclovir. A short course (800 mg tid for 2 days) is effective. Other treatment options include 800 mg PO bid for 5 days, generally started during the prodrome or within 2 days of onset of lesions. Famciclovir (Famvir) also is useful for treatment of recurrent genital herpes (dose is 125 mg q12h for 5 days in patients with normal renal function) started at the first sign of symptoms or valacyclovir (Valtrex) (dose is 500 mg q12h for 5 days in patients with normal renal function).
- Acyclovir-resistant mucocutaneous lesions in patients with HIV can be treated with foscarnet (40-60 mg/kg IV q8h in patients with normal renal function); cidofovir also has been reported to be effective in HSV infections resistant to acyclovir or foscarnet.
- Patients with six recurrences of genital herpes per year can be treated with valacyclovir 1 g qd, acyclovir 400 mg bid, or famciclovir 250 mg bid.

Herpes zoster

Definition: Herpes zoster is a disease caused by reactivation of the varicella-zoster virus. After the primary infection (chickenpox), the virus becomes latent in the dorsal root ganglia and reemerges when there is a weakening of the immune system (secondary to disease or advanced age).

DIAGNOSIS

- Pain generally precedes skin manifestation by 3 to 5 days and generally is localized to the dermatome that will be affected by the skin lesions.
- Constitutional symptoms are often present (malaise, fever, headache).
- The initial rash consists of erythematous maculopapules generally affecting one dermatome (thoracic region in most cases); some patients (<50%) may have scattered vesicles outside of the affected dermatome.
- The initial maculopapules evolve into vesicles and pustules by day 3 or 4.
- The vesicles have an erythematous base, are cloudy, and have various sizes (a distinguishing characteristic from herpes simplex in which the vesicles are of uniform size).
- The vesicles subsequently become umbilicated, then form crusts that generally fall off within 3 weeks; scarring may occur.
- Pain during and after the rash is generally significant.
- Secondary bacterial infection with *Staphylococcus aureus* or *Streptococcus pyogenes* may occur.
- Regional lymphadenopathy may occur.
- Herpes zoster may involve the trigeminal nerve (most frequent cranial nerve involved); involvement of the geniculate ganglion can cause facial palsy and a painful ear, with the presence of vesicles on the pinna and external auditory canal (Ramsay Hunt syndrome).

TREATMENT

- **Suppression of pain:** Gabapentin 300-600 mg bid is effective in the treatment of pain and sleep interference associated with postherpetic neuralgia.
- Lidocaine patch 5% (Lidoderm) also is effective in relieving postherpetic neuralgia. Patches are applied to intact skin to cover the most painful area for 12 hours within a 24-hour period.
- Oral antiviral agents can decrease acute pain, inflammation, and vesicle formation when treatment is begun within 48 hours of onset of rash. Treatment options are:

- Valacyclovir (Valtrex) 1000 mg tid for 7 days
- Famciclovir (Famvir) 500 mg tid for 7 days
- Immunocompromised patients should be treated with acyclovir 500 mg/m² or 10 mg/kg IV q8h in 1-hour infusions for 7 days, with close monitoring of renal function and adequate hydration; vidarabine (continuous 12-hour infusion of 10 mg/kg/day for 7 days) also is effective for treatment of disseminated herpes zoster in immunocompromised hosts.
- Patients with AIDS and transplant patients may develop acyclovir-resistant varicella zoster; these patients can be treated with foscarnet 40 mg/kg IV q8h continued for at least 10 days or until lesions are completely healed.
- Capsaicin cream (Zostrix) can be used for treatment of postherpetic neuralgia. It generally is applied three to five times daily for several weeks.
- Sympathetic blocks (stellate ganglion or epidural) with 0.25% bupivacaine and rhizotomy are reserved for severe cases unresponsive to conservative treatment.
- Corticosteroids should be considered in older patients if there are no contraindications. Initial dose is prednisone 60 mg/day tapered over 21 days. When used, there is a decrease in the use of analgesics and time to resumption of usual activities, but there is no effect on the incidence and duration of postherpetic neuralgia.

Hodgkin's disease

Definition: Malignant disorder of lymphoreticular origin, characterized histologically by the presence of multinucleated giant cells (Reed-Sternberg cells) usually originating from B lymphocytes in germinal centers of lymphoid tissue

DIAGNOSIS
- Symptomatic patients with Hodgkin's disease usually present with the following manifestations:
  - Fever and night sweats—fever in a cyclical pattern (days or weeks of fever alternating with afebrile periods) is known as *Pel-Ebstein fever*
  - Weight loss, generalized malaise
  - Persistent, nonproductive cough
  - Pain associated with alcohol ingestion, often secondary to heavy eosinophil infiltration of the tumor sites

- Pruritus
- **Others:** superior vena cava syndrome and spinal cord compression (rare)

- Diagnosis can be made with lymph node biopsy. There are four main histologic subtypes, based on the number of lymphocytes, Reed-Stemberg cells, and the presence of fibrous tissue:
  - Lymphocyte predominance
  - Mixed cellularity
  - Nodular sclerosis
  - Lymphocyte depletion
  - Nodular sclerosis is the most common type and occurs mainly in young adulthood, whereas the mixed cellularity type is more prevalent in patients >50 years old.
  - Staging for Hodgkin's disease follows the Ann Arbor staging *classification*
    - Stage I—involvement of a single lymph node region
    - Stage II—two or more lymph node regions on the same side of the diaphragm
    - Stage III—lymph node involvement on both sides of diaphragm, including spleen
    - Stage IV—diffuse involvement of external sites
    - Suffix A—no systemic symptoms
    - Suffix B—presence of fever, night sweats, or unexplained weight loss of ≥10% body weight over 6 months
    - Suffix X—indicates bulky disease >1/3 widening of mediastinum or >10 cm maximal dimension of nodal mass on a chest film.
  - Staging generally requires the following:
    - Detailed history (with documentation of "B symptoms" and physical examination)
    - Surgical biopsy
    - Laboratory evaluation (complete blood count, sedimentation rate, blood urea nitrogen, creatinine, alkaline phosphatase, liver function tests, albumin, lactate dehydrogenase, uric acid)
    - Bilateral bone marrow biopsy
    - Chest x-ray (posteroanterior and lateral)
    - CT of the chest (when abnormal findings are noted on chest x-ray) and of the abdomen and pelvis to visualize the mesenteric, hepatic, portal, and splenic hilar nodes.
    - Bipedal lymphangiography in selected patients to define periaortic and iliac lymph node involvement
    - Exploratory laparotomy and splenectomy (selected patients):
      - Decision to perform staging laparotomy depends on the therapeutic plan; it is generally not indicated in patients who have a

combined chemotherapy and radiation). Staging laparotomy also may not be required in patients with clinical stage I or who are unlikely to have abdominal disease (e.g., women with supra-diaphragmatic disease).
    ○ Exploratory laparotomy and splenectomy may be used for patients with clinical stage I-IIA or IIB.
    ○ It is useful in identifying patients who can be treated with irradiation alone with curative intent.
    ○ Polyvalent pneumococcal vaccine should be given prophylactically to all patients before splenectomy (increased risk of sepsis from encapsulated organisms in splenectomized patients).
  • Gallium scan

DIFFERENTIAL DIAGNOSIS
• Non-Hodgkin's lymphoma
• Sarcoidosis
• Infections (e.g., cytomegalovirus, Epstein-Barr virus, toxoplasmosis, HIV)
• Drug reaction

TREATMENT
• The main therapeutic modalities are radiotherapy and chemotherapy; the indication for each varies with pathologic stage and other factors.
    • **Stages I and II:** Radiation therapy alone is used, unless a large mediastinal mass is present (mediastinal-to-thoracic ratio ≥ 1.3); in the latter case, a combination of chemotherapy and radiation therapy is indicated.
    • **Stage IB or IIB:** Total nodal irradiation is often used, although chemotherapy is performed in many centers.
    • **Stage IIIA:** Treatment is controversial. It varies with the anatomic substage after splenectomy.
        • **Stage III$_1$A and minimum splenic involvement:** Radiation therapy alone may be adequate.
        • **Stage III$_2$ or III$_1$A with extensive splenic involvement:** There is disagreement whether chemotherapy alone or a combination of chemotherapy and radiation therapy is the preferred treatment modality.
        • **Stage IIIB and IVB:** The treatment of choice is chemotherapy with or without adjuvant radiotherapy.
• Various regimens can be used for combination chemotherapy. Most oncologists prefer the combination of doxorubicin plus bleomycin plus vincristine plus dacarbazine (ABVD). Other commonly used regimens are MOPP, MOPP-ABV, MOPP-ABVD, and MOPP-BAP.

Horner syndrome

Definition: The clinical triad of ipsilateral ptosis, miosis, and sometimes anhidrosis of the face. These physical findings are the result of disruption of the cervical sympathetic pathway along its course from the hypothalamus to the eye. Disruption of any of the three neurons involved in the pathway (central, preganglionic, or postganglionic) can cause Horner's syndrome.

DIAGNOSIS

- **Clinical presentation:**
  - Ptosis results from loss of sympathetic tone to eyelid muscles.
  - Miosis results from loss of sympathetic pupillodilator activity .The affected pupil reacts normally to light and accommodation. Anisocoria is greater in darkness.
  - The presence of anhidrosis varies and depends on the site of injury in the sympathetic pathway. Anhidrosis may occur with lesions affecting the central or preganglionic neurons.
  - Conjunctival or facial hyperemia may occur on the affected side because of loss of sympathetic vasoconstrictor activity.
  - In congenital Horner's syndrome, the iris on the affected side may fail to become pigmented, resulting in heterochromia of the iris, with the affected iris remaining blue-gray.
- **Imaging studies:**
  - Chest CT scan to rule out lung tumors
  - MRI of the head and neck to identify lesions affecting the central and cervical sympathetic pathway
  - Ultrasound, CT angiography, or magnetic resonance angiography to assess the vessels in the head and neck

ETIOLOGY

- Lesions affecting any of the neurons involved in the sympathetic pathway can cause Horner's syndrome.
  - **Mechanical:**
    - Syringomyelia
    - Trauma
    - Benign tumors
    - Malignant tumors (thyroid, Pancoast tumor)
    - Metastatic tumor
    - Lymphadenopathy
    - Neurofibromatosis
    - Cervical rib
    - Cervical spondylosis

malformation):
- Brainstem lesion—commonly occlusion of the posterior inferior cerebellar artery, but almost any of the vessels may be responsible (vertebral; superior, middle, or inferior lateral medullary arteries; superior or anterior inferior cerebellar arteries)
- Internal carotid artery aneurysm or dissection; injury of other major vessels (carotid artery, subclavian artery, ascending aorta) also can cause Horner's syndrome.
- Cluster headache, migraine

- **Miscellaneous:**
  - Congenital
  - Demyelination (multiple sclerosis)
  - Infection (apical tuberculosis, herpes zoster)
  - Pneumothorax
  - Iatrogenic (angiography; internal jugular/subclavian catheter, chest tube, surgery, epidural spinal anesthesia)
  - Radiation

TREATMENT
- Treatment depends on underlying cause.

CLINICAL PEARL
- Prognosis depends on underlying cause. Horner's syndrome is an uncommon presentation for malignancy. In one study, 60% of cases were idiopathic.

Huntington's chorea

Definition: An inherited neurodegenerative disorder characterized by involuntary movements, psychiatric disturbance, and cognitive decline

DIAGNOSIS
- Chorea refers to irregular rapid, flowing, nonstereotyped involuntary movements. When there is a writhing quality, it is referred to as *choreoathetosis*. Ninety percent of affected patients have chorea, but virtually any expression of basal ganglia dysfunction, including rigidity and dystonia, can be seen. Chorea is present early on and tends to decrease in end stages of disease.
- A Dancelike, lurching gait often is caused by chorea.
- Westphal variant includes cognitive dysfunction, bradykinesia, and rigidity. This variant is seen more commonly in juvenile-onset Huntington's disease.

- Oculomotor abnormalities are common early on and include increased latency of response and insuppressible eye blinking.
- Psychiatric disorders (can be present early on) include depression, obsessive-compulsive behaviors, and aggression associated with impaired impulse control.
- Confirm diagnosis by chromosome analysis.
- If chromosome analysis is normal, obtain complete blood count with smear, erythrocyte sedimentation rate, electrolytes, serum ceruloplasmin, 24-hour urinary copper excretion, thyroid function tests, antinuclear antibody, liver function tests, HIV, and antistreptolysin O titer. Consider paraneoplastic markers.
- CT or MRI shows atrophy most notably in the caudate and putamen. Cortex is involved to a lesser extent. A normal scan does not exclude the diagnosis.

ETIOLOGY

- Trinucleotide repeat disorder
- Unstable repeat results in CAG expansion
- Responsible gene is the Huntington gene located on chromosome 4; its function is not known.

TREATMENT

- Offer supportive counseling.
- Institute physical and occupational therapy.
- Arrange for home health care.
- Offer genetic counseling.
- Chorea does not need to be treated unless disabling.
- Chorea may be diminished by low doses of neuroleptics (e.g., haloperidol 1-10 mg/day).
- Give amantadine 300-400 mg tid.
- Tetrabenazine is a dopamine depleter that is not currently available in the United States. Side effects include parkinsonism and depression.
- Depression with suicidal ideation is common; this may improve with tricyclic antidepressants or selective serotonin reuptake inhibitors.

...cephalus, normal pressure (NPH)

Definition: A syndrome of symptomatic hydrocephalus in the setting of normal cerebrospinal fluid (CSF) pressure. The classic clinical triad of NPH includes gait disturbance, cognitive decline, and incontinence.

DIAGNOSIS

- **Gait difficulty** Patients often have difficulty initiating ambulation, and the gait may be broad-based and shuffling, with the appearance that the feet are stuck to the floor (i.e., "magnetic gait" or "frontal gait disorder").
- **Cognitive decline:** Mental slowing, forgetfulness, and inattention occur without agnosia, aphasia, or other "cortical" disturbances.
- **Incontinence:** Urinary urgency may be present initially; later incontinence develops. Occasionally fecal incontinence also occurs.
- Large-volume lumbar puncture:
- CT or MRI can be used to document ventriculomegaly. The distinguishing feature of NPH is ventricular enlargement out of proportion to sulcal atrophy.
- MRI has advantages over CT, including better ability to visualize structures in the posterior fossa, to visualize transependymal CSF flow, and to document extent of white matter lesions.

ETIOLOGY

- Approximately 50% of cases are idiopathic; remaining cases are from secondary causes, including prior subarachnoid hemorrhage, meningitis, trauma, or intracranial surgery.
- Symptoms are presumed to result from stretching of sacral motor and limbic fibers that lie near the ventricles, as dilation occurs.

TREATMENT

- Neurosurgical referral for shunting in appropriate patients. Factors that may predict positive outcome with surgery are:
  - NPH secondary to prior trauma, subarachnoid hemorrhage, or meningitis
  - History of mild impairment in cognition <2 years
  - Onset of gait abnormality before cognitive decline
  - Imaging shows hydrocephalus without sulcal enlargement
  - Transependymal CSF flow visualized on MRI

Hydronephrosis

Definition: Dilation of the renal pyelocalyceal system, most often as a result of impairment of urinary flow

DIAGNOSIS

- Pain is caused by distention of the collecting system or renal capsule and is related more to the rate of onset than the degree of obstruction. It can vary in location from flank to lower abdomen to testes/labia.
- Ultrasound is about 90% sensitive and specific for hydronephrosis and is noninvasive.
- Abdominal CT scan without intravenous contrast provides excellent localization of the site of obstruction.

ETIOLOGY

- **Mechanical impairments:**
  - **Congenital:** ureteropelvic junction narrowing, ureterovesical junction narrowing, ureterocele, retrocaval ureter, bladder neck obstruction, urethral valves, urethral stricture, meatal stenosis
  - **Acquired:**
    - Intrinsic to urinary tract—calculi, inflammation, trauma, sloughed papillae, ureteral tumor, blood clots, prostatic hypertrophy or cancer, bladder cancer, urethral stricture, phimosis
    - Extrinsic to urinary tract—gravid uterus, retroperitoneal fibrosis or tumor (e.g., lymphoma), aortic aneurysm, uterine fibroids, trauma (surgical or nonsurgical), pelvic inflammatory disease, pelvic malignancies (e.g., prostate, colorectal, cervical, uterine, bladder)
- **Functional impairments:**
  - Neurogenic bladder (often with adynamic ureter) can occur with spinal cord disease or diabetic neuropathy.
  - Pharmacologic agents, such as α-adrenergic antagonists and anticholinergic drugs, can inhibit bladder emptying.
  - Vesicoureteral reflux may occur.
  - Pregnancy can cause hydroureter and hydronephrosis (right more often than left) in the second month. Hormonal effects on ureteral tone combine with mechanical factors.

TREATMENT

- Urgent treatment is required if urinary tract obstruction is associated with urinary tract infection, acute renal failure, or uncontrollable pain.

venous antibiotics (if evidence of infection), and aggressive analgesia may be enough to treat acute unilateral urinary tract obstruction depending on the size (90% of stones <5 mm pass spontaneously).

- A urethral catheter is adequate to relieve most obstructions at or distal to the bladder, but occasionally a suprapubic catheter is required (e.g., impassable urethral stricture or urethral injury). Neurogenic bladder may require intermittent clean catheterization if frequent voiding and pharmacologic treatments are ineffective.
- A nephrostomy tube can be placed percutaneously to facilitate urinary drainage.
- Extracorporeal shock wave lithotripsy (ESWL) is used to fragment large stones to facilitate spontaneous passage or subsequent extraction. (*Note:* ESWL is contraindicated in pregnancy.)
- Nephroscopy is performed for extraction of proximal stones under direct vision.
- Cystoscopy with ureteroscopy is used for removal of distal ureteral stones using a loop or basket with or without fragmentation by ultrasonic or laser lithotripsy.
- Ureteral stents can be used for extrinsic and some intrinsic ureteral obstructions.
- Urethral dilation or internal urethrotomy can be used for urethral strictures.
- Nephrectomy or ureteral diversion may be required in severe cases (e.g., malignancy).
- Ureterovesical reimplantation can be used for reflux disease.
- Transurethral retrograde prostatectomy is used for severe obstruction from benign prostatic hypertrophy.
- Intravenous fluid and electrolyte replacement is needed; the patient must be monitored closely during the postobstructive diuresis (usually lasting several days to a week).

▬ Hyperaldosteronism

Definition: A clinical syndrome characterized by hypokalemia, hypertension, low plasma renin activity, and excessive aldosterone secretion

DIAGNOSIS
- In patients with hypokalemia and a low plasma renin activity, confirmatory tests for primary hyperaldosteronism include the following:

- Twenty-four-hour urine test for aldosterone and potassium levels (potassium >40 mEq and aldosterone >15 µg)
- Captopril test—administer 25-50 mg of captopril (angiotensin-converting enzyme [ACE] inhibitor), and measure plasma renin and aldosterone levels 1 to 2 hours later. A plasma aldosterone level >15 ng/dL confirms the diagnosis of primary aldosteronism. This test is more expensive and is best reserved for situations in which the 24-hour urine for aldosterone is ambiguous.
- Twenty-four-hour urinary tetrahydroaldosterone (<65 µg/24 hr) and saline infusion test (plasma aldosterone >10 ng/dL) also can be used in ambiguous cases.
- The renin-aldosterone stimulation test (posture test) is helpful in differentiating idiopathic hyperaldosteronism (IHA) from aldosterone-producing adenoma (APA). Patients with APA have a decrease in aldosterone levels at 4 hours, whereas patients with IHA have an increase in aldosterone levels.
- As a screening test for primary aldosteronism, an elevated plasma aldosterone-to-renin ratio (ARR), drawn randomly from patients on hypertensive drugs, is predictive of primary aldosteronism (positive predictive value 100% in one study). ARR is calculated by dividing plasma aldosterone value (ng/dL) by plasma renin activity (mg/mL/hr). ARR >100 is considered elevated.
- Bilateral adrenal venous sampling may be done to localize APA when adrenal CT scan is equivocal. In APA, ipsilateral/contralateral aldosterone level is >10:1, and ipsilateral venous aldosterone concentration is very high (>1000 ng/dL).
- Adrenal CT scans (with 3-mm cuts) may localize neoplasm.
- Adrenal scanning with iodocholesterol (NP-59) or 6-β-iodomethyl-19-norcholesterol after dexamethasone suppression—the uptake of tracer is increased in patients with aldosteronism and absent in patients with idiopathic aldosteronism and adrenal carcinoma.

ETIOLOGY

- APA (>60%)
- IHA (>30%)
- Glucocorticoid-suppressible hyperaldosteronism (<1%)
- Aldosterone-producing carcinoma (<1%)

TREATMENT

- Control of blood pressure and hypokalemia with spironolactone, amiloride, or ACE inhibitors.
- Surgery (unilateral adrenalectomy) for APA

Definition: Serum calcium level >10.3 mg/dL

DIAGNOSIS

- Initial laboratory studies should include serum calcium, albumin, PO_4^-, magnesium, alkaline phosphatase, electrolytes, blood urea nitrogen, creatinine, and 24-hour urine calcium collection.
- If the history suggests excessive intake of vitamin D (e.g., food faddists with intake of megadoses of fat-soluble vitamins), a serum vitamin D level (1,25-dihydroxyvitamin D) is indicated.
- The immunoassay for parathyroid hormone (PTH) distinguishes primary hyperparathyroidism from hypercalcemia caused by malignancy when the serum calcium level is >12 mg/dL; below this value there is considerable overlap, and the differentiation between these two major causes of hypercalcemia is extremely difficult.
- A very high level of urinary cyclic AMP strongly suggests primary hyperparathyroidism, although certain nonparathyroid malignancies also produce elevated levels of urinary cyclic AMP. PTH-like protein is increased in hypercalcemia associated with solid malignancies (e.g., squamous, breast, renal tumors).
- ECG shows shortening of the Q-T interval.

ETIOLOGY

- **Malignancy:** increased bone resorption via osteoclast-activating factors, secretion of PTH-like substances, prostaglandin E_2, direct erosion by tumor cells, transforming growth factors, colony-stimulating activity. Hypercalcemia is common in the following neoplasms:
  - Solid tumors—breast, lung, pancreas, kidneys, ovary
  - Hematologic cancers—myeloma, lymphosarcoma, adult T-cell lymphoma, Burkitt's lymphoma
- **Hyperparathyroidism:** increased bone resorption, gastrointestinal absorption, and renal absorption. Causes are as follows:
  - Parathyroid hyperplasia, adenoma
  - Hyperparathyroidism or renal failure with secondary hyperparathyroidism
- Granulomatous disorders—increased gastrointestinal absorption (e.g., sarcoidosis)
- Paget's disease—increased bone resorption, seen only during periods of immobilization
- Vitamin D intoxication, milk-alkali syndrome—increased gastrointestinal absorption
- Thiazides—increased renal absorption

• **Other causes:** familial hypocalciuric hypercalcemia, thyrotoxicosis, adrenal insufficiency, prolonged immobilization, vitamin A intoxication, recovery from acute renal failure, lithium administration, pheochromocytoma, disseminated systemic lupus erythematosus

TREATMENT

• **Acute severe hypercalcemia or symptomatic patient:**
  - Vigorous intravenous hydration with normal saline solution
  - Bisphosphonates—pamidronate 60-90 mg IV infusion over 24 hours or 60 mg in 500 mL of 0.9% saline infused over 4 hours. The serum calcium level is lowered to normal range within 2 to 5 days in approximately 75% of patients.
  - Calcitonin 4 U/kg q12h. Calcitonin is particularly useful in hypercalcemia associated with hyperphosphatemia because it also increases urinary phosphate excretion.
  - Mithramycin 25 µg/kg in 500 mL of 5% dextrose in water infused over 6 hours is a potent antihypercalcemic agent. It is generally used as a second-line agent.
    - It lowers serum calcium within 12 to 24 hours by inhibiting bone resorption.
    - Its use should be restricted to emergency treatment of severe hypercalcemia.
  - Zoledronic acid (Zometa) is also effective.
• **Chronic hypercalcemia:**
  - Identify and treat underlying disease (e.g. vitamin D intoxication, sarcoidosis).
  - Discontinue potential hypercalcemic agents (e.g. thiazide diuretics).
  - If hypercalcemia is caused by a parathyroid adenoma, parathyroidectomy is generally the treatment of choice.
  - Unless contraindicated, patients with chronic hypercalcemia should maintain a high daily intake of fluids (3-5 L/day) and of sodium chloride (>400 mEq/day) to increase renal calcium excretion.
  - **Medications:**
    - Glucocorticoids—hydrocortisone 3-5 mg/kg/day IV initially, then prednisone 30 mg PO bid
    - Oral phosphates 1-3 g/day in divided doses (e.g. Neutra-Phos 250-500 mg PO q6h)
    - Indomethacin (prostaglandin synthetase inhibitor) 75-150 mg/day is useful in prostaglandin-mediated hypercalcemia.

Definition: Plasma potassium concentration >4.9 mEq/L

DIAGNOSIS

- Stop all potassium intake (intravenous and oral).
- Rule out pseudohyperkalemia or laboratory error.
  - Repeat serum potassium level.
  - Obtain ECG; in patients with suspected pseudohyperkalemia secondary to hemolyzed specimen or thrombocytosis, the ECG does not show any manifestations of hyperkalemia.
  - In patients with thrombocytosis or severe leukocytosis, an accurate serum potassium can be determined by drawing a heparinized sample.
- In patients with true hyperkalemia and ECG or clinical manifestations, immediate intervention is indicated with one or more measures, depending on the severity of hyperkalemia.
- Check pH, and correct acidosis (if present).
- Check calcium, magnesium, glucose, electrolytes, blood urea nitrogen, and creatinine levels.
- Monitor ECG. ECG manifestations include the following:
  - Mild hyperkalemia—peaking or tenting of T waves, premature ventricular contractions
  - Severe hyperkalemia—peaking of T waves, widening of QRS complex, depressed ST segments, prolongation of P-R interval, sinus arrest, deep S wave, premature ventricular contractions, ventricular tachycardia, fibrillation, cardiac arrest

ETIOLOGY

- **Pseudohyperkalemia:**
  - Hemolyzed specimen
  - Severe thrombocytosis (platelet count >10^6 mL)
  - Severe leukocytosis (white blood cell count >10^5 mL)
  - Fist clenching during phlebotomy
- **Excessive potassium intake (often in setting of impaired excretion):**
  - Potassium replacement therapy
  - High-potassium diet
  - Salt substitutes with potassium
  - Potassium salts of antibiotics
- **Decreased renal excretion:**
  - Potassium-sparing diuretics (e.g., spironolactone, triamterene, amiloride)
  - Renal insufficiency

- Mineralocorticoid deficiency
- Hypovoninemic hypoaldosteronism (diabetes mellitus)
- Tubular unresponsiveness to aldosterone (e.g. systemic lupus erythematosus, multiple myeloma, sickle cell disease)
- Type 4 renal tubular acidosis
- Angiotensin-converting enzyme inhibitors
- Nonsteroidal antiinflammatory drugs
- Heparin administration
- Trimethoprim-sulfamethoxazole
- β-Blockers
- Pentamidine

Redistribution (excessive cellular release):

- Acidemia (each 0.1 decrease in pH increases the serum potassium by 0.4-0.6 mEq/L). Lactic acidosis and ketoacidosis cause minimal redistribution.
- Insulin deficiency
- Drugs (e.g. succinylcholine, markedly increased digitalis level, arginine, β-adrenergic blockers)
- Hypertonicity
- Hemolysis
- Tissue necrosis, rhabdomyolysis, burns
- Hyperkalemic periodic paralysis

TREATMENT

- Glucose 0.8 g IV bolus or IV infusion of 500 mL of 10% dextrose solution, plus 10 U of regular insulin IV—onset of action is 30 minutes and duration is 3 hours.
- Calcium gluconate (10% solution) 5-10 mL over 3 minutes—onset of action is <5 minutes, and duration is <1 hour.
- Sodium polystyrene sulfonate (Kayexalate), oral or via nasogastric tube, 20-50 g of Kayexalate plus 100-200 mL of 20% sorbitol. Retention enema 50 g of Kayexalate in 200 mL of water—onset of action is 1 to 2 hours, and duration is 3 hours.
- Sodium bicarbonate 1 ampule (44 mEq) over 5 minutes—onset of action is 30 minutes, and duration is 3 hours.
- Furosemide 40-160 mg IV over 30 minutes—onset of action is at start of diuresis.
- Dialysis (hemodialysis or peritoneal)—onset of action is 5 minutes after start of dialysis.

...ypermagnesemia

Definition: Plasma magnesium concentration >2.3 mg/dL

DIAGNOSIS
- Obtain a serum magnesium level.
- ECG manifestations include shortened P-R interval, heart block, peaked T waves, and increased QRS duration.
- Clinical manifestations include paresthesias, hypotension, confusion, decreased deep tendon reflexes, paralysis, coma, and apnea. Acute hypermagnesemia suppresses parathyroid hormone secretion and can produce hypocalcemia.

ETIOLOGY
- Renal failure (decreased glomerular filtration rate)
- Decreased renal excretion secondary to salt depletion
- Abuse of antacids and laxatives containing magnesium in patients with renal insufficiency
- Endocrinopathies (deficiency of mineralocorticoid or thyroid hormone)
- Increased tissue breakdown (rhabdomyolysis)
- Redistribution—acute diabetic ketoacidosis, pheochromocytoma
- **Other:** lithium, volume depletion, familial hypocalciuric hypercalcemia

TREATMENT
- Identify and correct underlying disorder.
- Intracardiac conduction abnormalities can be treated with intravenous calcium gluconate.
- Dialysis is indicated for severe hypermagnesemia.

Hypernatremia

Definition: Plasma sodium concentration >144 mEq/L

DIAGNOSIS
- Laboratory tests include serum electrolytes, blood urea nitrogen, creatinine, thyroid-stimulating hormone, and glucose.
- Clinical manifestations vary with degree of hypernatremia and rapidity of onset; they range from confusion and lethargy to seizures and coma.

ETIOLOGY

- Isovolemic (decreased total body water [TBW], normal total body sodium [TBNa] and extracellular fluid [ECF])
  - Diabetes insipidus (neurogenic and nephrogenic)
  - Skin loss (hyperhemia), iatrogenic, reset osmostat
- Hypervolemic (increased TBW, markedly increased TBNa and ECF)
  - Iatrogenic (administration of hypernatremic solutions)
  - Mineralocorticoid excess (Conn's syndrome, Cushing's syndrome)
  - Salt ingestion
- Hypovolemic: loss of water and Na$^+$ (water loss >Na$^+$)
  - Renal losses (e.g., diuretics, glycosuria)
  - Gastrointestinal, respiratory, and skin losses
  - Adrenal deficiencies

TREATMENT

- **Isovolemic hypernatremia:**
  - Fluid replacement with 5% dextrose in water. Correct only half of estimated water deficit in initial 24 hours. The rate of correction of serum sodium should not exceed 1 mEq/L/hr in acute hypernatremia or 0.5 mEq/L/hr in chronic hypernatremia.
  - Water deficit in hypernatremic patients: water deficit (in L) = 0.6 × body weight (kg) × ([measured serum sodium/normal serum sodium] − 1)
- **Hypovolemic hypernatremia:**
  - Fluid replacement with isotonic saline solution
  - Rate of correction of plasma osmolarity should not exceed 2 mOsm/kg/hr.
- **Hypervolemic hypernatremia:** Fluid replacement with 5% dextrose in water (to correct hypertonicity) is instituted after use of loop diuretics (to increase sodium excretion).

Hyperparathyroidism

Definition: An endocrine disorder caused by the excessive secretion of parathyroid hormone (PTH) from the parathyroid glands

DIAGNOSIS

- Physical examination may be normal. The presence of signs and symptoms varies with the rapidity of development and degree of hypercalcemia.
- Elevated serum ionized calcium level, low serum phosphorus, and normal or elevated alkaline phosphatase are present.

calcium levels seen in patients with familial hypocalciuric hypercalcemia.

- Serum PTH level is the best test for initial evaluation of confirmed hypercalcemia. The "intact" PTH (iPTH) is the best assay. The iPTH distinguishes primary hyperparathyroidism from hypercalcemia caused by malignancy when the serum calcium level is >12 mg/dL.
- ECG may reveal shortening of the Q-T interval secondary to hypercalcemia.

ETIOLOGY

- A single adenoma is found in 80% of patients. Ninety percent of adenomas are found within one of the parathyroid glands; the other 10% are in ectopic sites (e.g., lateral neck, thyroid, mediastinum, retroesophagus).
- Parathyroid gland hyperplasia occurs in 20% of patients.
- Primary hyperthyroidism is associated with multiple endocrine neoplasia I and II.

TREATMENT

- Unless contraindicated, patients should maintain a high intake of fluids (3-5 L/day) and sodium chloride (>400 mEq/day) to increase renal calcium excretion. Calcium intake should be 1000 mg/day.
- Potential hypercalcemic agents (e.g., thiazide diuretics) should be discontinued.
- Surgery is the only effective treatment for primary hyperparathyroidism.
- Asymptomatic elderly patients can be followed conservatively with periodic monitoring of serum calcium level and review of symptoms. Serum creatinine and PTH levels also should be obtained at 6- to 12-month intervals, and bone density (cortical and trabecular) should be determined yearly. Criteria for medical monitoring of patients with asymptomatic primary hyperparathyroidism are as follows:
  - Serum calcium level only mildly elevated
  - Asymptomatic patient
  - Normal bone status (no osteoporosis)
  - Normal kidney function and no urolithiasis or nephrocalcinosis
  - No previous episode of life-threatening hypercalcemia
- Acute severe hypercalcemia (serum calcium >13 mg/dL) or symptomatic patients can be treated with vigorous intravenous hydration with normal saline followed by intravenous furosemide. Calcitonin 4 IU/kg q12h is indicated when saline hydration and furosemide are ineffective or contraindicated. Bisphosphonates (pamidronate,

- etidronate), mithramycin, and gallium nitrate also are effective for severe hypercalcemia.
- Cinacalcet (Sensipar) is a newer, more powerful agent.

Hyperphosphatemia

Definition: Plasma phosphate concentration >5 mg/dL

DIAGNOSIS

- Serum electrolytes, blood urea nitrogen, creatinine, glucose, magnesium, calcium, creatine phosphokinase, lactate dehydrogenase, complete blood count, serum lipids
- Twenty-four-hour urine phosphate

ETIOLOGY

- Excessive phosphate administration
- Excessive oral intake or intravenous administration
- Laxatives containing phosphate (phosphate tablets, phosphate enemas)
- Decreased renal phosphate excretion
- Acute or chronic renal failure
- Hypoparathyroidism or pseudohypoparathyroidism
- Acromegaly, thyrotoxicosis
- Bisphosphonate therapy
- Tumor calcinosis
- Sickle cell anemia
- Transcellular shift out of cells
- Chemotherapy of lymphoma or leukemia, tumor lysis syndrome, hemolysis
- Acidosis
- Rhabdomyolysis, malignant hyperthermia
- Artifact (in vitro hemolysis)
- Pseudohyperphosphatemia (hyperlipidemia, paraproteinemia, hyperbilirubinemia)

TREATMENT

- Administer calcium carbonate (1 g with each meal, gradually increased to 8-12 g of calcium carbonate a day) to bind phosphate in the gut and prevent its absorption.
- Insulin and glucose infusion (to promote cell phosphate uptake) may be useful when a rapid decrease in phosphate is needed.
- Institute hemodialysis when renal failure is present.

hypersensitivity pneumonitis (HP)

Definition: A group of pulmonary diseases characterized by an immunologically induced inflammation of the lung parenchyma, which is due to intense or repeated inhalation of an organic agent or inorganic chemicals

DIAGNOSIS

- Clinical presentation varies depending on frequency and intensity of antigen exposure.
  - **Acute:** fever, cough, and dyspnea 4 to 6 hours after an intense exposure, lasting 18 to 24 hours
  - **Subacute:** insidious onset of productive cough, dyspnea on exertion, anorexia, and weight loss, usually from a heavy, sustained exposure
  - **Chronic:** gradually progressive cough, dyspnea, malaise, and weight loss, usually from low-grade or recurrent exposure
- Routine laboratory tests do not make the diagnosis, but typically the erythrocyte sedimentation rate, C-reactive protein, and leukocyte count are increased. The total IgG is elevated, and rheumatoid factor is often positive. Peripheral eosinophil count and serum IgE are generally normal.
- Pulmonary function tests typically show restrictive ventilatory patterns. Decreased forced expiratory volume in 1 second, decreased vital capacity, decreased diffusing capacity, and decreased static compliance are shown.
- Arterial blood gases show mild hypoxemia.
- Serum precipitin test is sensitive but not specific for HP (asymptomatic patients may have IgG antibodies in serum).
- Skin testing is unclear if helpful. Some clinicians believe it to be a safe, effective, and rapid procedure in the diagnosis and follow-up of patients with HP. Sensitivity is similar to that of the precipitin test, but the specificity is higher.
- Chest x-ray is nonspecific and may be normal in the early stage.
  - **Acute/subacute:** bilateral interstitial and alveolar nodular infiltrates in a patchy or homogeneous distribution. Apices often are spared.
  - **Chronic:** diffuse reticulonodular infiltrates and fibrosis. Honeycombing may develop.
- High-resolution chest CT scan has no pathognomonic features, but shows air-space and interstitial patterns in the acute and subacute stage. The chronic stage reveals honeycombing and bronchiectasis.
- **Diagnostic criteria:**

- **Major criteria:**
  - History of symptoms compatible with HP that seem to worsen within hours after antigen exposure
  - Confirmation of exposure to the offending agent by history, investigation of the environment, serum precipitin test, or bronchoalveolar lavage (BAL) antibody
  - Compatible changes on chest x-ray or high-resolution CT scan of the chest
  - BAL fluid lymphocytosis (if performed)
  - Compatible histologic changes by lung biopsy (if performed)
  - Positive natural challenge (reproduction of symptoms and laboratory abnormalities after exposure to the suspected environment) or by controlled inhalation challenge
- **Minor criteria:**
  - Basilar crackles
  - Decreased diffusion capacity
  - Arterial hypoxemia (either at rest or with exercise)

ETIOLOGY

- Numerous environmental agents, often encountered in occupational settings
- Common sources of antigens: "moldy" hay, silage, grain, or vegetables; bird droppings or feathers; low-molecular-weight chemicals (i.e., isocyanates), pharmaceutical products

TREATMENT

- Prednisone 0.5-1 mg/kg usually over 1 to 2 weeks, than tapered over 4 weeks. Glucocorticoids accelerate initial lung recovery but may have no long-term effect.

▬ Hypersplenism

Definition: Syndrome characterized by splenomegaly, cytopenia (decrease of one or more of the peripheral cell lines), and compensatory hyperplastic bone marrow

DIAGNOSIS

- Ultrasound is ordered to determine splenic size.
- CT or MRI is ordered to obtain structural information and rule out cysts, tumors, and infarcts.
- Complete blood count with differential shows neutrophilia (infection).
- Peripheral smear shows abnormal cells (malignancy, red blood cell [RBC] abnormalities) and organisms (bacteria, malaria, babesiosis).

_____ ...ematologic and infiltrative disorders.
- Tests to diagnose suspected cause of splenomegaly include liver
  function tests, hepatitis serology, HIV, rheumatoid factor, and antinuclear antibody. *Note:* RBC mass may be used to assess severity of
  anemia. If considering splenectomy secondary to severe anemia, RBC
  mass measurement differentiates true anemia (decrease in RBCs)
  from dilutional anemia (plasma volume expansion).

ETIOLOGY
- Splenomegaly increases the proportion of blood channeled through
  the red pulp, causing inappropriate splenic pooling of normal and
  abnormal blood cells. The size of the spleen determines the amount
  of cell sequestration. Ninety percent of platelets may be pooled in an
  enlarged spleen.
- Splenomegaly leads to increased destruction of RBCs. Platelets and
  white blood cells have about normal survival time even when
  sequestered and may be available if needed.
- Splenomegaly causes plasma volume expansion and exacerbates
  cytopenias by dilution.

TREATMENT
- Treat underlying disease.
- Splenectomy is considered for the following reasons:
  - Indicated for the management of the underlying cause
  - Persistent symptomatic disease (severe cytopenia) not responding
    to therapy
  - Necessary for diagnosis

CLINICAL PEARLS
- Thrombocytopenia is rarely of clinical consequence because of the
  ability to mobilize platelets slowly from the spleen if needed.
- Cytopenias are usually correctable with splenectomy; cell counts
  return to normal within a few weeks.

Hypertension

Definition: The Seventh Joint National Committee on Prevention, Detection, Evaluation, and Treatment of High Blood Pressure (JNC 7) classifies normal blood pressure in adults as <120 mm Hg systolic and <80 mm Hg diastolic. *Prehypertension* is defined as systolic blood pressure 120 to 139 mm Hg or diastolic blood pressure 80 to 89 mm Hg. *Stage 1 hypertension* is systolic blood pressure 140 to 159 mm Hg or diastolic blood pressure 90 to 99 mm Hg. *Stage 2 hypertension* is systolic blood pressure ≥160 mm Hg or diastolic blood pressure ≥100 mm Hg. *Malignant hypertension* is a potentially life-threatening condition that is secondary to elevated blood pressure. *Hypertensive emergencies* are situations that require rapid (within 1 hour) lowering of blood pressure to prevent end-organ damage. *Hypertensive urgencies* are significant blood pressure elevations that should be corrected within 24 hours of presentation.

DIAGNOSIS

- Physical examination may be normal except for the presence of hypertension.
- Laboratory tests include urinalysis, serum electrolytes, blood urea nitrogen, creatinine, fasting serum glucose, and lipid panel. If pheochromocytoma is suspected, 24-hour urine for metanephrines is warranted.
- On the ECG, check for presence of left ventricular hypertrophy with strain pattern.
- MRA or duplex ultrasound of the renal arteries should be ordered in suspected renovascular hypertension.

ETIOLOGY

- Essential (primary) hypertension (85%)
- Drug-induced or drug-related (5%)
- Renal hypertension (5%)
  - Renal parenchymal disease (3%)
  - Renovascular hypertension (<2%)
- Endocrine (4-5%)
  - Oral contraceptives (4%)
  - Primary aldosteronism (0.5%)
  - Pheochromocytoma (0.2%)
  - Cushing's syndrome and long-term steroid therapy (0.2%)
  - Hyperparathyroidism or thyroid disease (0.2%)
- Coarctation of the aorta (0.2%)

- **Lifestyle modifiications**
  - Lose weight if overweight.
  - Limit alcohol intake to ≤1 oz of ethanol per day in men or ≤0.5 oz in women.
  - Exercise (aerobic) regularly (at least 30 min/day, most days).
  - Reduce sodium intake to <100 mmol/day (<2.3 g of sodium).
  - Maintain adequate dietary potassium (>3500 mg/day) intake.
  - Stop smoking and reduce dietary saturated fat and cholesterol intake for overall cardiovascular health. Consume a diet rich in fruits and vegetables.
- **JNC 7 recommendations:**
  - Antihypertensive drug therapy should be initiated in patients with stage 1 hypertension. Diuretics or β-blockers are preferred for initial therapy because a reduction in morbidity and mortality has been shown and because of their lower cost.
  - Angiotensin-converting enzyme inhibitors, angiotensin receptor blockers, and calcium antagonists also are effective and generally well tolerated.
  - The choice of therapeutic agents in malignant hypertension varies with the cause. The initial goal of antihypertensive therapy is not to achieve a normal blood pressure, but rather to reduce the blood pressure gradually; cerebral hyperperfusion may occur if the mean blood pressure is lowered >40% in the initial 24 hours.
  - Nitroprusside is the drug of choice in hypertensive encephalopathy, hypertension and intracranial bleeding, malignant hypertension, hypertension and heart failure, and dissecting aortic aneurysm (used in combination with propranolol); its onset of action is immediate.
  - Fenoldopam is a newer vasodilator agent useful for the short-term (48 hours) management of severe hypertension when rapid but quickly reversible reduction of blood pressure is required.
  - Hypertensive urgencies can be treated effectively with oral clonidine 0.1 mg q20min (to a maximum of 0.8 mg); sedation is common.

Hyperthyroidism

Definition: Hypermetabolic state resulting from excess thyroid hormone

DIAGNOSIS
- **Clinical presentation:**
  - Patients with hyperthyroidism generally present with the following clinical manifestations: tachycardia, tremor, hyperreflexia, anxiety, irritability, emotional lability, panic attacks, heat intolerance, sweating, increased appetite, diarrhea, weight loss, and menstrual dysfunction (oligomenorrhea, amenorrhea). The presentation may be different in elderly patients.
  - Patients with Graves' disease may present with exophthalmos, lid retraction, and lid lag (Graves' ophthalmopathy). The following signs and symptoms of ophthalmopathy may be present: blurring of vision, photophobia, increased lacrimation, double vision, and deep orbital pressure. Clubbing of fingers associated with periosteal new bone formation in other skeletal areas (Graves' acropachy) and pretibial myxedema also may be noted.
- **Laboratory tests:**
  - Elevated free thyroxine
  - Elevated free triiodothyronine—generally not necessary for diagnosis
  - Low thyroid-stimulating hormone (TSH) (unless hyperthyroidism is a result of the rare hypersecretion of TSH from a pituitary adenoma)
  - Thyroid autoantibodies useful in selected cases to differentiate Graves' disease from toxic multinodular goiter (absent thyroid antibodies)
- **Imaging:**
  - Twenty-four-hour radioactive iodine (RAI) uptake is useful to distinguish hyperthyroidism from iatrogenic thyroid hormone synthesis (thyrotoxicosis factitia) and from thyroiditis.
  - An overactive thyroid shows increased uptake, whereas a normal underactive thyroid (iatrogenic thyroid ingestion, painless or subacute thyroiditis) shows normal or decreased uptake.
  - The RAI uptake results also vary with the etiology of the hyperthyroidism:
    - Graves' disease—increased homogeneous uptake
    - Multinodular goiter—increased heterogeneous uptake
    - Hot nodule—single focus of increased uptake

- Graves' disease (diffuse toxic goiter)—80% to 90% of all cases of hyperthyroidism
- Toxic multinodular goiter (Plummer's disease)
- Toxic adenoma
- Iatrogenic and factitious
- Transient hyperthyroidism (subacute thyroiditis, Hashimoto's thyroiditis)
- **Rare causes:** hypersecretion of TSH (e.g., pituitary neoplasms), struma ovarii, ingestion of large amount of iodine in a patient with preexisting thyroid hyperplasia or adenoma (Jod-Basedow phenomenon), hydatidiform mole, carcinoma of thyroid, amiodarone therapy

TREATMENT

- **Antithyroid drugs (thionamides):** Methimazole (Tapazole) inhibits thyroid hormone synthesis by blocking production of thyroid peroxidase. Adjunctive therapy to alleviate β-adrenergic symptoms of hyperthyroidism involves propranolol 20-40 mg PO q6h; dosage is increased gradually until symptoms are controlled.
- RAI is the treatment of choice for patients >21 years old and younger patients who have not achieved remission after 1 year of antithyroid drug therapy.
- Subtotal thyroidectomy is indicated in obstructing goiters, in any patient who refuses RAI and cannot be managed adequately with antithyroid medications (e.g., patients with toxic adenoma or toxic multinodular goiter), and in pregnant patients who cannot be managed adequately with antithyroid medication or develop side effects to them.

CLINICAL PEARL

- Elderly hyperthyroid patients may have only subtle signs (weight loss, tachycardia, fine skin, brittle nails). This form is known as *apathetic hyperthyroidism* and manifests with lethargy rather than hyperkinetic activity. An enlarged thyroid gland may be absent. Coexisting medical disorders (most commonly cardiac disease) also may mask the symptoms. These patients often have unexplained congestive heart failure or new-onset atrial fibrillation.

Hypoaldosteronism

Definition: Aldosterone deficiency or impaired aldosterone function

DIAGNOSIS

- **Initial laboratory tests:**
  - Increased potassium
  - Hyperchloremic metabolic acidosis (caused by the absence of hydrogen-secreting action of aldosterone)
  - Increased blood urea nitrogen and creatinine (secondary to renal disease)
  - Hyperglycemia (diabetes mellitus is common in these patients)
- **Workup:** Measurement of plasma renin activity after 4 hours of upright posture can differentiate hyporeninemic from hyperreninemic causes. Renin levels in the normal or low range identify cases that are renin-angiotensin dependent, whereas high renin levels identify cases that are renin-angiotensin independent. The diagnosis and etiology of hypoaldosteronism can be confirmed with the renin-aldosterone stimulation test:
  - Hyporeninemic hypoaldosteronism—low stimulated renin and aldosterone levels
  - End-organ refractoriness to aldosterone action—high stimulated renin and aldosterone levels
  - Adrenal gland abnormality—high stimulated renin and low aldosterone levels

ETIOLOGY

- **Hyporeninemic hypoaldosteronism (renin-angiotensin dependent):** decreased aldosterone production secondary to decreased renin production; the typical patient has renal disease secondary to various factors (e.g., diabetes mellitus, interstitial nephritis, multiple myeloma).
- **Hyperreninemic hypoaldosteronism (renin-angiotensin independent):** renin production by the kidneys is intact; the defect is in aldosterone biosynthesis or in the action of angiotensin II. Common causes of this form of hypoaldosteronism are medications (angiotensin-converting enzyme [ACE] inhibitors, heparin), lead poisoning, aldosterone enzyme defects, and severe illness.

TREATMENT

- Low-potassium diet with liberal sodium intake (at least 4 g of sodium chloride per day)
- Avoidance of ACE inhibitors and potassium-sparing diuretics

...cortisone 0.05-0.1 mg PO every morning in patients with aldosterone deficiency associated with deficiency of adrenal glucocorticoid hormones
- Furosemide 20-40 mg qd to correct hyperkalemia of hyporeninemic hypoaldosteronism

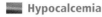 **Hypocalcemia**

Definition: Plasma calcium level <8.8 mg/dL

DIAGNOSIS
- **Laboratory tests:**
  - Serum albumin to rule out hypoalbuminemia
  - Blood urea nitrogen and creatinine to rule out renal failure
  - Serum magnesium to rule out severe hypomagnesemia
  - Serum PO_3^- and alkaline phosphatase to differentiate hypoparathyroidism from vitamin D deficiency
  - Serum parathyroid hormone (PTH) level by RIA should be ordered only if the diagnosis is uncertain with the preceding tests.
    - Markedly increased PTH—pseudohypoparathyroidism
    - Increased PTH—vitamin D deficiency
    - Decreased PTH—hypoparathyroidism
- **Clinical presentation:**
  - Neuromuscular irritability
    - *Chvostek's sign*—facial twitch after a gentle tapping over the facial nerve (can occur in 10-25% of normal adults)
    - *Trousseau's sign*—carpopedal spasm after inflation of blood pressure cuff above the patient's systolic blood pressure for 2 to 3 minutes
    - Tetany, paresthesias, myopathy, seizures, muscle spasm or weakness
  - Psychiatric disturbances—psychosis, depression, impaired cognitive function
  - Soft tissue calcifications, ocular cataracts
  - Cardiovascular—arrhythmias, congestive heart failure (caused by decreased myocardial contractility), increased Q-T interval, hypotension

ETIOLOGY
- **Renal insufficiency** hypocalcemia caused by
  - Increased calcium deposits in bone and soft tissue secondary to increased serum PO_4^- level

- Decreased production of 1,25-dihydroxyvitamin D
- Excessive loss of 25-hydroxyvitamin D (nephrotic syndrome)
- **Hypoalbuminemia:** Each decrease in serum albumin (g/L) decreases serum calcium by 0.8 mg/dL, but does not change free (ionized) calcium.
- **Vitamin D deficiency**
  - Inadequate intake
  - Malabsorption (most common cause)
  - Decreased production of 1,25-dihydroxyvitamin D (vitamin D–dependent rickets, renal failure)
  - Decreased production of 25-dihydroxyvitamin D (parenchymal liver disease)
  - Accelerated 25-hydroxyvitamin D catabolism (phenytoin, phenobarbital)
  - End-organ resistance to 1,25-dihydroxyvitamin D
- **Hypomagnesemia:** hypocalcemia caused by
  - Decreased PTH secretion
  - Inhibition of PTH effect on bone
- **Pancreatitis, hyperphosphatemia, osteoblastic metastases:** Hypocalcemia is secondary to increased calcium deposits (bone, abdomen).
- **Pseudohypoparathyroidism:** This autosomal recessive disorder is characterized by short stature, shortening of metacarpal bones, obesity, and mental retardation; the hypocalcemia is secondary to congenital end-organ resistance to PTH.
  - Idiopathic hypoparathyroidism, surgical removal of parathyroids (e.g., neck surgery)
  - **"Hungry bones syndrome":** rapid transfer of calcium from plasma into bones after removal of a parathyroid tumor
  - Sepsis
  - Massive blood transfusion (as a result of ethylenediamine tetraacetic acid in blood)

TREATMENT

- **Acute, severe symptomatic hypocalcemia caused by hypoparathyroidism or vitamin D deficiency** Give a slow intravenous bolus (over 15 minutes) of 10-30 mL of a 10% calcium gluconate solution followed by a infusion of 4 g of calcium gluconate in 500 mL of 5% dextrose in water over 4 hours (1 g calcium gluconate = 10 mL 10% calcium gluconate).
- **Hypoalbuminemia:**
  - Improve nutritional status.
  - Calcium replacement is not indicated because the free (ionized) calcium is normal.

correct the magnesium deficiency.

- Severe hypomagnesemia (serum magnesium level <0.8 mEq/L)—give 1 g (8 mEq) IV of a 10% magnesium sulfate solution slowly (over 15 minutes).
- Moderate-to-severe hypomagnesemia (serum magnesium level 0.8-1.3 mEq/L)—give one 2-mL ampule of a 50% magnesium solution intramuscularly; may repeat q4-6h.
- **Chronic hypocalcemia caused by hypoparathyroidism or vitamin D deficiency**
  - Calcium supplementation—give 1-4 g/day of elemental calcium (e.g., calcium carbonate 650 mg PO qid provides 1 g of elemental calcium/day).
  - Vitamin D replacement (e.g., calcitriol 0.25 μg/day)
- **Chronic hypocalcemia caused by renal failure:**
  - Reduction of hyperphosphatemia with phosphate-binding antacids
  - Vitamin D and oral calcium supplementation (as noted earlier)

▰ Hypoglycemia

Definition: Hypoglycemia can be defined arbitrarily as a plasma glucose level <50 mg/dL. To establish the diagnosis, the following three criteria are necessary:

- Presence of symptoms:
  - Adrenergic—sweating, anxiety, tremors, tachycardia, palpitations
  - Neuroglycopenic—seizures, fatigue, syncope, headache, behavior changes, visual disturbances, hemiplegia
- Low plasma glucose level in symptomatic patient
- Relief of symptoms after ingestion of carbohydrates

DIAGNOSIS

- In a normal person, when the plasma glucose level is low (e.g., fasting state), the plasma insulin level also is low. Any patient presenting with fasting hypoglycemia of unexplained cause should have the following tests drawn during the hypoglycemic episode:
  - Plasma insulin level and proinsulin level
  - C-peptide (connecting peptide)
  - Plasma and urine sulfonylurea levels
- Factitious hypoglycemia should be considered, especially if the patient has ready access to insulin or sulfonylureas (e.g., medical or paramedical personnel, family members who are diabetic or in the medical profession).

- To diagnose factitious hypoglycemia secondary to sulfonylureas, screen serum and urine to determine the presence of sulfonylureas.
- To diagnose factitious hypoglycemia secondary to insulin, the following tests may be obtained:

  Insulin level is markedly increased after exogenous insulin injection; proinsulin level is decreased.

  C-peptide levels are elevated in patients with insulinoma and sulfonylureas but not after exogenous insulin injection.
- Pancreatic islet cell neoplasms (insulinomas) are usually small (<3 cm), single, insulin-producing adenomas. Measurement of inappropriately elevated serum insulin levels despite an extremely low plasma glucose level after prolonged fasting (24-72 hours) is pathognomonic for these neoplasms.
- The insulinoma should be located by selective pancreatic arteriography and removed surgically.

ETIOLOGY

Reactive hypoglycemia:

- Hypoglycemia usually occurs 2 to 4 hours after a carbohydrate-rich meal.
- These patients never have symptoms in the fasting state and rarely experience loss of consciousness secondary to hypoglycemia.
- Patients who have had subtotal gastrectomy rapidly absorb carbohydrates, causing an early and very high plasma glucose level followed by a late insulin surge that reaches its peak when most of the glucose has been absorbed and that results in hypoglycemia.
- Type 2 (non—insulin-dependent) diabetics can experience hypoglycemia 3 to 4 hours postprandially secondary to a delayed and prolonged second phase of insulin secretion.
- Congenital deficiencies of enzymes necessary for carbohydrate metabolism and functional (idiopathic) hypoglycemia are additional causes of reactive hypoglycemia.

Fasting hypoglycemia:

- Symptoms usually appear in the absence of food intake (at night or during early morning).
- Etiologies include insulinoma, mesenchymal tumors that synthesize insulin-like hormones, adrenal failure, glycogen storage disorders, severe liver disease, and renal disease.
- **Iatrogenic or drug-induced:** hypoglycemic drugs, excessive insulin replacement, factitious, ethanol-induced hypoglycemia

- Treatment varies depending on etiology of hypoglycemia.

■ Hypokalemia

Definition: Plasma potassium concentration <3.3 mEq/L

DIAGNOSIS

- Distinguish true potassium depletion from redistribution (e.g., alkalosis, insulin administration).
- Measure 24-hour urinary potassium excretion while patient is receiving a regular dietary sodium intake.
  - <20 mEq—consider extrarenal potassium loss
  - >20 mEq—renal potassium loss
- If renal potassium wasting is suspected, the following steps are indicated:
  - Measure 24-hour urine chloride.
    - >10 mEq—diuretics, Bartter's syndrome, mineralocorticoid excess (chloride unresponsive)
    - <10 mEq—vomiting, gastric drainage (chloride responsive)
  - Measure blood pressure; if elevated, consider mineralocorticoid excess.
  - Measure serum HCO_3^-; a low level suggests renal tubular acidosis.
- ECG manifestations
  - Mild hypokalemia—flattening of T waves, ST segment depression, premature ventricular contractions, prolonged Q-T interval
  - Severe hypokalemia—prominent U waves, atrioventricular conduction disturbances, ventricular tachycardia or fibrillation

ETIOLOGY

- **Cellular shift (redistribution) and undetermined mechanisms:**
  - Alkalosis (each 0.1 increase in pH decreases serum potassium by 0.4-0.6 mEq/L)
  - Insulin administration
  - Vitamin B_{12} therapy for megaloblastic anemias, acute leukemias
  - Hypokalemic periodic paralysis—rare familial disorder manifested by recurrent attacks of flaccid paralysis and hypokalemia
  - β-Adrenergic agonists (e.g., terbutaline), decongestants, bronchodilators, theophylline, caffeine
  - Barium poisoning, toluene intoxication, verapamil intoxication, chloroquine intoxication
  - Correction of digoxin intoxication with digoxin antibody fragments (Digibind)

- **Increased renal excretion:**
  - Drugs—diuretics, including carbonic anhydrase inhibitors (e.g., acetazolamide), amphotericin B, high-dose sodium penicillin, nafcillin, ampicillin, carbenicillin, cisplatin, aminoglycosides, corticosteroids, mineralocorticoids, foscarnet sodium
  - Renal tubular acidosis—distal (type 1) or proximal (type 2)
  - Diabetic ketoacidosis, ureteroenterostomy
  - Magnesium deficiency
  - Postobstruction diuresis, diuretic phase of acute tubular necrosis
  - Osmotic diuresis (e.g., mannitol)
  - Bartter's syndrome—hyperplasia of juxtaglomerular cells leading to increased renin and aldosterone, metabolic alkalosis
  - Increased mineralocorticoid activity (primary or secondary aldosteronism), Cushing's syndrome
  - Chronic metabolic alkalosis from loss of gastric fluid (increased renal potassium secretion)
- **Gastrointestinal loss:** vomiting, nasogastric suction
  - **Diarrhea:**
  - Villous adenoma
  - Laxative abuse
  - Fistulas
  - Inadequate dietary intake (e.g., anorexia nervosa)
  - Cutaneous loss (excessive sweating)
  - High dietary sodium intake, excessive use of licorice

TREATMENT

- Institute potassium replacement.
  - Oral potassium replacement is preferred.
  - Intravenous infusion should not exceed 20 mEq/hr.
- Monitor ECG and urinary output.
- Identify underlying cause, and treat accordingly.
- Administer intravenous normal saline solution in chloride-responsive hypokalemia.

Hypomagnesemia

Definition: Plasma magnesium concentration <1.8 mg/dL.

DIAGNOSIS

- Laboratory tests include serum magnesium, phosphorus, calcium, electrolytes, blood urea nitrogen, creatinine, and glucose.
- Obtain 24-hour urine magnesium and creatinine values.

...clude prolonged Q-T interval, T wave flattening, prolonged P-R interval, atrial fibrillation, and torsades de pointes.

- **Clinical and laboratory manifestations:**
  - Neuromuscular—weakness, hyperreflexia, fasciculations, tremors, convulsions, delirium, coma
  - Cardiovascular—cardiac arrhythmias
  - Hypokalemia refractory to potassium replacement
  - Hypocalcemia refractory to calcium replacement

ETIOLOGY

- **Gastrointestinal and nutritional:**
  - Defective gastrointestinal absorption (malabsorption)
  - Inadequate dietary intake (e.g., alcoholics)
  - Parenteral therapy without magnesium
  - Chronic diarrhea, villous adenoma, prolonged nasogastric suction, fistulas (small bowel, biliary)
- **Excessive renal losses:**
  - Diuretics
  - Renal tubular acidosis
  - Diuretic phase of acute tubular necrosis
  - Endocrine disturbances (diabetic ketoacidosis, hyperaldosteronism, hyperthyroidism, hyperparathyroidism), syndrome of inappropriate secretion of antidiuretic hormone, Bartter's syndrome, hypercalciuria, hypokalemia
  - Cisplatin, alcohol, cyclosporine, digoxin, pentamidine, mannitol, amphotericin B, foscarnet, methotrexate
  - Antibiotics (gentamicin, ticarcillin, carbenicillin)
- **Redistribution:** hypoalbuminemia, cirrhosis, administration of insulin and glucose, theophylline, epinephrine, acute pancreatitis, cardiopulmonary bypass
- **Miscellaneous:** sweating, burns, prolonged exercise, lactation, "hungry bones" syndrome

TREATMENT

- Correct magnesium deficiency.
  - Mild—magnesium oxide 600 mg PO provides 35 mEq of magnesium; dosage is 1-2 tablets qd.
  - Moderate—50% solution magnesium sulfate (each 2-mL ampule contains 8 mEq or 96 mg of elemental magnesium); dosage is one 2-mL ampule of 50% magnesium solution q6h as needed.
  - Severe (serum magnesium level <1 mg/dL) and symptomatic patient (seizures, tetany)—2 g magnesium in 20 mL 5% dextrose in water (D5W) IV over 60 minutes; monitor ECG, blood pressure, pulse, respiration, deep tendon reflexes, and urinary output. An alternative regimen is the administration of 6 g of magnesium

sulfate (49 mEq) in 1000 mL of D5W over 3 hours, followed by 10 g of magnesium sulfate in 2000 mL of D5W over 24 hours.
- Identify and correct underlying disorder.

Hyponatremia

Definition: Plasma sodium concentration <134 mEq/L

DIAGNOSIS

- Serum electrolytes, blood urea nitrogen, creatinine, glucose, uric acid, serum osmolality, thyroid-stimulating hormone
- Urine sodium, urine osmolality

ETIOLOGY

- **Isovolemic:**
  - Syndrome of inappropriate secretion of antidiuretic hormone (SIADH)
    - Water intoxication (e.g., schizophrenic patients, primary polydipsia; sodium-free irrigant solutions, multiple tap-water enemas, dilute infant formulas). These entities are rare and often associated with a deranged antidiuretic hormone axis
    - Renal failure
    - Reset osmostat (e.g., chronic active tuberculosis, carcinomatosis)
    - Glucocorticoid deficiency (hypopituitarism)
    - Hypothyroidism
    - Thiazide diuretics, nonsteroidal antiinflammatory drugs, carbamazepine, amitriptyline, thioridazine, cyclophosphamide, colchicine, tolbutamide, chlorpropamide, angiotensin-converting enzyme inhibitors, clofibrate, oxytocin, selective serotonin reuptake inhibitors, amiodarone. With these medications, various drug-induced mechanisms are involved.
- **Hypovolemic:**
  - Renal losses—diuretics, partial urinary tract obstruction, salt-losing renal disease
  - Extrarenal losses—gastrointestinal (vomiting, diarrhea), extensive burns, third spacing (peritonitis, pancreatitis)
  - Adrenal insufficiency
- **Hypervolemic:**
  - Congestive heart failure
  - Nephrotic syndrome
  - Cirrhosis
  - Pregnancy
  - Isotonic hyponatremia (normal serum osmolality)

(increased serum lipids and serum proteins). Newer sodium assays eliminate this problem.

- Isotonic infusion (e.g., glucose, mannitol)
- Hypertonic hyponatremia (increased serum osmolality)
- Hyperglycemia—each 100 mg/dL increment in blood glucose above normal decreases plasma sodium concentration by 1.6 mEq/L
- Hypertonic infusions (e.g., glucose, mannitol)

TREATMENT

- **Isovolemic hyponatremia:**
  - SIADH—fluid restriction unless acutely symptomatic
  - Acute symptomatic patient—hypertonic 3% or 5% saline solution infusion; give 200-500 mL slowly, followed by fluid restriction to 750 mL/day for 24 to 48 hours. Hypertonic saline can be combined with furosemide to limit treatment-induced expansion of the extra-cellular fluid volume.
- **Hypovolemic hyponatremia:** 0.9% saline solution infusion
- **Hypervolemic hyponatremia:** sodium and water restriction. The combination of captopril and furosemide is effective in patients with hyponatremia resulting from congestive heart failure.
- **Chronic hyponatremia:** Correction of chronic hyponatremia should be kept at a rate <10 mEq/L (mmol/L) in any 24-hour period to prevent myelinolysis, a neurologic disorder that can occur after rapid correction of hyponatremia. Initially named *central pontine myelinolysis*, this disease now is known also to affect extrapontine brain areas. Manifestations of myelinolysis usually evolve several days after correction of hyponatremia. Typical features are disorders of upper motor neurons, spastic quadriparesis and pseudobulbar palsy, and mental disorders ranging from mild confusion to coma. Death may occur. The motor and localizing signs of myelinolysis differ from the generalized encephalopathy that is caused by untreated hyponatremia.

CLINICAL PEARLS

- Generally the serum sodium should be corrected only halfway to normal in the initial 24 hours (but not >1 mEq/L/hr) to prevent complications from rapid correction (cerebral edema, myelinolysis, seizures). A slower correction rate is indicated in patients with chronic hyponatremia.
- In symptomatic patients with hyponatremia, an increase in the serum sodium concentration of 2 mEq/L/hr to a level of 120 to 130 mEq/L is considered safe by some experts; however, less rapid correction may be indicated in patients with severe or chronic hyponatremia.

Hypophosphatemia

Definition: Plasma phosphate concentration <2.5 mg/dL

DIAGNOSIS
- Serum phosphate, calcium, glucose, electrolytes, blood urea nitrogen, creatinine
- Twenty-four-hour urine phosphate, creatinine

ETIOLOGY
- Decreased intake (prolonged starvation [alcoholics], hyperalimentation, or intravenous infusion without phosphorus)
- Malabsorption
- Phosphate-binding antacids
- **Renal loss:**
  - Renal tubular acidosis
  - Fanconi syndrome, vitamin D–resistant rickets
  - Acute tubular necrosis (diuretic phase)
  - Hyperparathyroidism (primary or secondary)
  - Familial hypophosphatemia
  - Hypokalemia, hypomagnesemia
  - Acute volume expansion
  - Glycosuria, idiopathic hypercalciuria
  - Acetazolamide
- **Transcellular shift into cells:**
  - Alcohol withdrawal
  - Diabetic ketoacidosis (recovery phase)
  - Glucose-insulin or catecholamine infusion
  - Anabolic steroids
  - Total parenteral nutrition
  - Theophylline overdose
  - Severe hyperthermia; recovery from hypothermia
  - "Hungry bones" syndrome

TREATMENT
- Mild-to-moderate hypophosphatemia (>1 mg/dL)—Neutra-Phos capsules (250 mg per capsule) 2 capsules tid
- Severe symptomatic hypophosphatemia (<1 mg/dL)—intravenous administration of phosphate salts (0.08-0.16 mmol/kg over 6 hours) repeated every 6 hours until serum phosphate level is >1.5 mg/dL

hypothermia

Definition: *Hypothermia* is a rectal temperature <35°C (95.8°F). *Accidental hypothermia* is an unintentionally induced decrease in core temperature in the absence of preoptic anterior hypothalamic conditions.

DIAGNOSIS

- The clinical presentation varies with the severity of hypothermia. Shivering may be absent if body temperature is <33.3°C (92°F) or in patients taking phenothiazines.
- Hypothermia may masquerade as cerebrovascular accident, ataxia, or slurred speech, or the patient may appear comatose or clinically dead.
- Physiologic stages of hypothermia are as follows:
  - **Mild hypothermia (32.2-35°C [90-95°F]):** arrhythmias, ataxia
  - **Moderate hypothermia (28-32.2°C [82.4-90°F]):** progressive decrease of level of consciousness, pulse, cardiac output, and respiration; fibrillation, dysrhythmias (increased susceptibility to ventricular tachycardia); elimination of shivering mechanism for thermogenesis
  - **Severe hypothermia (≤28°C [82.4°F]):** absence of reflexes or response to pain, decreased cerebral blood flow, decreased carbon dioxide, increased risk of ventricular fibrillation or asystole
- Laboratory tests show the following: Metabolic and respiratory acidosis are usually present. K^+ is decreased initially, then increases with increasing hypothermia; extreme hyperkalemia indicates a poor prognosis. Decreased hematocrit is caused by hemoconcentration. Leukocytes and platelets (caused by splenic sequestration) are decreased. Clotting time is increased.
- Chest x-ray generally is not helpful; it may reveal evidence of aspiration (e.g., intoxicated patient with aspiration pneumonia).
- ECG may show prolonged P-R, Q-T, and QRS segments; depressed ST segments; inverted T waves; atrioventricular block; and hypothermic J waves (Osborn waves) at <28°C (82.4°F). The ECG is characterized by notching of the junction of the QRS complex and ST segments.

TREATMENT

- Secure an airway before warming all unconscious patients; precede endotracheal intubation with oxygenation (if possible) to minimize the risk of arrhythmias during the procedure.
- Peripheral vasoconstriction may impede placement of a peripheral intravenous catheter; consider femoral venous access as an alternative to the jugular or subclavian sites to avoid ventricular stimulation.

- A Foley catheter should be inserted, and urinary output should be monitored and maintained >0.5 to 1 mL/kg/hr with intravascular volume replacement.
- Continuous ECG monitoring of patients is recommended; ventricular arrhythmias can be treated with bretylium; lidocaine is generally ineffective, and procainamide is associated with an increased incidence of ventricular fibrillation in hypothermic patients.
- Correct severe acidosis and electrolyte abnormalities.
- Hypothyroidism, if present, should be treated promptly (see "Myxedema Coma").
- If clinical evidence suggests adrenal insufficiency, administer intravenous methylprednisolone.
- In patients unresponsive to verbal or noxious stimuli or with altered mental status, 100 mg of thiamine, 0.4 mg of naloxone, and 1 ampule of 50% dextrose may be given.
- Warm (40-45°C [104-113°F]), humidified oxygen also should be given if it is available.
- **Specific treatment**
  - **Mild hypothermia (rectal temperature <32.3°C [90°F]:**
    Passive external rewarming is indicated. Place the patient in a warm room (temperature >21°C [69.8°F]), and cover with insulating material after gently removing wet clothing; recommended rewarming rates vary from 0.5°C/hr to 20°C/hr, but should not exceed 0.55°C/hr in elderly persons.
  - **Moderate-to-severe hypothermia:** Deliver heat via fluids, including warm gastrointestinal irrigation (with saline enemas and via nasogastric tube), intravenous fluids (usually 5% dextrose in normal saline without potassium) warmed to 40°C to 42°C (104-107.6°F), and peritoneal dialysis with dialysate heated to 40°C to 42°C (104 to 107.6°F), and inhalation of heated humidified oxygen. Consider immersion in a bath of warm water (40°C [104°F]); active external rewarming may produce shock because of excessive peripheral vasodilation. Ideal candidates are previously healthy, young patients with acute immersion hypothermia. Extracorporeal blood warming with cardiopulmonary bypass seems to be an efficacious rewarming technique in young, otherwise healthy persons.

Definition: Disorder caused by the inadequate secretion of thyroid hormone

DIAGNOSIS
- **Clinical presentation:**
  - Skin—dry, coarse, thick, cool, sallow (yellow color caused by carotenemia); nonpitting edema in skin of eyelids and hands (myxedema) secondary to infiltration of subcutaneous tissues by a hydrophilic mucopolysaccharide substance
  - Hair—brittle and coarse; loss of outer one third of eyebrows
  - Facies—dulled expression, thickened tongue, thick slow-moving lips
  - Thyroid gland—may or may not be palpable (depending on the cause of the hypothyroidism)
  - Heart sounds—distant, possible pericardial effusion
  - Pulse—bradycardia
  - Neurologic—delayed relaxation phase of the deep tendon reflexes, cerebellar ataxia, hearing impairment, poor memory, peripheral neuropathies with paresthesia
  - Musculoskeletal—carpal tunnel syndrome, muscular stiffness, weakness
- **Laboratory tests:**
  - Increased thyroid-stimulating hormone (TSH)—TSH may be normal if the patient has secondary or tertiary hypothyroidism, the patient is receiving dopamine or corticosteroids, or the level is obtained after severe illness
  - Decreased free thyroxine (T_4)
  - Other common laboratory abnormalities—hyperlipidemia, hyponatremia, and anemia
  - Increased antimicrosomal and antithyroglobulin antibody titers—useful when autoimmune thyroiditis is suspected as the cause of hypothyroidism

ETIOLOGY
- **Primary hypothyroidism (thyroid gland dysfunction):** The cause of >90% of the cases of hypothyroidism
  - Hashimoto's thyroiditis—the most common cause of hypothyroidism after 8 years of age
  - Idiopathic myxedema—nongoitrous form of Hashimoto's thyroiditis
  - Previous treatment of hyperthyroidism (radioactive iodine therapy, subtotal thyroidectomy)

- Subacute thyroiditis
- Radiation therapy to the neck (usually for malignant disease)
- Iodine deficiency or excess
- Drugs (lithium, aminosalicylic acid, sulfonamides, phenylbutazone, amiodarone, thiourea)
- Congenital—approximately 1 case per 4000 live births
- Prolonged treatment with iodides
- **Secondary hypothyroidism:** pituitary dysfunction, postpartum necrosis, neoplasm, infiltrative disease causing deficiency of TSH
- **Tertiary hypothyroidism:** hypothalamic disease (granuloma, neoplasm, or irradiation causing deficiency of thyrotropin-releasing hormone)
- **Tissue resistance to thyroid hormone:** rare

TREATMENT

- Start replacement therapy with levothyroxine 25-100 µg/day, depending on the patient's age and the severity of the disease. The dose may be increased every 6 to 8 weeks, depending on the clinical response and serum TSH level. Elderly patients and patients with coronary artery disease should be started with 12.5-25 µg/day (higher doses may precipitate angina).

CLINICAL PEARLS

- Periodic monitoring of TSH level is an essential part of treatment. The patient should be evaluated initially with office visit and TSH levels every 6 to 8 weeks until the patient is clinically euthyroid and the TSH level is normalized.
- For monitoring therapy in patients with central hypothyroidism, measurement of serum free T_4 level is appropriate and should be maintained in the upper half of the normal range.
- Pregnant patients also have increased requirements. Women with hypothyroidism should increase levothyroxine dose by approximately 30% as soon as pregnancy is confirmed.

Immune thrombocytopenic purpura (ITP)

Definition: Autoimmune disorder characterized by a low platelet count and mucocutaneous bleeding

DIAGNOSIS

- **Clinical presentation:** The presentation of ITP is different in

petechiae from severe thrombocytopenia

- In adults, the presentation is insidious. A history of prolonged purpura may be present. Many patients are diagnosed incidentally on the basis of automated laboratory tests that now routinely include platelet counts.
- The physical examination may be normal.
- Patients with severe thrombocytopenia may have petechiae, purpura, epistaxis, or heme-positive stool from gastrointestinal bleeding.
- Splenomegaly is unusual; its presence should alert to the possibility of other etiologies of ITP.
- The presence of dysmorphic features (skeletal anomalies, auditory abnormalities) may indicate a congenital disorder as the etiology of ITP.
- **Laboratory tests:**
  - Order complete blood count, platelet count, and peripheral smear. Platelets are decreased but are normal in size or may appear larger than normal. Red blood cells and white blood cells have a normal morphology.
  - Additional tests may be ordered to exclude other etiologies of thrombocytopenia when clinically indicated (e.g., HIV, antinuclear antibody, thyroid-stimulating hormone, liver enzymes, bone marrow examination).
  - The direct assay for the measurement of platelet-bound antibodies has an estimated positive predictive value of 80% to 83%. A negative test cannot be used to rule out the diagnosis.
- **Imaging:** Obtain CT scan of abdomen in patients with splenomegaly to exclude other disorders causing thrombocytopenia.

ETIOLOGY

- Increased platelet destruction caused by autoantibodies to platelet-membrane antigens

TREATMENT

- Treatment varies with the platelet count, patient's age, and bleeding status.
- Observation and frequent monitoring of platelet count are needed in asymptomatic patients with platelet counts >30,000/mm^3.
- Methylprednisolone 30 mg/kg/day IV infused over 20 to 30 minutes (maximum dose 1 g/day for 2-3 days) plus intravenous immunoglobulin 1 g/kg/day for 2 to 3 days and infusion of platelets should be given to patients with neurologic symptoms, patients with internal bleeding, and patients undergoing emergency surgery.

- Prednisone 1-2 mg/kg qd, continued until the platelet count is normalized, then slowly tapered, is indicated in adults with platelet counts <20,000/mm³ and adults who have platelet counts <50,000/mm³ and significant mucous membrane bleeding. Response rates range from 50% to 75%, and most responses occur within the first 3 weeks.
- High-dose immunoglobulins (IgG 0.4 g/kg/day IV infused on 3-5 consecutive days) or high-dose parenteral glucocorticoids (methylprednisolone 30 mg/kg/day) are used in children with platelet counts <20,000/mm³ and significant bleeding or adults with severe thrombocytopenia or bleeding.
- Rituximab, a monoclonal antibody directed against the CD20 antigen, has been reported useful for ITP patients resistant to conventional treatment and may help prevent serious or fatal bleeding.
- Platelet transfusion is needed only in case of life-threatening hemorrhage.

CLINICAL PEARL

- Splenectomy should be considered in adults with platelet counts <30,000/mm³ after 6 weeks of medical treatment or after 6 months if <10-20 mg of prednisone per day is required to maintain a platelet count <30,000/mm³. In children, splenectomy generally is reserved for persistent thrombocytopenia (<1 year) and clinically significant bleeding. Appropriate immunizations (pneumococcal vaccine in adults and children, Haemophilus influenzae vaccine and meningococcal vaccine in children) should be administered before splenectomy.

Impetigo

Definition: Superficial skin infection generally secondary to Staphylococcus aureus or Streptococcus or both

DIAGNOSIS

- Multiple lesions with golden yellow crusts and weeping areas often are found on the skin around the nose, mouth, and limbs (nonbullous impetigo).
- Vesicles are present that enlarge rapidly to form bullae with contents that vary from clear to cloudy. There is subsequent collapse of the center of the lesion. The peripheral areas may retain fluid, and a honey-colored crust may appear in the center. As the lesions enlarge and become contiguous with the others, a scaling border replaces the fluid-filled rim (bullous impetigo). There is minimal erythema

- **S. aureus coagulase positive:** the dominant microorganism
- **Streptococcus pyogenes (group A beta-hemolytic strepto-cocci):** M-T serotypes of this organism associated with acute nephritis are 2, 49, 55, 57, and 60

TREATMENT
- Remove crusts by soaking with wet cloth compresses (crusts block the penetration of antibacterial creams).
- Apply 2% mupirocin ointment (Bactroban) three times daily for 10 days to the affected area or until all lesions have cleared.
- Oral antibiotics are used in severe cases. Commonly used agents are dicloxacillin 250 mg qid for 7 to 10 days, cephalexin 250 mg qid for 7 to 10 days, or azithromycin 500 mg on day 1 and 250 mg on days 2 through 5.

CLINICAL PEARLS
- Impetigo can be prevented by prompt application of mupirocin or triple antibiotic ointment (bacitracin, polymyxin B/bacitracin [Polysporin], and neomycin) to sites of skin trauma.
- Patients who are carriers of S. aureus in their nares should be treated with mupirocin ointment applied to the nares twice daily for 5 days.
- Fingernails should be kept short, and patients should be advised not to scratch any lesions to avoid spread of infection.

■ Inclusion body myositis

Definition: Inflammatory myopathy with distinctive clinical and pathologic features

DIAGNOSIS
- **Physical findings and clinical presentation:**
  - Onset is insidious (>6 years from the onset of symptoms to diagnosis).
  - Steadily progressive asymmetric and painless muscle weakness and atrophy occur affecting the finger or wrist flexors (commonly the flexor pollicis longus), knee extensor (quadriceps), and foot dorsiflexion. Over time, weakness spreads to involve other muscles.
  - A common complaint is difficulty with ambulation and frequent falls (due to buckling of knees caused by knee extensor weakness).
  - Fatigue and reduced tolerance of exertion are common.
  - Dysphagia is common (60%).

- Classic appearance is a scooped-out medial aspect of forearms and thin, atrophic quadriceps muscles.
- Facial and neck weakness can be seen.
- Early loss of patellar reflexes occurs.
- **Workup:**
  - **Electromyography:** Active myopathic changes (fibrillation potentials; positive sharp waves; and short-duration, low-amplitude, polyphasic motor unit action potentials) are seen. Mixed myopathic and neurogenic changes also can be seen.
  - **Nerve conduction studies:** Occasionally sensory nerve conduction studies are abnormal (if there is an associated neuropathy).
  - **Muscle biopsy:** Findings include small angular atrophic and denervated fibers, CD8 cytotoxic T-cell endomysial infiltration, and intracytoplasmic rimmed vacuoles and cytoplasmic tubofilamentous inclusions on electromicrosopic examination of the affected muscle fiber.
- **Laboratory tests:**
  - Creatine phosphokinase (normal to increased 3-5 times normal)
  - Thyroid function test to rule out thyroid disease
  - Antinuclear antibody, rheumatoid factor, double-stranded DNA, erythrocyte sedimentation rate, scl-70, anti-Ro, and anti-La to rule out other autoimmune diseases

TREATMENT

- Corticosteroids, cyclophosphamide, chlorambucil, azathioprine, cyclosporine, methotrexate, and intravenous immunoglobulin have been used, but without evidence of benefit.
- Intravenous immunoglobulin might provide some benefit for patients with dysphagia.
- Interferon beta has been used, but further studies are needed.
- Oxandrolone (a synthetic anabolic steroid) use resulted in muscle strength improvement, but further studies are needed.
- A several-month trial of prednisone (0.6 mg/kg) is usually recommended.
- Exercise therapy includes isotonic training program of weak muscles.
- Nutritional assessment is indicated if dysphagia is present.

Definition: A chronic disorder of the gastrointestinal tract of undetermined etiology. IBD encompasses numerous chronic relapsing inflammatory disorders of the gastrointestinal tract. Classically IBD can be subdivided into two major groups:

• Crohn's disease
• Ulcerative colitis or proctitis

DIAGNOSIS

• Endoscopic examination to establish the presence of mucosal inflammation is the primary means of diagnosing IBD.
• Laboratory tests may reveal anemia, hypoalbuminemia, vitamin B_{12} deficiency, folate deficiency (more common in Crohn's disease), and electrolyte abnormalities.

TREATMENT

• **Medical therapy:**
  ◦ Avoid oral feedings during acute exacerbation to decrease colonic activity; a low-roughage diet may be helpful in *early* relapse. Total parenteral nutrition (TPN) with bowel rest may be necessary in severe cases.
  ◦ Aminosalicylates are the primary therapies for mild-to-moderate IBD. These agents should be selected principally on the basis of disease location.
    ▫ Sulfasalazine (Azulfidine) is the oldest, least expensive, and least tolerated of the 5-aminosalicylic acid (ASA) compounds. It is effective in ulcerative colitis and in Crohn's disease confined to the colon; dosage is 500 mg PO bid initially, increased as tolerated until therapeutic dosages of 4-6 g/day are achieved. Patients with sulfa allergies should avoid sulfasalazine. Folate supplementation is recommended because sulfasalazine inhibits folate absorption.
    ▫ Mesalamine (Rowasa) is useful for mild-to-moderate ulcerative colitis/proctitis. It can be administered as an enema (40 mg once daily at bedtime for 3-6 weeks) and suppository (500 mg bid) for patients with distal colonic disease. Oral forms in which the 5-ASA is in a slow-release or pH-dependent matrix (mesalamine [Pentasa 1 g PO qid and Asacol 800 mg PO tid]) can deliver therapeutic concentrations to the more proximal small bowel or distal ileum, and although they are approved for the treatment of ulcerative colitis, they often also are used for Crohn's disease.

- Olsalazine (Dipentum) is useful for maintenance of remission of ulcerative colitis in patients intolerant to sulfasalazine. Usual dose is 500 mg bid taken with food.

- Balsalazide (Colazal) is indicated for mild to moderately active ulcerative colitis. Usual dose is three 750-mg capsules tid.

- Corticosteroids are commonly used when 5-ASA compounds are inadequate. They can be administered orally, rectally, or intravenously. Oral corticosteroids are useful for outpatient therapy of moderately severe ulcerative colitis. Methylprednisolone or prednisone (e.g., prednisone 40-60 mg/day) steroid-retention enemas may be useful in patients with ulcerative colitis limited to the rectum and accompanied by severe tenesmus. Hydrocortisone 100 mg IV q6h is useful for remission induction therapy in acute severe ulcerative colitis.

- Steroid analogues are locally active corticosteroids that target specific areas of inflammation in the gastrointestinal tract. Budesonide (Entocort EC) is available as a controlled-ileal-release formulation and is approved for mild to moderately active Crohn's disease involving the ileum or ascending colon or both. Adult dose is 9 mg qd for maximum of 8 weeks.

- The immunosuppressants azathioprine (Imuran) and its active metabolite mercaptopurine (Purinethol) can be used in patients with severe IBD that is refractory to the preceding measures or in whom the corticosteroid dose cannot be tapered or discontinued. They are not useful for induction therapy (effectiveness is not evident for several weeks). Methotrexate is effective for the treatment of Crohn's disease, particularly when attempting to taper off steroids. It is used long-term in patients who do not respond to or cannot tolerate azathioprine or mercaptopurine in patients with Crohn's disease who enter remission after treatment with methotrexate, a low dose of methotrexate (15 mg IM weekly) is effective in maintaining remission. Folic acid 1 mg/day should be given to all patients receiving methotrexate.

- The antibiotics metronidazole and ciprofloxacin are effective in treating perianal complications in patients with active Crohn's disease (e.g., perianal fistulas).

- Intravenous cyclosporine blocks lymphocyte activation and is useful for the treatment of severe ulcerative colitis in hospitalized patients Cyclosporine usually is added after an initial 7- to 10-day trial of intravenous corticosteroids. Prophylaxis against *Pneumocystis carinii* pneumonia is advised in all patients taking cyclosporine.

...nal antibody targeting tumor necrosis factor-α, can induce clinical improvement in 80% of patients with Crohn's disease refractory to other agents. It also is effective in promoting closure of fistulas. Its mechanism of action is incompletely understood. It is very costly. A purified protein derivative test should be done before using infliximab.

- Natalizumab, a selective adhesion-molecule inhibitor, has been reported to be effective in increasing the rate of remission and response in active Crohn's disease.
- Erythropoietin is useful in patients with anemia refractory to treatment with iron and vitamins.

- **Treatment of complications:**
  - Fulminant colitis or toxic megacolon (midtransverse colon ≥6 cm in diameter)
    - Intravenous corticosteroids
    - Broad-spectrum intravenous antibiotics (e.g., cefoxitin plus gentamicin)
    - Vigorous intravenous hydration, correction of any electrolyte abnormalities, and TPN
    - Nasogastric suction
    - Correct anemia and metabolic and nutritional abnormalities
    - Surgical intervention if there is no marked improvement with preceding measures
  - Anal fistulas and other perineal diseases
    - Intravenous metronidazole (Flagyl) 20 mg/kg/day in divided doses
    - Surgical repair
    - Extensive bowel resection if patient develops recurrent retrovaginal or rectovesicular fistulas
  - Intestinal obstruction
    - Nasogastric suction
    - Intravenous hydration
    - Intravenous steroids and intravenous antibiotics
    - Surgical intervention if no improvement
  - Abscess formation
    - Intravenous antibiotics
    - Intravenous steroids
    - Intravenous hydration
- **Surgical therapy:** Surgery is indicated in patients with ulcerative colitis who fail to respond to intensive medical therapy. Proctocolectomy with end ileostomy is usually curative in these patients, and it eliminates the high risk of developing adenocarcinoma of the colon (10-20% of patients develop adenocarcinoma after 10 years with the

disease). Newer surgical techniques allow for preservation of the sphincter. In Crohn's disease, surgery generally is not curative (postoperative recurrence rate >50%); it is generally reserved for treatment of severe complications (e.g. intractable recurrent rectovaginal or rectovesicular fistulas or intractable obstruction).

CLINICAL PEARLS

Psychotherapy is useful for situational adjustment crises. A trusting and mutually understanding relationship and referral to self-help groups are crucial because of the chronicity of IBD and the relatively young age of the patients.

Because of the increased risk of colon carcinoma, colonoscopic surveillance and multiple biopsies should be instituted approximately 10 years after diagnosis in all patients with IBD.

Interstitial nephritis

Definition: Group of disorders primarily affecting the interstitium and renal tubules; interstitial nephritis may be acute or chronic

DIAGNOSIS

- Renal biopsy is the only definitive method of establishing the diagnosis of interstitial nephritis. All other laboratory tests provide supportive evidence of interstitial nephritis.
- Complete blood count shows anemia and eosinophilia.
- Blood urea nitrogen and creatinine are elevated and typically represent the first clue of interstitial nephritis.
- Urinalysis reveals hematuria and pyuria.
- Eosinophiluria by Hansen stain suggests allergic interstitial nephritis.
- Proteinuria <3 g/24 hr
- Renal biopsy in acute interstitial nephritis reveals infiltration of inflammatory cells into the interstitium with interstitial edema and sparing of the glomeruli. In chronic interstitial nephritis, fibrotic scar tissue replaces the cellular infiltrate.
- Ultrasound of the kidneys shows normal size kidneys in acute interstitial nephritis and small, contracted kidneys in chronic interstitial nephritis.

- **Clinical presentation:**
  - **Acute interstitial nephritis:**
    Patients usually asymptomatic and found to have a sudden decrease in renal function

infection or initiation of a new medication

- Classic triad—fever, rash, and arthralgias
- Lumbar flank pain
- Gross hematuria
- Usually oliguric

- **Chronic interstitial nephritis:**
  - Usually present with symptoms related to the underlying cause (e.g., sarcoidosis, multiple myeloma, urate nephropathy)
  - Symptoms of renal failure (e.g., weakness, nausea, pruritus)
  - Hypertension

ETIOLOGY

- Acute interstitial nephritis usually is caused by drugs or infection or is associated with immune or neoplastic disorders.
- Common drugs include penicillin, methicillin, rifampin, cephalosporins, trimethoprim-sulfamethoxazole, ciprofloxacin, non-steroidal antiinflammatory drugs, thiazides, furosemide, triamterene, allopurinol, phenytoin, captopril, and cimetidine.
- Infective organisms include *Streptococcus*, *Legionella*, *Corynebacterium diphtheriae*, *Yersinia*, *Salmonella*, HIV, Epstein-Barr virus, cytomegalovirus, *Mycoplasma*, *Rickettsia*, and *Mycobacterium tuberculosis*.
- Autoimmune causes of acute interstitial nephritis include Sjögren's syndrome, systemic lupus erythematosus, and Wegener's granulomatosis.
- Common causes of chronic interstitial nephritis include polycystic kidney disease, urate nephropathy, analgesic nephropathy, sarcoidosis, multiple myeloma, lead nephropathy, hypercalcemia, and Balkan nephropathy.

TREATMENT

- Treat with low-protein, low-potassium, low-sodium diet; correction of underlying electrolyte abnormalities; and intravenous hydration for hypercalcemia.
- Corticosteroids 1 mg/kg/day are used in patients with drug-induced acute interstitial nephritis not responding to withdrawal of the medication within 3 to 4 days. Therapy is continued for 4 to 6 weeks.
- Cyclophosphamide 2 mg/kg/day is added as a second agent for patients not responding to corticosteroids.
- Combined therapy is continued for 6 weeks.
- Treatment of chronic interstitial nephritis is directed at the underlying cause (e.g., corticosteroids for sarcoidosis, ethylenediamine tetraacetic acid in lead nephropathy).

- Other therapeutic measures include blood pressure control and reducing uric acid and calcium levels if indicated.

Irritable bowel syndrome (IBS)

Definition: Chronic functional disorder manifested by alteration in bowel habits and recurrent abdominal pain and bloating. The modified ROME criteria define IBS as the presence of ≥12 weeks of continuous or recurrent abdominal pain or discomfort that cannot be explained by structural or biochemical abnormalities and the presence of at least two of the following three features:

- Pain is relieved with defecation.
- Onset of pain is associated with a change in the frequency of bowel movement.
- Onset of pain is associated with a change in the form of the stool.

DIAGNOSIS

- The clinical presentation of IBS consists of abdominal pain and abnormalities of defecation, which may include loose stools usually after meals and in the morning, alternating with episodes of constipation. Diagnostic workup is aimed primarily at excluding the conditions listed in the differential diagnosis. It is important to identify "red flags" of other diseases, such as weight loss, rectal bleeding, onset in patients 50 years old, fever, nocturnal pain, and family history of malignancy.
- The criteria for diagnosis of IBS are >3 months of symptoms *including* abdominal pain that is relieved by a bowel movement, *or* pain accompanied by a change in bowel pattern, *and* abnormality in bowel movement 25% of the time, characterized by the following features:
  - Abdominal distention
  - Abnormal consistency
  - Abnormal defecation (e.g., straining, sense of incomplete evacuation)
  - Abnormal frequency
  - Mucus with bowel movement

TREATMENT

- The patient should be encouraged to maintain a high-fiber diet and to eliminate foods that aggravate symptoms. Avoidance of dietary caffeine and dietary excesses is helpful.
- Behavioral therapy is recommended, particularly in younger patients if social stressors are important triggers of IBS.

be stressed.

- Patients should be instructed that there might be some increased bloating on initiation of fiber supplementation, which should resolve within 2 to 3 weeks. It is important that patients take these fiber products on a regular basis and not only as needed.
- Antispasmodics-anticholinergics may be useful in refractory cases (e.g., dicyclomine [Bentyl] 10-20 mg tid).
- Patients who appear anxious can benefit from use of sedatives and anticholinergics, such as chlordiazepoxide-clidinium (Librax) or selective serotonin reuptake inhibitors. Tricyclic antidepressants in low doses also are effective in some patients with IBS.
- Loperamide is effective for diarrhea. Alosetron (Lotronex), a serotonin type 3 receptor antagonist previously withdrawn because of severe constipation and ischemic colitis, has been reintroduced with limited availability. It is indicated only for women with severe chronic, diarrhea-predominant IBS unresponsive to conventional therapy and not due to anatomic or metabolic abnormality. Starting dose is 1 mg qd.
- Tegaserod (Zelnorm), a 5-HT$_4$ receptor partial agonist, increases gastrointestinal motility and can be used to relieve symptoms in patients whose predominant symptom is constipation. Usual dose is 2-6 mg PO bid before meals. Tegaserod is contraindicated in patients with severe renal insufficiency, moderate-to-severe hepatic impairment, intestinal adhesions, or a history of bowel obstruction.

Korsakoff's psychosis

Definition: A disorder of learning and memory, out of proportion to other cognitive functions, associated with thiamine deficiency. It is classically seen in alcoholics and may follow the presentation of Wernicke's encephalopathy.

DIAGNOSIS
- There is impairment of ability to remember new material.
- Remote memory is said to be retained, but is almost universally diminished on careful testing.
- Confabulation may occur.
- Serum pyruvate is elevated.
- Whole blood or erythrocyte transketolase are decreased; there is rapid resolution to normal in 24 hours with thiamine repletion.
- MRI may show diencephalic and mesencephalic lesions acutely, but there is no definitive radiologic study for diagnosis.

ETIOLOGY
- Thiamine deficiency, commonly in alcoholics or other malnourished populations, although it may be iatrogenic from prolonged infusion of dextrose-containing fluids without thiamine repletion

TREATMENT
- Thiamine 100 mg IV or IM should be given immediately. Typical duration of intravenous treatment is 3 to 5 days.
- Thiamine given acutely during Wernicke's phase (disorders of extraocular movements, confusion, and ataxia) may prevent the development of Korsakoff's psychosis.

▪ Labyrinthitis

Definition: A peripheral vestibulopathy characterized by acute onset of vertigo usually associated with nausea and vomiting; it may or may not be associated with hearing loss

DIAGNOSIS
- Vertigo, nausea, and vomiting occur with onset over several hours.
- Symptoms usually peak within 24 hours, then resolve gradually over several weeks.
- During the first day, the patient usually has difficulty focusing the eyes because of spontaneous nystagmus.
- Imaging studies usually are not necessary, but enhancement of the bony labyrinth may be seen by MRI after injection of contrast material. Head CT with fine cuts through temporal bones is recommended if history of trauma or suspect cholesteatoma. MRI of the brain with and without contrast with fine cuts through the internal auditory canal is recommended if abnormal cranial nerve examination or eighth cranial nerve tumor suspected.
- Laboratory tests are not helpful.

ETIOLOGY
- Often preceded 1 to 2 weeks by a viral-like illness

TREATMENT
- Phenergan or other antiemetics are effective.
- The vestibular suppressant, meclizine 12.5-25 mg qid, often is used. A scopolamine patch also is effective.
- Methylprednisolone 100 mg/day × 3 days is given with slow taper over 3 weeks.

- Labyrinthitis usually has a benign course, with complete recovery within 1 to 3 months, although older patients may have intractable dizziness that persists for many months.

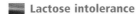 Lactose intolerance

Definition: Insufficient concentration of lactase enzyme, leading to fermentation of malabsorbed lactose by intestinal bacteria with subsequent production of intestinal gas and various organic acids

DIAGNOSIS
- **Lactose breath hydrogen test:** An increase in breath hydrogen >20 ppm within 90 minutes of ingestion of 50 g of lactose is positive for lactase deficiency. This test is positive in 90% of patients with lactose malabsorption. Common causes of false-negative results are recent use of oral antibiotics or recent high colonic enema.
- The lactose tolerance test is an older and less accurate testing modality (20% rate of false-positive and false-negative results). The patient is given an oral dose of 1-1.5 g of lactose/kg body weight. Blood glucose level is measured hourly for 3 hours. The test is considered positive if the patient develops intestinal symptoms, and the blood glucose level rises <20 mg/dL above the fasting baseline level.
- The diagnosis usually can be made on the basis of the history and improvement with dietary manipulation.
- Clinical presentation includes abdominal tenderness and cramping, bloating, flatulence, and diarrhea about 2 hours after ingestion of lactose.
- Physical examination may be normal.

ETIOLOGY
- **Congenital lactase defiiciency** common in premature infants; rare in full-term infants and generally inherited as a chromosomal recessive trait
- **Secondary lactase intolerance:** usually a result of injury of the intestinal mucosa (Crohn's disease, viral gastroenteritis, AIDS enteropathy, cryptosporidiosis, Whipple's disease, sprue)

TREATMENT
- A lactose-free diet generally results in prompt resolution of symptoms. Lactose is found primarily in dairy products, but may be present as an ingredient or component of common foods and beverages. Possible sources of lactose are breads, candies, cold cuts, dessert mixes, cream soups, bologna, commercial sauces and gravies,

chocolate, drink mixes, and medications. Labels should be read carefully to identify sources of lactose.

- Addition of a lactase enzyme supplement (LactAid tablets, Dairy Ease) before the ingestion of milk products may prevent symptoms in some patients. It is not effective, however, for all lactose-intolerant patients.
- Lactose-intolerant patients must ensure adequate calcium intake. Calcium supplementation is recommended to prevent osteoporosis.

CLINICAL PEARLS

- There is great variability in signs and symptoms in patients with lactose intolerance depending on the degree of lactase deficiency.
- Most patients with lactose intolerance can ingest 12 oz of milk daily without symptoms.
- Nondairy synthetic drinks (e.g., Coffee-Mate) and rice milk are well tolerated.

Lambert-Eaton syndrome

Definition: A disorder of neuromuscular transmission caused by antibodies directed against presynaptic voltage-gated P/Q calcium channels on motor and autonomic nerve terminals. There are two forms: *paraneoplastic* (most common) and *nonparaneoplastic* (autoimmune).

DIAGNOSIS

- Weakness with diminished or absent muscle stretch reflexes
- Proximal lower extremity muscles affected most
- Ocular and bulbar muscles less commonly affected
- Transient strength improvement with brief exercise
- Autonomic dysfunction common (dry mouth in 75%, sexual dysfunction, blurred vision, constipation, orthostasis)
- Confirm diagnosis by characteristic electrodiagnostic (electromyography/nerve conduction studies) findings:
  - Reduced motor amplitudes with normal sensory studies
  - Less than 10% decrement in motor amplitudes on slow repetitive nerve stimulation (RNS) at 2 to 3 Hz, with >100% increment on fast RNS (20-30 HZ) or immediately after 10 seconds of maximum exercise (postexercise facilitation)

TREATMENT

- Anticholinesterase agents (pyridostigmine 30-60 mg q4-6h) may yield some improvement.

3-day intervals.

- Plasma exchange (200-250 mL/kg over 10-14 days) or intravenous immunoglobulins (2 g/kg over 2-5 days) often produce significant, temporary improvement.
- Prednisone 1-1.5 mg/kg/day can be tapered gradually over months to minimal effective dose.
- Azathioprine can be given alone or in combination with prednisone. Give 2.5 mg/kg/day. If the patient is intolerant of this, administer cyclosporine 3 mg/kg/day instead.
- 3,4-Diaminopyridine 10-20 mg PO qid (maximum 100 mg/day) may improve muscle strength and reduce autonomic symptoms in 85% of patients in uncontrolled series. It is available in Europe, but limited to research studies in the United States.

CLINICAL PEARL

- Screen for an underlying malignancy. Presentation with Lambert-Eaton syndrome may precede diagnosis of small cell lung cancer by 5 years. Chest x-ray or CT scan of the chest may be required every 6 to 12 months for small cell lung cancer.

Lead poisoning

Definition: Multisystem abnormalities resulting from excessive lead exposure

DIAGNOSIS

- **Check venous blood lead level:** normal level <10 µg/dL; levels of 50 to 70 µg/dL indicate moderate toxicity; levels >70 µg/dL associated with severe poisoning
- Mild anemia with basophilic stippling on peripheral smear
- Elevated zinc protoporphyrin levels or free erythrocyte protoporphyrin level
- An increased body burden of lead with previous high-level exposure in patients with occupational lead poisoning can be shown by measuring the excretion of lead in urine after premedication with calcium ethylenediamine tetraacetic acid (EDTA) or another chelating agent.

ETIOLOGY

- Chronic repeated exposure to paint containing lead, plumbing, storage of batteries, pottery, or lead soldering

TREATMENT

- For children with blood levels of 10 to 19 µg/dL, the Centers for Disease Control and Prevention (CDC) recommends adequate amounts of calcium, iron, zinc, and protein in the patient's diet and family education on sources of lead exposure and potential adverse health effects.
- For children with blood levels of 20 to 44 µg/dL, the CDC recommends case management by a qualified social worker, clinical management, environmental assessment, and lead hazard control.
- Chelation therapy should be considered in children with refractory blood lead levels.
- Chelation therapy is indicated in children with blood lead levels of 45 µg/dL.
- Succimer 10 mg/kg PO q8h for 5 days, then q12h for 2 weeks can be used in patients with levels of 45 to 70 µg/dL.
- EDTA and dimercaprol are effective in patients with severe toxicity.
- Use of EDTA and succimer is indicated in children with blood levels < 70 µg/dL.
- Penicillamine (Cuprimine) also can be used for lead poisoning, but it is not approved by the Food and Drug Administration for this condition.

CLINICAL PEARLS

- Lead poisoning is most common in children age 1 to 5 years (17,000 cases/100,000 persons). The highest rates are among blacks, individuals with low income, and urban children.
- Patients with mild-to-moderate toxicity generally improve without any residual deficits. The presence of encephalopathy at diagnosis is a poor prognostic sign. Residual neurologic deficits may persist in these patients.

Leukemia, chronic lymphocytic (CLL)

Definition: Lymphoproliferative disorder characterized by proliferation and accumulation of mature neoplastic-appearing lymphocytes

DIAGNOSIS

- Proliferative lymphocytosis (≥15,000/dL) of well-differentiated lymphocytes is the hallmark of CLL.
- There is monotonous replacement of the bone marrow by small lymphocytes (marrow contains ≥30% of well-differentiated lymphocytes).

... and elevated lactate dehydrogenase may be present at the time of diagnosis.

- Anemia or thrombocytopenia, if present, indicates poor prognosis.
- Clinical presentation varies according to stage of the disease. Some patients come to medical attention because of weakness and fatigue (secondary to anemia) or lymphadenopathy. Many cases are diagnosed on the basis of laboratory results obtained after routine physical examination.
- **Staging:**
  - Rai et al divided CLL into five clinical stages:
    - Stage 0—characterized by lymphocytosis only ($\geq$15,000/mm^3 on peripheral smear, bone marrow aspirate $\geq$40% lymphocytes). The coexistence of lymphocytosis and other factors increases the clinical stage.
    - Stage 1—lymphadenopathy
    - Stage 2—lymphadenopathy/hepatomegaly
    - Stage 3—anemia (hemoglobin <11 g/mm^3)
    - Stage 4—thrombocytopenia (platelets <100,000/mm^3)
  - Another well-known staging system developed by Binet divides CLL into three stages:
    - Stage A—hemoglobin $\geq$10 g/dL, platelets $\geq$100,000/mm^3, and fewer than three areas involved (cervical, axillary, and inguinal lymph nodes [whether unilaterally or bilaterally]; spleen; and liver)
    - Stage B—hemoglobin $\geq$10 g/dL, platelets $\geq$100,000/mm^3, and three or more areas involved
    - Stage C—hemoglobin <10 g/dL, low platelets (<100,000/mm^3), or both (independent of the areas involved)

TREATMENT

- Observation is appropriate for patients in Rai stage 0 or Binet stage A.
- **Symptomatic patients in Rai stages I and II or Binet stage B:** chlorambucil; local irradiation for isolated symptomatic lymphadenopathy and lymph nodes that interfere with vital organs
- **Fludarabine** is an effective treatment for CLL that does not respond to initial treatment with chlorambucil. Reports indicate that when used as the initial treatment for CLL, fludarabine yields higher response rates and a longer duration of remission and progression-free survival than chlorambucil; overall survival is not enhanced, however.
- **Rai stages III and IV, Binet stage C:** chlorambucil chemotherapy with or without prednisone
  - Fludarabine; CAP (cyclophosphamide, Adriamycin, prednisone); or cyclophosphamide, doxorubicin, vincristine, and prednisone

(mini-CHOP) can be used in patients who respond poorly to chlorambucil.
- Splenic irradiation can be used in selected patients with advanced disease.
- Hypogammaglobulinemia is frequent in CLL and is the chief cause of infections. Immune globulin 250 mg/kg IV q4wk may prevent infections, but has no effect on survival. Infections should be treated with broad-spectrum antibiotics. Patients should be monitored for opportunistic infections.
- Recombinant hematopoietic cofactors (e.g., granulocyte-macrophage colony-stimulating factor and granulocyte colony-stimulating factor) may be useful to overcome neutropenia related to treatment.
- Erythropoietin may be used to treat anemia that is unresponsive to other measures.

CLINICAL PEARLS
- Trisomy 12 is the most common chromosomal abnormality, followed by 14 q+, 13 q, and 11 q; these all indicate a poor prognosis.
- The patient's prognosis is directly related to the clinical stage (e.g. the average survival in patients in Rai stage 0 or Binet stage A is >120 months, whereas for Rai stage 4 or Binet stage C, it is approximaely 30 months). Overall 5-year survival is 60%.

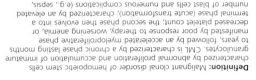

Leukemia, chronic myelogenous (CML)

Definition: Malignant clonal disorder of hemopoietic stem cells characterized by abnormal proliferation and accumulation of immature granulocytes. CML is characterized by a chronic phase lasting months to years, followed by an accelerated myeloproliferative phase manifested by poor response to therapy, worsening anemia, or decreased platelet count, the second phase then evolves into a terminal phase (acute transformation), characterized by an elevated number of blast cells and numerous complications (e.g., sepsis, bleeding).

DIAGNOSIS
- An elevated white blood count (generally >100,000/mm^3) is present with broad spectrum of granulocytic forms.
- Bone marrow shows hypercellularity with granulocytic hyperplasia, increased ratio of myeloid cells to erythroid cells, and increased number of megakaryocytes. Blasts and promyelocytes constitute

... is markedly decreased (used to distinguish CML from other myeloproliferative disorders).
- Anemia and thrombocytosis are often present.
- Common complaints at the time of diagnosis are weakness or discomfort secondary to an enlarged spleen (abdominal discomfort or pain). Splenomegaly is present in 40% of patients at the time of diagnosis. Forty percent of patients are asymptomatic, and diagnosis is based solely on an abnormal blood count.

ETIOLOGY

- Chromosome translocation t (9; 22) (q34;q11.2). This translocation is present in >95% of patients. The remaining patients have a complex or variant translocation involving additional chromosomes that have the same end result (fusion of the *BCR* [break point cluster region] gene on chromosome 22 to *ABL* [Ableson leukemia virus] gene on chromosome 9).

TREATMENT

- Imatinib mesylate (Gleevec), an oral tyrosine kinase inhibitor, is effective and indicated as first-line treatment for CML myeloid blast crisis, accelerated phase, or CML in its chronic phase. More than 60% of patients have major cytogenetic response (<35% Philadelphia chromosome—positive cells in the marrow), and >80% have progression-free survival after 24 months. Complete hematologic response usually occurs in <1 month.
- Symptomatic hyperleukocytosis (e.g., central nervous system symptoms) can be treated with leukapheresis and hydroxyurea; allopurinol should be started to prevent urate nephropathy after the rapid lysis of the leukemia cells.
- Cytotoxic chemotherapy with hydroxyurea has largely replaced busulfan as the standard cytotoxic drug.
- Allogeneic stem cell transplantation (SCT) (after intense chemotherapy with busulfan and cyclophosphamide or combined chemotherapy with cyclophosphamide and fractionated total body irradiation to destroy residual leukemic cells) is the only curative treatment for CML in chronic phase unresponsive to imatinib. Generally, only 20% of patients are candidates for SCT given the limitations of age or lack of HLA-matched related donors.
  - SCT should be considered in young patients (increased survival in patients <55 years old) with compatible siblings.
  - Early SCT is important for patient's survival.
  - Transplantation of marrow from an HLA-matched, unrelated donor is now recognized as safe and effective therapy for selected patients with CML.

CLINICAL PEARL

- Philadelphia chromosome (which results from the reciprocal translocation between the long arms of chromosomes 9 and 22) is present in >95% of patients with CML; its presence (Ph[1]) is a major prognostic factor because survival rate of patients with Philadelphia chromosome is approximately eight times better than that of patients without it.

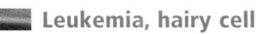

Leukemia, hairy cell

Definition: Lymphoid neoplasm characterized by the proliferation of mature B cells with prominent cytoplasmic projections ("hairs")

DIAGNOSIS

- Pancytopenia involving erythrocytes, neutrophils, and platelets is common; anemia is usually present and varies from minimal to severe.
- Hairy cells can account for 5% to 80% of cells in the peripheral blood. The cytoplasmic projections on the cells are redundant plasma membranes.
- Leukemic cells stain positively for tartrate-resistant acid phosphatase stain.
- Bone marrow may result in a "dry tap" (because of increased marrow reticulin).
- Physical examination shows splenomegaly (present in >90% of cases) secondary to tumor cell infiltration.

TREATMENT

- Drugs of choice are the purine analogues cladribine or pentostatin. They induce complete remissions in 85% of patients and partial responses in 5% to 25%.
- Cladribine 0.14 mg/kg qd × 7 days has minimal toxicity and induces complete durable responses with a single course of therapy.
- Interferon alfa produces a partial remission in 30% to 70% of patients and complete remission, often of short duration, in 5% to 10% of patients.
- The anti-CD22 recombinant immunotoxin BL22 can induce complete remission in patients with hairy cell leukemia that is resistant to treatment with purine analogues.

CLINICAL PEARL

- Approximately 8% to 10% of patients are asymptomatic and have minimal splenomegaly and minor cytopenia. These patients usually
  . . . . . . routine laboratory evaluation and do not require

disease progression.

Lyme disease

Definition: Multisystem disease caused by a spirochete (*Borrelia burgdorferi*) transmitted by the bite of an *Ixodes* tick (most commonly *Ixodes scapularis*)

DIAGNOSIS

- Diagnosis is made primarily on clinical grounds and confirmed by serologic testing.
- Only one third of patients remember a tick bite.
- More than 90% of symptomatic patients develop the rash of erythema chronicum migrans (ECM).
- Serologic tests should be used only to support a clinical diagnosis of Lyme disease, not as the primary basis for making diagnostic or treatment decisions. Serologic testing is performed with ELISA. False-negative results may be seen in the initial 2 to 4 weeks of infection and may be caused by early treatment of ECM; serologic testing is not useful early in the course of Lyme disease. False-positive results can occur with other spirochetal infections and in patients with various autoimmune disorders (e.g., systemic lupus erythematosus, rheumatoid arthritis). In addition, there is significant lack of standardization among laboratories or test kits.
- The clinical manifestations of Lyme disease vary with the stage of the disease and include several presentations:
  - **Stage I (localized early infection):** usually manifested by a characteristic expanding annular skin lesion (ECM); it typically occurs 3 to 30 days after the tick bite as a centrifugally expanding, erythematous annular patch with a bull's-eye appearance
  - **Stage II (disseminated infection):** follows stage I by days or weeks; patients may experience attacks of joint swelling and pain in large joints, neurologic complications (aseptic meningitis, encephalitis, cranial neuritis), cardiac abnormalities (atrioventricular block, myocarditis), and various other multisystem manifestations
  - **Stage III (persistent infection):** follows stage II by ≥1 years and is manifested by inflammatory arthritis affecting large joints (particularly the knee) and chronic cutaneous and neurologic sequelae; chronic Lyme arthritis is associated with HLA-DR4 and HLA-DR2 alleles.

TREATMENT

- Give doxycycline 100 mg bid for 14 days. There is no clear evidence that treatment with >2 weeks of antibiotics improves the prognosis. A single 200-mg dose of doxycycline given within 72 hours after an *I. scapularis* tick bite has been reported to be effective in preventing the development of Lyme disease.
- Alternative antibiotics are amoxicillin 500 mg qid for 14-21 days, cefuroxime 500 mg bid for 14-21 days, and ceftriaxone 2 g/day IV for 14-21 days.

Meningitis, bacterial

Definition: Inflammation of the meninges secondary to bacterial infection

DIAGNOSIS

- **Lumbar puncture:** The classic findings on cerebrospinal fluid (CSF) examination are elevated white blood cell (WBC) count (predominantly polymorphonuclear leukocytes), decreased glucose, elevated protein, and positive Gram stain.
- **Laboratory tests:** WBC count usually reveals leukocytosis with shift to the left; however, leukopenia can also be present. Peripheral lymphocytosis usually suggests a viral cause (aseptic meningitis). Blood cultures are appropriate; however, antibiotic therapy should not be delayed until all cultures are obtained if patient is very ill.
- **Clinical presentation:** The classic presentation consists of fever, headache, lethargy, confusion, and nuchal rigidity; these manifestations are not always present, particularly in infants, elderly patients, and immunocompromised patients.
- **Physical examination:**
  - **Kernig's sign:** pain in the lower back or posterior thigh when the knee is extended while the patient is lying in the supine position, and the hip is flexed at a right angle
  - **Brudzinski's sign:** rapid flexion of the neck elicits involuntary flexing of the knees in a supine position
  - Altered mental status (confusion, lethargy)
  - Bulging fontanelle, poor feeding, vomiting, and respiratory distress in infants
  - Petechial-purpuric rash that develops on the trunk, lower extremities, mucous membranes, conjunctiva, and occasionally on the palms and soles suggests meningococcal meningitis, but also can be present in viral meningitis and other bacterial meningitis/

abscess or mass lesion.

- Seizures may occur in 40% of patients in the first week of illness, but they are an unusual initial presentation; cranial nerve palsies (most notably sensorineural hearing loss) also may be present early in the course of illness.

ETIOLOGY

- The type of infecting organism varies with the age of the patient and several predisposing factors:
  - *Streptococcus pneumoniae* is common in adults and elderly patients; predisposing factors include blunt head trauma, otitis media, pneumonia, sickle cell disease, and CSF leaks; mortality rate is 30%; permanent neurologic sequelae occur in 50% of survivors.
  - *Neisseria meningitidis* is common in young adults and children, especially those with complement deficiencies.
  - *Haemophilus influenzae* is seen in preschool-age children; predisposing factors in adults include head trauma, otitis media, and sinusitis.
  - *Listeria monocytogenes* occurs in elderly and immunosuppressed patients (lymphoma, corticosteroids, dialysis patients, organ transplant recipients).
  - Gram-negative bacilli usually are seen in neonates (acquired in passage through birth canal), elderly debilitated patients, and neutropenic patients and in postcranial surgery.
  - *Staphylococcus aureus* is seen in diabetic patients and patients with *S. aureus* pneumonia or cancer.

TREATMENT

- Intravenous antibiotic therapy should be based on the results of the Gram stain. Empiric therapy in adults (18-50 years old) consists of a third-generation cephalosporin (cefotaxime or ceftriaxone). In older adults (>50 years old), ampicillin should be added to the third-generation cephalosporin. In children 3 months to 18 years old, use of a third-generation cephalosporin or meropenem is recommended.
- The American Academy of Pediatrics recommends dexamethasone in the treatment of *H. influenzae* meningitis in previously healthy infants and children >2 months old. Dexamethasone is given in four divided doses of 0.6 mg/kg/day IV for the first 4 days of antimicrobial therapy. Dexamethasone also may benefit children with pneumococcal meningitis and should be given within the first 2 days of illness.
- Dexamethasone 10 mg IV q6h should be given in most adults with suspected pneumococcal meningitis. It can be given with or just before the first dose of the antibiotic. It is not indicated in patients who already have received antimicrobial therapy.

Mesenteric venous thrombosis

Definition: Thrombotic occlusion of the mesenteric venous system involving major trunks or smaller branches and leading to intestinal infarction in its acute form

DIAGNOSIS
- **Abdominal CT scan (diagnostic in 90%):** bowel wall thickening, venous dilation, venous thrombus
- **Symptoms:** abdominal pain in 90% of patients, typically out of proportion to the physical findings. Nausea and vomiting occur in 50%, and gastrointestinal bleeding occurs in 50% (occult) and 15% (gross).
- **Physical findings:**
  - Early—abdominal tenderness, decreased bowel sounds, abdominal distention
  - Later—guarding and rebound tenderness, fever, and septic shock
- **Laboratory tests:** complete blood count (leukocytosis), electrolytes (metabolic acidosis [lactic] indicates bowel infarction), elevated amylase, tests for hypercoagulable status

ETIOLOGY
- Hypercoagulable states
- Portal hypertension
- Inflammation
- Pancreatitis
- Peritonitis (e.g., appendicitis, diverticulitis, perforated viscus)
- Inflammatory bowel disease
- Pelvic or intraabdominal abscess
- Intraabdominal cancer
- Postoperative state or trauma
- Blunt abdominal trauma
- Postoperative states (abdominal surgery)
- Thrombosis may begin in small mesenteric branches (e.g., in hypercoagulable states) and propagate to the major venous mesenteric trunks or begin in large veins (e.g., in cirrhosis, intraabdominal cancer, surgery) and extend distally. If collateral drainage is inadequate, the intestine becomes congested, edematous, cyanotic, and hemorrhagic and eventually may infarct.

TREATMENT
- Anticoagulation or thrombolytic therapy
- Laparotomy if intestinal infarction is suspected
  - **Short ischemic segment:** resection

- Nonviable—resection or close
- Viable—intraarterial papaverine or thrombectomy followed by second-look intervention

Metabolic syndrome

Definition: Combination of four conditions: abdominal obesity, hypertension, dyslipidemia, and diabetes

DIAGNOSIS
- Guidelines from the National Cholesterol Education Program define the metabolic syndrome as the presence of any three of the following:
  - **Abdominal obesity:** waist circumference >102 cm (40 inches) in men and >88 cm (35 inches) in women
  - **Hypertriglyceridemia:** ≥150 mg/dL (1.69 mmol/L)
  - **Low high-density lipoprotein cholesterol:** <40 mg dL in men and <50 mg dL in women
  - **High blood pressure:** ≥130/85 mm Hg
  - **High fasting glucose:** ≥110 mg/dL (6.1 mmol/L)

TREATMENT
- Prescribe dietary modifications aimed at weight loss.
- Instruct patient to increase physical activity.
- Treat hypertension.
  - Blood pressure goal is <130/80 mm Hg.
  - Angiotensin converting enzyme inhibitors may be preferred as initial drug.
- Treat hyperlipidemia.
  - Low-density lipoprotein (LDL) goal is <100 mg/dL, or if patient has coronary heart disease (CHD) or CHD risk equivalents (peripheral arterial disease, abdominal aortic aneurysm, symptomatic carotid artery disease, diabetes, or an estimated 10-year CHD risk >20%), LDL goal is <70 mg/dL.
  - HMG CoA reductase inhibitors (statins) commonly are used as first-line agents.
  - Patients with high (200-499 mg/dL) or very high (>500 mg/dL) triglycerides may benefit from the addition of fibrates. Hypothyroidism must be ruled out.
- Treat diabetes.
  - Fasting blood glucose goal is <130 mg/dL.
  - Metformin and thiazolidinediones are used as first-line agents to improve insulin sensitivity.

- Treat cardiovascular risk factors.
- Prescribe aspirin therapy in patients with coronary artery disease.
- Risk can be lowered with weight loss, exercise, blood pressure control, and treatment of hyperlipidemia.

Milk-alkali syndrome

Definition: Consumption of large amounts of calcium and alkali resulting in the triad of hypercalcemia, metabolic alkalosis, and renal insufficiency

DIAGNOSIS

Symptoms range from asymptomatic (diagnosis made by the incidental finding of hypercalcemia and renal failure) to symptomatic hypercalcemia including nausea, vomiting, anorexia, fatigue, vague abdominal pain, nephrolithiasis, and constipation. In more chronic cases, polyuria and polydipsia may be reported.

- **Laboratory tests:**
  - Elevated plasma calcium (wide variation reported)
  - Renal insufficiency
  - Elevated plasma bicarbonate and arterial pH
  - Parathyroid hormone, usually suppressed, may be elevated, particularly if checked after treatment has begun
  - Phosphate level variable

ETIOLOGY

- Overconsumption of supplemental calcium bicarbonate with reported ranges of 2.5 to 20 g/day.

TREATMENT

- Discontinuation of calcium bicarbonate supplements
- Hydration and furosemide if symptomatic hypercalcemia
- Monitor for rebound hypocalcemia as a result of elevation of parathyroid hormone with treatment
- Patient education regarding appropriate calcium supplementation

CLINICAL PEARL

- Hypercalcemia and symptoms resolve with withdrawal of excess calcium supplementation and treatment of hypercalcemia. Patients initially presenting with renal failure may have residual renal insufficiency.

Definition: Retrograde blood flow through the left atrium secondary to an incompetent mitral valve; eventually there is an increase in left atrial and pulmonary pressures, which may result in right ventricular failure

DIAGNOSIS

- **Physical findings:**
  - Hyperdynamic apex, often with palpable left ventricular lift and apical thrill
  - Holosystolic murmur at apex with radiation to base or to left axilla; poor correlation between the intensity of the systolic murmur and the degree of regurgitation
  - Apical early diastolic to middiastolic rumble (rare)
- **Echocardiography:**
  - Enlarged left atrium, hyperdynamic left ventricle (erratic motion of the leaflet is seen in patients with ruptured chordae tendineae). Doppler echocardiography shows evidence of MR. The most important aspect of the echocardiogram is the quantification of left ventricular systolic performance.

ETIOLOGY

- Papillary muscle dysfunction (as a result of ischemic heart disease)
- Ruptured chordae tendineae
- Infective endocarditis
- Calcified mitral valve annulus
- Left ventricular dilation
- Rheumatic valvulitis
- Primary or secondary mitral valve prolapse
- Hypertrophic cardiomyopathy
- Idiopathic myxomatous degeneration of the mitral valve
- Myxoma
- Systemic lupus erythematosus
- Fenfluramine, dexfenfluramine

TREATMENT

- **Medical:**
  - Give digitalis for inotropic effect and to control ventricular response if atrial fibrillation with fast ventricular response is present.
  - Afterload reduction (to decrease the regurgitant fraction and to increase cardiac output) may be accomplished with nifedipine,

hydralazine plus nitrates, or angiotensin-converting enzyme inhibitors.
- Anticoagulants are indicated if atrial fibrillation occurs.
- Antibiotic prophylaxis is needed before dental and surgical procedures.
- **Surgical:**
- Surgery is the only definitive treatment for MR.
- The timing of surgical repair is controversial; generally, surgery should be considered early in symptomatic patients despite optimal medical therapy and in patients with moderate-to-severe MR and minimal symptoms if there is echocardiographic evidence of rapidly progressive increase in left ventricular end-diastolic and end-systolic dimension (echocardiographic evidence of systolic failure includes end-systolic dimension >55 mm and fractional shortening <31%).
- Surgery also is indicated in asymptomatic patients with preserved ventricular function if there is a high likelihood of valve repair, or if there is evidence of pulmonary hypertension or recent atrial fibrillation.

Mitral stenosis

Definition: A narrowing of the mitral valve orifice. The cross section of a normal orifice measures 4 to 6 cm². A murmur becomes audible when the valve orifice becomes <2 cm². When the orifice approaches 1 cm², the condition becomes critical, and symptoms become more evident.

DIAGNOSIS
- **Physical findings:**
  - Prominent jugular A waves are present in patients with normal sinus rhythm.
  - Opening snap occurs in early diastole; a short (<0.07 second) A_2 to opening snap interval indicates severe mitral stenosis.
  - Apical middiastolic or presystolic rumble that does not radiate is present.
  - Accentuated S_1 (because of delayed and forceful closure of the valve) is present.
  - If pulmonary hypertension is present, there may be an accentuated P_2 or a soft, early diastolic decrescendo murmur (Graham Steell murmur) caused by pulmonary regurgitation (it is best heard along the left sternal border and may be confused with aortic regurgitation).

... heave may be present at the left
sternal border.
- Patients with mitral stenosis usually have symptoms of left-sided
  heart failure, including dyspnea on exertion, paroxysmal nocturnal
  dyspnea, and orthopnea.
- Right ventricular dysfunction (in late stages) may be manifested by
  peripheral edema, enlarged and pulsatile liver, and ascites.
- **Echocardiogram:** The characteristic finding on echocardiogram is a
  markedly diminished E-to-F slope of the anterior mitral valve leaflet
  during diastole; there is also fusion of the commissures, resulting in
  anterior movement of the posterior mitral valve leaflet during diastole (calcification in the valve also may be noted).

ETIOLOGY
- Progressive fibrosis, scarring, and calcification of the valve
- Rheumatic fever (still a common cause in underdeveloped countries); heart valves most frequently affected in rheumatic heart
  disease (in descending order of occurrence) are mitral, aortic, tricuspid, and pulmonary
- Congenital defect (parachute valve)
- **Rare causes:** endomyocardial fibroelastosis, malignant carcinoid
  syndrome, systemic lupus erythematosus

TREATMENT
- **Medical:**
  - If the patient is in atrial fibrillation, control the rate response with
    diltiazem, digitalis, or esmolol. Although digitalis is the drug of
    choice for long-term heart rate control, intravenous diltiazem or
    esmolol may be preferable when a rapid decrease in heart rate is
    required.
  - If the patient has persistent atrial fibrillation (because of large left
    atrium), permanent anticoagulation is indicated to decrease the
    risk of serious thromboembolism.
  - Treat congestive heart failure with diuretics and sodium restriction.
  - Give antibiotic prophylaxis with dental and surgical procedures.
- **Surgical:**
  - Valve replacement is indicated when the valve orifice is <0.7 to
    0.8 cm^2 or if symptoms persist despite optimal medical therapy;
    commissurotomy may be possible if the mitral valve is noncalci-
    fied and if there is pure mitral stenosis without significant sub-
    valvular disease.
  - Percutaneous transvenous mitral valvotomy is becoming the
    therapy of choice for many patients with mitral stenosis responding
    poorly to medical therapy, particularly patients who are poor surgi-
    cal candidates and whose valve is not heavily calcified; balloon

valvotomy gives excellent mechanical relief, usually resulting in prolonged benefit.

Mitral valve prolapse (MVP)

Definition: The posterior bulging of interior and posterior leaflets in systole. *MVP syndrome* refers to a constellation of MVP and associated symptoms (e.g., autonomic dysfunction, palpitations) or other physical abnormalities (e.g., pectus excavatum).

DIAGNOSIS
- **Clinical presentation:**
  - The usual patient is a young woman with narrow anteroposterior chest diameter, low body weight, and low blood pressure.
  - Mid to late click is heard best at the apex.
  - Crescendo middiastolic to late diastolic murmur is heard.
  - Findings are accentuated in the standing position.
  - Most patients with MVP are asymptomatic; symptoms (if present) consist primarily of chest pain and palpitations.
  - Neurologic abnormalities (e.g., transient ischemic attack or stroke) are rare.
  - Patients also may complain of anxiety, fatigue, and dyspnea.
- **Echocardiography:** Echocardiography shows the anterior and posterior leaflets bulging posteriorly in systole.

ETIOLOGY
- Myxomatous degeneration of connective tissue of mitral valve
- Congenital deformity of mitral valve and supportive structures
- Secondary to other disorders (e.g., Ehlers-Danlos syndrome, pseudoxanthoma elasticum)

TREATMENT
- The empiric use of antiarrhythmic drugs to prevent sudden death in patients with uncomplicated MVP is not advisable. β-blockers may be tried in symptomatic patients (e.g., palpitations, chest pain); they decrease the heart rate, decreasing the stretch on the prolapsing valve leaflets.
- Antibiotic prophylaxis for infective endocarditis when undergoing dental, gastrointestinal, or genitourinary procedures is indicated only in patients with MVP who have a systolic murmur and echocardiographic evidence of mitral regurgitation.

The incidence of complications of MVP is low (<1%/yr) and generally associated with an increase in mitral leaflet thickness to ≥5 mm; young patients (<45 years old) with absence of mitral systolic murmur or mitral regurgitation on Doppler echocardiography are at low risk for any complications.

Multifocal atrial tachycardia

Definition: Chaotic, irregular atrial activity at rates of 100 to 180 beats/min

DIAGNOSIS
- **ECG:**
  - Variable P-P intervals are seen.
  - Morphology of the P wave varies from beat to beat (Fig. 12) with a minimum of three different forms of P wave besides those from the sinus node.
  - Each QRS complex is preceded by a P wave.
  - Atrial rate is 100 to 150 beats/min.

ETIOLOGY
- Chronic obstructive pulmonary disease (COPD)
- Metabolic disturbances (hypoxemia, hypokalemia, hypomagnesemia)
- Sepsis
- Theophylline toxicity
- Congestive heart failure (CHF)
- Acute myocardial infarction

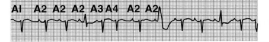

FIGURE 12. Multifocal atrial tachycardia. Letter designations A1, A2, A3, and A4 show premature contractions from varying foci. The 4th, 8th, and 11th QRS complexes are aberrant. (From Goldberger E: Treatment of Cardiac Emergencies, 5th ed. St Louis, Mosby, 1990.)

TREATMENT

- Treat the underlying cause (e.g., improve oxygenation, correct electrolyte abnormalities).
- Give verapamil 5 mg IV at a rate of 1 mg/min (may repeat after 20 minutes). Calcium gluconate 1 g IV given 5 minutes before treatment with verapamil may reduce drug-induced hypotension without affecting the antiarrhythmic effect.
- Metoprolol or esmolol also has been used in the absence of COPD, CHF, or bronchospasm.
- Amiodarone may be useful in refractory cases.

Multiple endocrine neoplasia (MEN)

Definition: Familial syndrome that occurs in an autosomal dominant pattern; the endocrine "neoplasms" may be expressed as hyperplasia, adenoma, or carcinoma and may develop synchronously or metachronously

CLASSIFICATION

- **MEN I (Werner's syndrome):**
  - Tumors or hyperplasia of anterior pituitary, enteropancreatic neuroendocrine system (insulinoma, gastrinoma, glucagonoma), parathyroid, and other tissues
  - **Possible associated conditions:**
    - Adrenocortical adenoma or hyperplasia
    - Thyroid adenoma or hyperplasia
    - Renal cortical adenoma
    - Carcinoid tumors
    - Gastrointestinal polyps
    - Skin angiofibromas and skin collagenomas
  - **Clinical manifestations:**
    - Peptic ulcer and its complications
    - Hypoglycemia
    - Hypercalcemia or nephrocalcinosis or both
    - Headache, visual field defects, secondary amenorrhea
    - Multiple subcutaneous lipomas
    - **Other:** flushing, acromegaly, Cushing's syndrome, hyperthyroidism
- **MEN II (Sipple's syndrome, MEN IIA):**
  - Associated with medullary thyroid carcinoma (MTC), pheochromocytoma, and hyperparathyroidism

- Neck mass (caused by MTC)
  - Hypertension
  - Headache, palpitations, sweating
  - Hypercalcemia, nephrocalcinosis, osteitis fibrosa cystica
- Relatives of affected persons should be screened to detect MTC at an early stage; screening can be accomplished with:
  - Pentagastrin test—unreliable because it does not distinguish C-cell hyperplasia from small carcinomas
  - DNA analysis—new and highly reliable method for identification of MEN II A gene carriers
- **MEN III (multiple mucosal neuroma syndrome, MEN IIB):**
  - Associated with MTC, pheochromocytoma, and multiple mucosal neuromas
  - **Possible associated conditions:** intestinal ganglioneuromatosis, marfanoid habitus
  - **Clinical manifestations:**
    - Neck mass (caused by MTC)
    - Headache, palpitations, sweating, hypertension
    - Mucosal neuromas (initially noted as whitish, yellow-pink nodules involving lips and anterior third of tongue)
    - Marfan-like habitus (with absence of cardiovascular abnormalities and lens subluxation)
    - Peripheral neuropathy (caused by neuromatous plaques overlying the posterior columns of the spinal cord, cauda equina, and sciatic nerve)

Multiple myeloma

Definition: A malignancy of plasma cells characterized by overproduction of intact monoclonal immunoglobulin or free monoclonal kappa or lambda chains

DIAGNOSIS
- **Clinical presentation:** The patient usually comes to medical attention because of one or more of the following:
  - Bone pain (back, thorax) or pathologic fractures caused by osteolytic lesions
  - Fatigue or weakness because of anemia secondary to bone marrow infiltration with plasma cells
  - Recurrent infections as a result of impaired neutrophil function and deficiency of normal immunoglobulins
  - Nausea and vomiting caused by constipation and uremia

- Delirium secondary to hypercalcemia
- Neurologic complications, such as spinal cord or nerve root compression, blurred vision from hyperviscosity
- **Laboratory tests:**
  - Normochromic, normocytic anemia; rouleaux formation on peripheral smear
  - Hypercalcemia is present in 15% of patients at diagnosis
  - Elevated blood urea nitrogen, creatinine, uric acid, and total protein
  - Proteinuria secondary to overproduction and secretion of free monoclonal kappa or lambda chains (Bence Jones protein)
  - Tall homogeneous monoclonal spike (M spike) on protein immunoelectrophoresis in approximately 75% of patients
  - Hyponatremia, reduced ion gap resulting from the positive charge of the M protein serum hyperviscosity (more common with production of IgA)
  - **Bone marrow examination:** usually shows nests or sheets of plasma cells, which comprise >30% of the bone marrow, and ≥10% are immature

TREATMENT

- Newly diagnosed patients with stage II or III myeloma and good performance status are best treated with autologous stem cell transplantation.
- Chemotherapeutic agents effective in multiple myeloma are:
  - Melphalan and prednisone: The rates of response to this treatment range from 40% to 60%. Adding continuous low-dose interferon to standard melphalan-prednisone therapy does not improve response rate or survival; however, response duration and plateau phase duration are prolonged by maintenance therapy with interferon.
  - Vincristine, doxorubicin (Adriamycin), and dexamethasone (VAD) can be used in patients not responding or relapsing after treatment with melphalan and prednisone; methylprednisolone is substituted for dexamethasone (VAMP) in some centers.
  - High-dose chemotherapy (HDCT) with vincristine, melphalan, cyclophosphamide, and prednisone (VMCP) alternating with vincristine, carmustine, doxorubicin, and prednisone (BVAP) combined with bone marrow transplantation improves response rate, event-free survival, and overall survival in patients with myeloma.
  - Thalidomide, an agent with antiangiogenic properties, is useful to induce responses in patients with multiple myeloma refractory to chemotherapy.

toxic for multiple myeloma. It is indicated for treatment of refractory multiple myeloma.

CLINICAL PEARLS

- Monthly infusions of the bisphosphonate pamidronate provide significant protection against skeletal complications and improve the quality of life of patients with advanced multiple myeloma. Zoledronic acid (Zometa) also can be used for treatment of hypercalcemia of malignancy.
- Current HDCT regimens with autologous stem cell support achieve complete response in approximately 20% to 30% of patients, with best results seen in good-risk patients, defined as young patients (<50 years old) with good performance status and a low tumor burden (β_2-microglobulin ≤2.5 mg/L).

Multiple sclerosis (MS)

Definition: Chronic demyelinating disease of unknown cause, characterized pathologically by zones of demyelinization (plaques) scattered throughout the white matter

DIAGNOSIS

- MRI of the brain with gadolinium can identify lesions 3 to 4 mm and is frequently diagnostic in suspected cases; it also can be used to assess disease load, activity, and progression. MRI typically reveals multiple, predominantly periventricular plaques; however, a normal MRI study cannot be used conclusively to exclude MS.
- Lumbar puncture is particularly useful when MRI is inconclusive because Lyme disease, acute disseminated encephalopathy, and hypertensive changes may mimic MS.
  - In MS, the cerebrospinal fluid (CSF) may show increased gamma globulin (mostly IgG, but often IgA and IgM).
  - Agarose electrophoresis discloses discrete "oligoclonal" bands in the gamma region in approximately 90% of patients, including some with normal IgG levels.
  - Other possible CSF abnormalities are increased total protein, increased mononuclear white blood cells, and presence of myelin basic protein (elevated in acute attacks, indicates active myelin destruction).
- Measurement of visual evoked response is useful to assess nerve fiber conduction (myelin loss or destruction slows conduction velocity).

Clinical presentation:

Visual abnormalities:

- Paresis of medial rectus muscle on lateral conjugate gaze (internuclear ophthalmoplegia) and horizontal nystagmus of the adducting eye
- Central scotoma, decreased visual acuity (optic neuritis)
- Marcus Gunn pupil (pupil that paradoxically dilates with direct light), indicating damage to the optic nerve anterior to the chiasm, is frequently present
- Nystagmus

Abnormalities of reflexes

- Increased deep tendon reflexes
- Positive Hoffmann's sign, positive Babinski's sign
- Decreased abdominal skin reflex, decreased cremasteric reflex
- **Lhermitte's sign.** flexion of the neck while the patient is lying down elicits an electrical sensation extending bilaterally down the arms, back, and lower trunk
- **Charcot's triad**: nystagmus, scanning speech, and intention tremor
- Impaired recognition of objects by touch alone (astereognosis)

TREATMENT

- Treatment should be given at the earliest stages, when inflammation predominates and before substantial, irreversible axonal loss occurs. Initial pharmacologic treatment is aimed at ameliorating acute exacerbations with high-dose intravenous methylprednisolone (5-day course at a dose of 1000 mg/day; an alternative dose is 15 mg/kg/day)
- Immunomodulators have been shown to slow progression of the disease. Currently available disease-modifying drugs for MS are interferon beta-1a (Avonex, Rebif), interferon beta-1b (Betaseron), and glatiramer acetate (Copaxone).
- Natalizumab, an α₄ integrin antagonist, has been shown to reduce the number for inflammatory brain lesions and relapses in patients with relapsing MS.
- Fatigue is a common complaint in patients with MS; it can be treated with amantadine 100 mg bid for 2 to 3 weeks before deciding whether it is effective. Pemoline also can be used when amantadine is not effective. Modafinil, a stimulant approved for narcolepsy, also has been reported as effective.
- Control of spasticity may be achieved with baclofen (Lioresal), dantrolene, or lorazepam.
- Pain is a frequent complaint and can be treated with gabapentin.
- ... e is helpful for relief of spasticity Carbamazepine,

...ery drugs also may be effective. ~~...steroidal antiinflamma-~~

- Depression is frequent (20% of patients) and can be treated with antidepressants and referral to a psychotherapist or psychiatrist if severe.
- Urinary urgency can be treated with oxybutinin or propantheline.
- Tremor generally can be controlled with clonazepam 0.5 mg bid.
- Referral for physical therapy or occupational therapy is recommended after exacerbations.

▰ Myasthenia gravis (MG)

Definition: Acquired autoimmune disorder of neuromuscular transmission characterized by the presence of a gamma globulin antibody (AChR-ab) directed against the nicotinic acetylcholinic receptor (AChR) of the neuromuscular junction, resulting in reduction in postsynaptic response to acetylcholine

DIAGNOSIS
- **Clinical manifestations:**
  - The hallmark of mg is weakness that is made worse with exercise and improved by rest. Symptoms fluctuate and are often better in the morning.
  - More than 50% of patients present initially with ptosis, ocular muscle weakness, or both.
  - Difficulty in chewing, abnormal smile, dysarthria, and dysphagia are common.
  - Involvement of the respiratory muscles may require intubation and assisted ventilation.
  - Pain may occur in fatigued muscles (e.g., neck muscles).
- **Physical examination:**
  - Clinical manifestations are reproducible with exercise. Observation of the patient performing repetitive muscle contractions of involved muscles shows rapidly developing weakness.
  - Physical examination may be normal at rest.
  - Patients with complaints of ptosis show fatigue weakness and ptosis when asked to sustain upward gaze for >3 minutes without interruption.
- **Diagnostic evaluation:**
  - Improvement of symptoms after use of anticholinesterase medications—edrophonium chloride (Tensilon) or pyridostigmine bromide (Mestinon)
  - Elevated level of AChR-ab (present in 90% of patients with generalized mg and 60% of patients with ocular myasthenia)—this sero-

logic test should be performed only if testing with anti-cholinesterase drugs supports the diagnosis of MG. Generally, AchR-ab titers do not correlate with clinical severity.

- Single-fiber electromyography—highly accurate in confirming MG in suspected patients with normal conventional repetitive stimulation
- Evaluate for presence of associated diseases.
  - MRI or CT of anterior mediastinum to rule out thymoma (found in 12% of patients with MG)
  - Thyroid-stimulating hormone to rule out thyroid disease (found in 3-15% of patients with MG)
  - Vitamin B_{12} level to rule out pernicious anemia
  - Antinuclear antibody, rheumatoid factor (increased association with systemic lupus erythematosus, rheumatoid arthritis)

TREATMENT

- Give cholinesterase inhibitors. Pyridostigmine dose is 30-60 mg PO q4-6h initially; onset of effect is 30 minutes, and duration is 4 hours. A longer acting preparation (Mestinon Timespan 180 mg) can be given once or twice daily; however, absorption may be erratic. Major side effects are gastrointestinal upset and increased salivation and bronchial secretions.
- Corticosteroids are useful for long-term immunosuppression. Initial dose is generally 40-80 mg/day as a single dose, adjusted over several weeks on the basis of patient response. Maintenance doses range from 5 mg qod to 100 mg qd, depending on patient response; most patients require steroid therapy indefinitely. Slowly tapering steroids when control is achieved and switching to alternate-day doses should be attempted.
- Immunosuppressants include azathioprine (Imuran) 2-3 mg/kg/day and cyclosporine 5 mg/kg/day. They are often used in patients with severe generalized weakness and may reduce the need for corticosteroids. Most patients require lifelong immunosuppressive therapy.
- Plasma exchange is indicated in severely ill patients (myasthenic crisis with respiratory failure, significant bulbar involvement) and preoperatively in thymectomy candidates.
- Thymectomy is indicated in all patients with thymoma. thymectomy in the absence of thymoma is more controversial—generally recommended for mg patients age 18 (postpubertal) to 60, particularly patients not responding well to medical treatment.

Myelodysplastic Syndrome

Definition: A group of acquired clonal disorders affecting the hematopoietic stem cells and characterized by cytopenias with hypercellular bone marrow and various morphologic abnormalities in the hematopoietic cell lines. Myelodysplasia encompasses several heterogeneous syndromes. The French-American-British classification of myelodysplastic syndromes includes the following: refractory anemia, refractory anemia with ringed sideroblasts, refractory anemia with excess blasts, chronic myelomonocytic leukemia, and refractory anemia with excess blasts in transformation.

DIAGNOSIS
- **Laboratory tests:**
  - Anemia with variable mean corpuscular volume (normal or increased)
  - Reduced reticulocyte count (in relation to the degree of anemia)
  - Hypogranular or agranular neutrophils
  - Thrombocytopenia or normal platelet count
  - Hypogranular platelets may be present
  - Hypercellular bone marrow, with frequent clonal chromosomal abnormalities
- **Imaging studies:** Abdominal CT scan may reveal hepatosplenomegaly

TREATMENT
- Red blood cell transfusions are given to patients with severe symptomatic anemia.
- Results of chemotherapy are generally disappointing.
- The role of myeloid growth factors (granulocyte colony-stimulating factor, granulocyte-macrophage colony-stimulating factor) and immunotherapy is undefined. In one trial, 34% of patients treated with antithymocyte globulin (40 mg/kg for 4 days) became transfusion independent. Response also was associated with a statistically significantly longer survival.
- Allogeneic stem cell transplantation should be considered in patients <60 years old because this is the established procedure with cure potential.

CLINICAL PEARLS
- Cure rates in young patients with allogeneic bone marrow transplantations approach 30% to 50%.
- The risk of transformation to acute myelogenous leukemia varies with the percentage of blasts in the bone marrow.

- Advanced age, male sex, and deletion of chromosomes 5 and 7 are associated with a poor prognosis.
- According to the International Myelodysplastic Syndrome Risk Analysis Workshop, the most important variables in disease outcome are the specific cytogenetic abnormalities, the percentage of blasts in the bone marrow, and the number of hematopoietic lineages involved in the cytopenias.

Myocarditis

Definition: An inflammatory condition of the myocardium

DIAGNOSIS

Clinical presentation:

- Persistent tachycardia out of proportion to fever
- Faint S_1, S_2 sounds on auscultation
- Murmur of mitral regurgitation
- Pericardial friction rub if associated with pericarditis
- Signs of biventricular failure (hypotension, hepatomegaly, peripheral edema, distention of neck veins, S_3)
- Patients may present with a history of a recent flulike syndrome (fever, arthralgias, malaise)

Laboratory tests:

- Elevated cardiac troponin T suggests myocarditis in patients with clinically suspected myocarditis. A normal level does not rule out the diagnosis.
- Increased creatine kinase (with elevated MB fraction, lactate dehydrogenase) and aspartate aminotransferase secondary to myocardial necrosis
- Increased erythrocyte sedimentation rate (nonspecific but may be of value in following the progress of the disease and the response to therapy)
- Increased white blood cell count (increased eosinophils if parasitic infection)
- Viral titers (acute and convalescent)
- Cold agglutinin titer, antistreptolysin O titer, blood cultures
- Lyme disease antibody titer

Imaging:

- Chest x-ray—enlargement of cardiac silhouette
- Echocardiogram—dilated and hypokinetic chambers, segmental wall motion abnormalities
- Cardiac catheterization and angiography in selected patients—to detect coronary artery disease and valvular disease

nspecific ST-T wave changes; inter-
ventricular conduction defects and bundle branch block may be
present. Lyme disease and diphtheria cause all degrees of heart
block. Changes of acute myocardial infarction can occur with focal
necrosis.

ETIOLOGY

- **Infection:**
  - Viral (coxsackie B virus, cytomegalovirus, echovirus, poliovirus, ade-
    novirus, mumps, HIV, Epstein-Barr virus)
  - Bacterial (*Staphylococcus aureus, Clostridium perfringens,* diphthe-
    ria, any severe bacterial infection)
  - *Mycoplasma*
  - Mycotic (*Candida, Mucor, Aspergillus*)
  - Parasitic (*Trypanosoma cruzi, Trichinella, Echinococcus,* ameba,
    Toxoplasma)
  - *Rickettsia rickettsii*
  - Spirochetal (*Borrelia burgdorferi* [Lyme carditis])
- Rheumatic fever
- Secondary to drugs (e.g., cocaine, emetine, doxorubicin, sulfon-
  amides, isoniazid, methyldopa, amphotericin B, tetracycline, phenylbu-
  tazone, lithium, 5-fluorouracil, phenothiazines, interferon alfa, tricyclic
  antidepressants, cyclophosphamides)
- Toxins (carbon monoxide, ethanol, diphtheria toxin, lead, arsenicals)
- Collagen vascular disease (systemic lupus erythematosus, sclero-
  derma, sarcoidosis, Kawasaki syndrome)
- Sarcoidosis
- Radiation
- Postpartum

TREATMENT

- Treat underlying cause (e.g., use specific antibiotics for bacterial
  infection).
- Treat congestive heart failure (CHF) with diuretics, angiotensin-
  converting enzyme inhibitors, and salt restriction. A β-blocker may be
  added when clinical stability has been achieved. Digoxin should be
  used wtih caution and only at low doses.
- If ventricular arrhythmias are present, treat with quinidine or
  procainamide.
- Provide anticoagulation to prevent thromboembolism.
- Use preload and afterload reducing agents to treat cardiac
  decompensation.
- Corticosteroid use is contraindicated in early infectious myocarditis;
  it may be justified in only selected patients with intractable CHF,
  severe systemic toxicity, and severe life-threatening arrhythmias.

- Immunosuppressive drugs (prednisone with cyclosporine or azathioprine) do not have any significant effect on the prognosis of myocarditis and should not be used in the routine treatment of patients with myocarditis. Immunosuppression may be unnecessary because treatment of myocarditis from systemic autoimmune disease (e.g., systemic lupus erythematosus, scleroderma) and in patients with idiopathic giant cell myocarditis.

CLINICAL PEARLS

- A right ventricular endomyocardial biopsy can confirm the diagnosis, although a negative biopsy result does not exclude myocarditis. Studies have shown that myocardial biopsy may be unnecessary because immunosuppression therapy based on biopsy results is generally ineffective.
- Nearly 50% of patients with myocarditis die within 5 years of diagnosis. Prognosis is best for patients with "fulminant" lymphocytic myocarditis (severe hemodynamic compromise, rapid onset of symptoms, or high fever). These patients tend to have complete recovery with total resolution of myocarditis on repeat biopsy.

Myxedema coma

Definition: A life-threatening complication of hypothyroidism characterized by profound lethargy or coma and usually accompanied by hypothermia

DIAGNOSIS

- ### Clinical presentation:
  - Profound lethargy or coma
  - Hypothermia (rectal temperature <$35°C$ [$95°F$]); often missed by using ordinary thermometers graduated only to $34.5°C$ or because the mercury is not shaken below $36°C$
  - Bradycardia, hypotension (secondary to circulatory collapse)
  - Delayed relaxation phase of deep tendon reflexes, areflexia
  - Myxedema facies
  - Alopecia, macroglossia, ptosis, periorbital edema, nonpitting edema, doughy skin
  - Bladder dystonia and distention
- ### Laboratory tests:
  - Markedly increased thyroid-stimulating hormone (if primary hypothyroidism), decreased serum free thyroxine
  - Complete blood count with differential; urine and blood cultures

calcium, glucose

- Arterial blood gases to rule out hypoxemia and carbon dioxide retention
- Cortisol level to rule out adrenal insufficiency
- Elevated creatine phosphokinase
- Hyperlipidemia

ETIOLOGY
- Decompensation of hypothyroidism secondary to:
  - Sepsis
  - Exposure to cold weather
  - Central nervous system depressants (sedatives, narcotics, antidepressants)
  - Trauma, surgery

TREATMENT
- Give levothyroxine 5-8 µg/kg (300-500 µg) IV infused over 15 minutes, then 100 µg IV q24h.
- Glucocorticoids also should be administered until coexistent adrenal insufficiency can be ruled out. Hydrocortisone hemisuccinate 100 mg IV bolus is given initially, followed by 50 mg IV q12h or 25 mg IV q6h until initial plasma cortisol level is confirmed normal.
- Intravenous hydration with 5% dextrose in normal saline is used to correct hypotension and hypoglycemia (if present); avoid overhydration and possible water intoxication because clearance of free water is impaired in these patients.

CLINICAL PEARL
- If the diagnosis is suspected, initiate treatment immediately without waiting for confirming laboratory results.

▰ Nephrotic syndrome

Definition: Syndrome characterized by high urine protein excretion (>3.5 g/1.73 m^2/24 hr), peripheral edema, and metabolic abnormalities (hypoalbuminemia, hypercholesterolemia)

DIAGNOSIS
- **Clinical presentation:**
  - Peripheral edema
  - Ascites, anasarca
  - Hypertension
  - Pleural effusion

- Typically patients present with severe peripheral edema, exertional dyspnea, and abdominal fullness secondary to ascites. There is a significant amount of weight gain in most patients.
- **Laboratory tests:**
  - Urinalysis reveals proteinuria. The presence of hematuria, cellular casts, and pyuria suggests nephrotic syndrome. Oval fat bodies (tubular epithelial cells with cholesterol esters) also are found in the urine in patients with nephrotic syndrome.
  - Twenty-four-hour urine protein excretion is >3.5 g/1.73 m³/24 hr.
  - Abnormalities of blood chemistries include serum albumin <3 g/dL, decreased total protein, elevated serum cholesterol, elevated glucose, and azotemia.
  - Additional tests in patients with nephrotic syndromes, depending on the history and physical examination, are antinuclear antibody, serum and urine immunoelectrophoresis, C3, C4, CH-50, lactate dehydrogenase, liver enzymes, alkaline phosphatase, hepatitis B and C screening, and HIV.
- **Imaging:**
  - CT scan or ultrasound of kidneys
  - Chest x-ray

ETIOLOGY

- Idiopathic (may be secondary to the following glomerular diseases: minimal change disease [nil disease, lipoid nephrosis], focal segmental glomerular sclerosis, membranous nephropathy, membranoproliferative glomerular nephropathy)
- Associated with systemic diseases (diabetes mellitus, systemic lupus erythematosus, amyloidosis); amyloidosis and dysproteinemias should be considered in patients >40 years old
- Most children with nephrotic syndrome have minimal change disease (this form also associated with allergy, nonsteroidals, and Hodgkin's disease).
- Focal glomerular disease can be associated with HIV infection and heroin abuse. A more severe form of nephrotic syndrome associated with rapid progression to end-stage renal failure within months also can occur in HIV-seropositive patients and is called *collapsing glomerulopathy.*
- Membranous nephropathy can occur with Hodgkin's lymphoma, carcinomas, systemic lupus erythematosus, and gold therapy.
- Membranoproliferative glomerulonephropathy often is associated with upper respiratory infections.

TREATMENT

- Treat with bed rest as tolerated, avoidance of nephrotoxic drugs, low-

... protein loss exceeds 10 g/24 hr (some patients may require additional dietary protein to prevent negative nitrogen balance and significant protein malnutrition).

- Improved urinary protein excretion and serum lipid changes have been observed with a low-fat soy protein diet providing 0.7 g of protein/kg/day. Because of increased risk of malnutrition, many nephrologists recommend normal protein intake.
- Strict sodium restriction helps manage peripheral edema.
- Monitor patients closely for development of peripheral venous thrombosis and renal vein thrombosis because of hypercoagulable state secondary to loss of antithrombin III and other proteins involved in the clotting mechanism.
- Furosemide is useful for severe edema.
- Use of angiotensin-converting enzyme inhibitors to reduce proteinuria is generally indicated even in normotensive patients.
- Anticoagulant therapy should be administered as long as patients have nephrotic proteinuria, an albumin level <20 g/L, or both.
- The mainstay of therapy is treatment of the underlying disorder.
  - Minimal change disease generally responds to prednisone 1 mg/kg/day. Relapses can occur when steroids are discontinued. In these patients, cyclophosphamide and chlorambucil may be useful.
  - For focal and segmental glomerulosclerosis, steroid therapy is also recommended. Response rate is approximately 35% to 40%, and most patients progress to end-stage renal disease within 3 years.
  - For membranous glomerulonephritis, prednisone 2 mg/kg/day may be useful in inducing remission. Cytotoxic agents can be added if there is poor response to prednisone.
  - Most patients with membranoproliferative glomerulonephritis are treated with steroid therapy and antiplatelet drugs. Despite treatment, most patients progress to end-stage renal disease within 5 years.

CLINICAL PEARL

- Patients should be monitored for azotemia and should be treated aggressively for hypertension and hyperlipidemia. Furosemide is useful for severe edema. Anticoagulants may be necessary for thromboembolic events. Prophylactic anticoagulation should be considered in patients with membranous glomerulonephritis.

▨ Neuroleptic malignant syndrome (NMS)

Definition: Disorder characterized by hyperthermia, muscular rigidity, autonomic dysfunction, and depressed and fluctuating levels of arousal that evolve over 24 to 72 hours. NMS occurs as an idiosyncratic adverse reaction most commonly to dopamine-receptor antagonists (especially D2/4 receptor) or sudden withdrawal from a dopaminergic agent or agonist, such as antiparkinsonian medications.

DIAGNOSIS
- **Clinical presentation:**
  - Muscle rigidity (hypertonia, cogwheeling, or "lead pipe" rigidity)
  - Hyperthermia (38.6-42.3°C, usually <40°C [104°F])
  - Autonomic symptoms (diaphoresis, sialorrhea, skin pallor, urinary incontinence)
  - Tachycardia, tachypnea
  - Labile blood pressure (hypertension or postural hypotension)
  - Mental status changes (agitation, catatonia, fluctuating consciousness, obtundation)
- **Laboratory tests:**
  - Elevated creatine phosphokinase (in 71% of patients, with a mean value of 3700 U/L)
  - Urinary myoglobin
  - Leukocytosis (usually 10,000-40,000 mm³)
  - Electrolytes and renal function
  - Blood gases
  - Drug levels

ETIOLOGY
- The etiology is unknown. Impaired thermoregulation in hypothalamus and limbic cortex may occur as a result of relative lack of dopamine activity (central dopamine-blockade hypothesis—most accepted).
- Neuroleptic drugs have different potencies for inducing NMS.
  - **Typical neuroleptics:** high potency, haloperidol; medium potency, chlorpromazine, fluphenazine; low potency, levomepromazine, loxapine
  - **Atypical neuroleptics:** low potency, risperidone, olanzapine, clozapine, quetiapine

TREATMENT
- Stop all neuroleptic agents, and reinstitute any recently discontinued

- Give intravenous benzodiazepines (e.g., diazepam 2-10 mg, with total daily dose of 10-60 mg) to relax muscles and control agitation.
- Bromocriptine, a dopamine receptor agonist, is the mainstay of therapy for patients with NMS. Initial doses of 2.5-10 mg are given IV q8h and are increased by 5 mg/day until clinical improvement is seen. The drug should be continued for at least 10 days after the syndrome has been controlled, then tapered slowly.
- Amantadine, an *N*-methyl-d-aspartate receptor antagonist with possible dopaminergic properties, administered orally at doses of 100-200 mg PO bid, has been shown to reduce mortality compared with supportive therapy alone.
- Dantrolene therapy is also effective. Initially, patients can be given 0.25 mg/kg IV q6-12h, followed by a maintenance dose of 3 mg/kg/day. After 2 to 3 days, patients may be given the drug orally (25-600 mg in divided doses). Oral dantrolene therapy (50-600 mg/day) may be continued for several days afterward.
- Electroconvulsive therapy with neuromuscular blockage is indicated in pharmacologically refractory cases. Succinylcholine should not be used because it may cause hyperkalemia and cardiac arrhythmias in patients with rhabdomyolysis or dysautonomia.

▩ Nonalcoholic fatty liver disease

Definition: Liver disease occurring in patients who do not abuse alcohol and manifested histologically by mononuclear cells or polymorphonuclear cells (or both), hepatocyte ballooning, and spotty necrosis

DIAGNOSIS
- Diagnosis usually is suspected on the basis of hepatomegaly, asymptomatic elevations of transaminases, or "fatty liver" on abdominal ultrasound in obese patients with little or no alcohol use. Liver biopsy confirms the diagnosis and provides prognostic information. The diagnosis should be considered in patients with suspected advanced liver fibrosis (presence of obesity or type 2 diabetes, aspartate aminotransferase-to-alanine aminotransferase [AST/ALT] ratio 1, age 45 years).
- **Laboratory tests:**
  - ALT and AST are elevated; AST/ALT ratio is usually <1, but can increase as fibrosis advances.

- Serology is negative for infectious hepatitis and generally normal for γ-glutamyl transpeptidase and serum alkaline phosphatase.
- Hyperlipidemia (primarily hypertriglyceridemia) may be present.
- Elevated glucose levels may be present.
- Prolonged prothrombin time, hypoalbuminuria, and elevated bilirubin may be present in advanced stages.
- Elevated serum ferritin and increased transferrin saturation may be found in 10% of patients; however, hepatic iron index and hepatic iron level are normal.
- Liver biopsy specimen may show a wide spectrum of liver damage, ranging from simple steatosis to advanced fibrosis and cirrhosis.

- **Imaging:**
- Ultrasound generally reveals diffuse increase in echogenicity compared with that of the kidneys; CT scan reveals diffuse low-density hepatic parenchyma.
- Occasionally, patients may have focal rather than diffuse steatosis, which may be misinterpreted as a liver mass on ultrasound or CT; use of MRI in these cases identifies focal fatty infiltration.

ETIOLOGY

- Insulin resistance is the most reproducible factor in the development of nonalcoholic fatty liver disease.
- Risk factors are obesity (especially truncal obesity), diabetes mellitus, and hyperlipidemia.

TREATMENT

- Weight reduction is indicated in all obese patients (500 g/wk in children and 1600 g/wk in adults is preferred).
- No medications have been proved directly to improve liver damage from nonalcoholic fatty liver disease.
- Medications to control hyperlipidemia (e.g., fenofibrates for elevated triglycerides) and hyperglycemia (e.g., metformin) can lead to improvement in abnormal liver test results.

CLINICAL PEARL

- The presence of steatohepatitis or advanced fibrosis on liver biopsy is associated with a worse prognosis.

Non-Hodgkin's lymphoma (NHL)

Definition: Heterogeneous group of malignancies of the lymphoreticular system

DIAGNOSIS

- Initial laboratory evaluation may reveal only mild anemia and elevated lactate dehydrogenase (LDH) and erythrocyte sedimentation rate (ESR). Proper diagnostic and staging of NHL requires the following:
  - Thorough history, physical examination, and adequate biopsy
  - Routine laboratory evaluation (complete blood count, ESR, urinalysis, LDH, blood urea nitrogen, creatinine, serum calcium, uric acid, liver function tests, serum protein electrophoresis)
  - Chest x-ray (posteroanterior and lateral)
  - Bone marrow evaluation (aspirate and full bone core biopsy)
  - CT scan of abdomen and pelvis; CT scan of chest if chest x-ray films abnormal
  - Bone scan (particularly in patients with histiocytic lymphoma)
- Depending on the histopathology, the results of the above-listed studies, and the planned therapy, some other tests may be performed, including gallium scan (e.g., in patients with high-grade lymphomas), liver/spleen scan, positron emission tomography scan, lymphangiography, and lumbar puncture.
- β₂-Microglobulin levels should be obtained initially (prognostic value) and serially in patients with low-grade lymphomas (useful to monitor therapeutic response of the tumor).

ETIOLOGY

- The etiology is unknown.

TREATMENT

- The therapeutic regimen varies with the histologic type and pathologic stage.
- **Low-grade NHL (nodular, poorly differentiated):**
  - Local radiotherapy for symptomatic obstructive adenopathy
  - Deferment of therapy and careful observation in asymptomatic patients
  - Single-agent chemotherapy with cyclophosphamide or chlorambucil and glucocorticoids
  - Combination chemotherapy alone or with radiotherapy: generally indicated only when the lymphoma becomes more invasive, with poor response to less aggressive treatment. Commonly used regimens are CVP, CHOP, CHOP-BLEO, COPP, BACOP; addition of

recombinant interferon alfa at low doses to chemotherapy prolongs remission duration in patients with low-grade NHL.

- Monoclonal antibodies directed against B-cell surface antigens also can be used to treat follicular lymphomas that are resistant to conventional therapy. The anti-CD20 monoclonal antibody rituximab is a targeted, minimally toxic treatment effective against low-grade NHL. In patients who have not received previous treatment, The addition of rituximab to CHOP is generally well tolerated; however, additional studies may be necessary to clarify the role of CHOP plus rituximab in patients with indolent NHL.
  - Ibritumomab tiuxetan (Zevalin), an immunoconjugate that combines the linker-chelator tiuxetan with the monoclonal antibody ibritumomab, can be used as part of a two-step regimen for treatment of patients with relapsed or refractory low-grade, follicular, or transformed B-cell NHL, refractory to rituximab.
- New purine analogues (FLAMP, cladribine) can be used in salvage treatment of refractory lymphomas. They all have activity in follicular lymphomas.

- **Intermediate-grade and high-grade NHL (diffuse histiocytic lymphoma):**
  - Combination chemotherapy regimens (e.g., CHOP, PRO-MACE-CYTABOM, MACOP-B, M-BACOD): An anthracycline-containing regimen (e.g., CHOP) given in standard doses and schedule is generally best for treatment of older patients with advanced-stage, aggressive-histology lymphoma who do not have significant comorbid illness.
  - High-dose sequential therapy is superior to standard-dose MACOP-B for patients with diffuse large cell lymphoma of the B-cell type. Dose-modified chemotherapy should be considered for most HIV-infected patients with lymphoma. Compared with treatment with standard doses of cytotoxic chemotherapy (M-BACOD), reduced doses cause significantly fewer hematologic toxic effects, yet have similar efficacy in patients with HIV-related lymphoma.
  - Three cycles of CHOP followed by involved-field radiotherapy may be superior to eight cycles of CHOP alone in patients with localized intermediate-grade and high-grade NHL.
  - The addition of rituximab against CD20 B-cell lymphoma to the CHOP regimen increases the complete response rate and prolongs event-free and overall survival in elderly patients with diffuse large B-cell lymphoma without a clinically significant increase in toxicity.
  - Granulocyte-colony stimulating factor may be effective in reducing the risk of infection in patients with aggressive lymphoma undergoing chemotherapy.

...ine 131 anti-B1 antibody therapy for NHL, either alone or in combination with other treatments, may be effective.

- Treatment with high-dose chemotherapy and autologous bone marrow transplant compared with conventional chemotherapy increases event-free and overall survival in patients with chemotherapy-sensitive NHL in relapse.

CLINICAL PEARLS

- Patients often present with asymptomatic lymphadenopathy.
- Approximately one third of NHL originates extranodally. Involvement of extranodal sites can result in unusual presentations (e.g., gastrointestinal tract involvement can simulate peptic ulcer disease).
- NHL cases associated with HIV occur predominantly in the brain.
- Pruritus, fever, night sweats, and weight loss are less common than in Hodgkin's disease.

▰ Nonketotic hyperosmolar syndrome

Definition: State of extreme hyperglycemia, marked dehydration, serum hyperosmolarity, altered mental status, and absence of ketoacidosis

DIAGNOSIS

- **Clinical presentation:**
  - Evidence of extreme dehydration (poor skin turgor, sunken eyeballs, dry mucous membranes)
  - Neurologic defects (reversible hemiplegia, focal seizures)
  - Orthostatic hypotension, tachycardia
  - Evidence of precipitating factors (pneumonia, infected skin ulcer)
  - Coma (25% of patients), delirium
- **Laboratory tests:**
  - Hyperglycemia—serum glucose usually >600 mg/dL
  - Hyperosmolarity—serum osmolarity usually >340 mOsm/L
  - Serum sodium—may be low, normal, or high; if normal or high, the patient is severely dehydrated because an elevated glucose draws fluid from the intracellular space, decreasing the serum sodium; the corrected sodium can be obtained by increasing the serum sodium concentration by 1.6 mEq/dL for every 100 mg/dL increase in the serum glucose level over normal
  - Serum potassium—may be low, normal, or high; regardless of the initial serum level, the total body deficit is approximately 5 to 15 mEq/kg

- Serum bicarbonate—usually <12 mEq/L (average 17 mEq/L)
- Arterial pH—usually >7.2 (average 7.26); serum bicarbonate and arterial pH may be lower if lactic acidosis is present
- Blood urea nitrogen (BUN)—azotemia (prerenal) is usually present (BUN generally 60-90 mg/dL)
- Phosphorus—hypophosphatemia (average deficit 70-140 mm
- Calcium—hypocalcemia (average deficit 50-100 mEq)
- Magnesium—hypomagnesemia (average deficit 50-100 mEq)
- Complete blood count with differential, urinalysis, and blood and urine cultures should be performed to rule out infectious etiology.

ETIOLOGY

- Infections—20% to 25% (e.g., pneumonia, urinary tract infection, sepsis)
- New or previously unrecognized diabetes—30% to 50%
- Reduction or omission of patient medication
- Stress (myocardial infarction, cerebrovascular accident)
- Drugs (diuretics [dehydration], phenytoin, diazoxide [impaired insulin secretion])

TREATMENT

- Institute vigorous fluid replacement. The volume and rate of fluid replacement are determined by renal and cardiac function. Typically, infuse 1000-1500 mL/hr for the initial 1-2 L, then decrease the rate of infusion to 500 mL/hr and monitor urinary output, blood chemistries, and blood pressure. Use 0.9% normal saline (isotonic solution) if the patient is hypotensive or serum osmolarity is <320 mOsm/L; otherwise use 0.45% normal saline solution. A slower infusion rate may be used initially in patients with compromised cardiovascular or renal status. Replace electrolytes, and monitor serum levels frequently (e.g., serum sodium and potassium q2h for the first 12 hours). Serum potassium chloride (KCl) replacement in patients with normal renal function and adequate urinary output is started when the serum potassium level is <5.2 mEq/L (e.g., 10 mEq KCl/hr if potassium level is <5.2 mEq/L). Continuous ECG monitoring and hourly measurement of urinary output are recommended.
- Correct hyperglycemia. The goal is for plasma glucose to decline by at least 75 to 100 mg/dL/hr.
- Vigorous intravenous hydration decreases the serum glucose level in most patients by 80 mg/dL/hr; a regular intravenous bolus (10 U) is often not necessary.
- Begin low-dose insulin infusion at 1-2 U/hr (e.g., 25 U of regular insulin in 250 mL of 0.9% saline solution at 20 mL/hr) until the serum glucose level approaches 300 mg/dL; then the patient is started on regular subcutaneous insulin with sliding scale

hours despite adequate fluid administration and urine output, consider doubling the hourly insulin dose.
- Glucose should be monitored q1-2h in the initial 12 hours.
- In the absence of renal failure, phosphate can be administered at a rate of 0.1 mmol/kg/hr (5-10 mmol/hr) to a maximum of 80 to 120 mmol in 24 hours. Magnesium replacement, in the absence of renal failure, can be administered intramuscularly (0.05-0.10 mL/kg of 20% magnesium sulfate) or as intravenous infusion (4-8 mL of 20% magnesium sulfate [0.08-0.16 mEq/kg]). Repeat magnesium, phosphate, and calcium levels should be obtained after 12 to 24 hours.

CLINICAL PEARL
- The typical patient presenting with hyperosmolar coma is an elderly or bed-confined diabetic with impaired ability to communicate thirst who is evaluated after an interval of 1 to 2 weeks of prolonged osmotic diuresis.

 Osteomyelitis

Definition: Infection involving the bones and bone marrow

DIAGNOSIS
- **Clinical presentation:**
  - Classic presentation consists of bone pain, fever, chills, and generalized malaise.
  - There is significant tenderness over the bone and limitations of movement of the involved extremity.
- **Laboratory tests:**
  - Blood cultures
  - White blood cell count—peripheral leukocytosis usually present
  - Erythrocyte sedimentation rate (ESR)—a normal value does not rule out osteomyelitis; an initially elevated ESR may be useful in following the course of the disease
  - Multiple deep cultures of a draining sinus, bony curettage, and débrided bed of any involved bones should be obtained. Aspirate and culture any joint effusions.
  - The definitive diagnosis of osteomyelitis rests on the isolation of the infective organism from bone or joint fluid obtained either by surgery or by multiple percutaneous needle biopsies.

Imaging:

- Initial x-rays may be normal because radiologic changes lag behind the clinical manifestations. Positive radiographic findings usually become apparent at about 4 weeks.
- Initial changes consist of subperiosteal elevation and soft tissue swelling; these are followed by lytic changes generally 3 to 4 weeks after the onset of disease.
- Radionuclide scanning (technetium-99m scan) can detect osteomyelitis early in its course; however, neoplasms, trauma, and other inflammatory processes also may produce positive radionuclide scans. Negative scans in documented osteomyelitis generally are caused by impaired blood supply in the infected area. Twenty-four-hour nuclear scanning with indium-labeled leukocytes is useful to diagnose osteomyelitis in diabetic foot ulcers.
- MRI is the most expensive, but also the most accurate imaging study for osteomyelitis; it has the highest sensitivity, has good specificity, and allows differentiation from soft tissue infection. It is especially useful in cases of axial osteomyelitis to assess the extent of vertebral, paravertebral, and soft tissue involvement. It also is useful in distinguishing bone tumor or infarction from osteomyelitis and in distinguishing normal from abnormal areas in planning surgery for diabetic patients with osteomyelitis.
- Doppler studies are useful in patients with peripheral vascular disease to determine vascular adequacy.

ETIOLOGY

- *Staphylococcus aureus* is the most common causative agent.
- Gram-negative bacilli include *Salmonella*, *Escherichia coli*, *Pseudomonas*, and *Klebsiella*.
- *Salmonella* often is seen in patients with sickle cell disease.
- *Pseudomonas* is more frequent in intravenous drug addicts; puncture wounds in sneakers also occur.
- *Haemophilus influenza* generally is seen in infants and children.
- Coagulase-negative staphylococci or *Propionibacterium* is seen in foreign body—associated infection.
- Anaerobes often involve the sacrum (associated with infected decubitus ulcers), skull, and hands (after human bites) and diabetic foot lesions.
- *Bartonella henselae* is seen in HIV infection.
- *Pasteurella multocida* or *Eikenella corrodens* is seen in human or animal bites.
- **Others:** streptococci, *Mycobacterium tuberculosis* (generally involves spine and results in compression fractures), fungi (*Candida albicans*, *Aspergillus*).

- The choice of antibiotic depends on the suspected likely pathogen. Nafcillin or oxacillin 2 g IV q4h and cefazolin 2 g IV q8h are preferred as initial agents in adults with *S. aureus* osteomyelitis from hematogenous spread. Vancomycin 1 g IV q12h is an alternative agent. In suspected *Pseudomonas* osteomyelitis, use ceftazidime plus aminoglycoside.
- Oral ciprofloxacin is an effective and inexpensive choice in osteomyelitis caused by Enterobacteriaceae. Because of reports of the development of resistance, careful monitoring of patients is necessary when ciprofloxacin is used as monotherapy in *Pseudomonas* osteomyelitis.
- Perform surgical débridement of all devitalized bone and tissue.
- Immobilize affected bone (e.g., plaster, traction) if the bone is unstable after débridement or removal of prosthesis.

Paget's disease of bone

Definition: Nonmetabolic disease of bone characterized by repeated episodes of osteolysis and excessive attempts at repair that result in a weakened bone of increased mass. *Monostotic* (solitary lesion) and *polyostotic* (numerous lesions) disease are described.

DIAGNOSIS
- Plain x-rays reflect the characteristic radiolucency and opacity.
- Bone scanning usually reflects the activity and extent of the disease.
- Laboratory tests show increased serum alkaline phosphatase and normal serum calcium and phosphorus levels.
- Symptoms result mainly from the effects of complications.
  - Skeletal pain, especially hip and pelvis
  - Bowing of long bones, sometimes leading to pathologic fracture
  - Increased heat of extremity (resulting from increased vascularity)
  - Skull enlargement and spinal involvement caused by characteristic bone enlargement, which can produce neurologic complications (vision loss, hearing loss, radicular pain, and cord compression)
  - Thoracic kyphoscoliosis
  - Secondary osteoarthritis, especially of hip
  - Heart failure as a result of chest and spine deformity and blood shunting

TREATMENT
- Calcitonin
- Bisphosphonates

- Nonsteroidal antiinflammatory drugs for pain relief
- General indications for treatment
  - All symptomatic patients
  - Asymptomatic patients with high level of metabolic activity or patients at risk for deformity
- Preoperative, if surgery involves pagetic bone

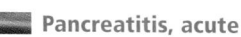

Pancreatitis, acute

Definition: An inflammatory process of the pancreas with intrapancreatic activation of enzymes that also may involve peripancreatic tissue or remote organ systems or both

DIAGNOSIS

- **Clinical presentation:**
  - Epigastric tenderness and guarding; pain usually developing suddenly, reaching peak intensity within 10 to 30 minutes, severe and lasting several hours without relief
  - Hypoactive bowel sounds (secondary to ileus)
  - Tachycardia, shock (secondary to decreased intravascular volume)
- **Laboratory tests:**
  - Amylase is increased, usually elevated in the initial 3 to 5 days of acute pancreatitis. Isoamylase determinations (separation of pancreatic cell isoenzyme components of amylase) are useful in excluding occasional cases of salivary hyperamylasemia.
  - Urinary amylase determinations are useful to diagnose acute pancreatitis in patients with lipemic serum, to rule out elevated serum amylase secondary to macroamylasemia, and to diagnose acute pancreatitis in patients whose serum amylase is normal.
  - Serum lipase levels are elevated in acute pancreatitis; the elevation is less transient than serum amylase; concomitant evaluation of serum amylase and lipase increases diagnostic accuracy of acute pancreatitis. An elevated lipase-to-amylase ratio suggests alcoholic pancreatitis.
  - Complete blood count reveals leukocytosis. Hematocrit may be increased initially secondary to hemoconcentration; decreased hematocrit may indicate hemorrhage or hemolysis.
  - Blood urea nitrogen (BUN) is increased secondary to dehydration.
  - Elevation of serum glucose in a previously normal patient correlates with the degree of pancreatic malfunction.
  - Liver panel shows aspartate aminotransferase (AST) and lactate dehydrogenase (LDH) are increased secondary to tissue necrosis; bilirubin and alkaline phosphatase may be increased secondary to

alanine aminotransferase concentrations is an excellent indicator (95% probability) of biliary pancreatitis.

- Serum calcium is decreased secondary to saponification, precipitation, and decreased parathyroid hormone response.
- Arterial blood gases show PaO_2 may be decreased secondary to adult respiratory distress syndrome or pleural effusion; pH may be decreased secondary to lactic acidosis, respiratory acidosis, and renal insufficiency.
- Serum electrolytes show potassium may be increased secondary to acidosis or renal insufficiency; sodium may be increased secondary to dehydration.
- **Imaging:**
  - Abdominal plain film is useful to distinguish other conditions that may mimic pancreatitis (perforated viscus); it may reveal localized ileus (sentinel loop), pancreatic calcifications (chronic pancreatitis), blurring of left psoas shadow, dilation of transverse colon, or calcified gallstones.
  - Chest x-ray may reveal elevation of one or both diaphragms, pleural effusions, basilar infiltrates, or platelike atelectasis.
  - Abdominal ultrasound is useful to detect gallstones (sensitivity of 60-70% for detecting stones associated with pancreatitis). It also is useful for detecting pancreatic pseudocysts; its major limitation is the presence of distended bowel loops overlying the pancreas.
  - CT is superior to ultrasonography in identifying pancreatitis and defining its extent, and it plays a role in diagnosing pseudocysts (they appear as a well-defined area surrounded by a high-density capsule). Gastrointestinal fistula or infection of a pseudocyst can be identified by the presence of gas within the pseudocyst. Sequential contrast-enhanced CT is useful to detec pancreatic necrosis. CT also can grade the severity of pancreatitis.

ETIOLOGY

- **In >90% of cases:** biliary tract disease (calculi or sludge) or alcohol
- Drugs (thiazides, furosemide, corticosteroids, tetracycline, estrogens, valproic acid, metronidazole, azathioprine, methyldopa, pentamidine, ethacrynic acid, procainamide, sulindac, nitrofurantoin, angiotensin-converting enzyme inhibitors, danazol, cimetidine, piroxicam, gold, ranitidine, sulfasalazine, isoniazid, acetaminophen, cisplatin, opiates, erythromycin)
- Abdominal trauma
- Surgery
- Endoscopic retrograde cholangiopancreatography
- Infections (predominantly viral infections)

- Peptic ulcer (penetrating duodenal ulcer)
- Pancreas divisum (congenital failure of fusion of dorsal or ventral pancreas)
- Idiopathic
- Pregnancy
- Vascular (vasculitis, ischemic)
- Hypolipoproteinemia (types I, IV, and V)
- Hypercalcemia
- Pancreatic carcinoma (primary or metastatic)
- Renal failure
- Hereditary pancreatitis
- Occupational exposure to chemicals (methanol, cobalt, zinc, mercuric chloride, creosol, lead, organophosphates, chlorinated naphthalenes)
- **Others:** scorpion bite, obstruction at ampulla region (neoplasm, duodenal diverticula, Crohn's disease), hypotensive shock

TREATMENT

- **General measures:**
  - Maintain adequate intravascular volume with vigorous intravenous hydration.
  - Patient should remain nothing-per-mouth status until clinically improved, stable, and hungry.
  - Nasogastric suction is useful in severe pancreatitis to decompress the abdomen in patients with ileus.
  - **Control pain:** Oral analgesics may cause spasms of the sphincter of Oddi (meperidine may produce less constriction than other analgesics; however, clear evidence regarding this claim is lacking, and metabolites may cause significant neurotoxic effects, such as seizures, myoclonus, or tremors).
  - Correct metabolic abnormalities (e.g., replace calcium and magnesium as necessary).
  - Total parenteral nutrition may be necessary in prolonged pancreatitis.
- **Specific measures:**
  - Intravenous antibiotics should not be used prophylactically; their use is justified if the patient has evidence of septicemia, pancreatic abscess, or pancreatitis secondary to biliary calculi.
  - Surgical therapy has a limited role in acute pancreatitis; it is indicated in the following:
    - Gallstone-induced pancreatitis; cholecystectomy when acute pancreatitis subsides
    - Perforated peptic ulcer
    - Excision or drainage of necrotic or infected foci

- Prognosis varies with the severity of pancreatitis; overall mortality in acute pancreatitis is 5% to 10%; poor prognostic signs are the following (Ranson criteria):
  - Age >55 years old
  - Fluid sequestration >6000 mL
  - Laboratory abnormalities on admission: white blood cell count >16,000/mm^3, blood glucose >200 mL/dL, serum LDH >350 IU/L, AST >250 IU/L
  - Laboratory abnormalities during the initial 48 hours: decreased hematocrit >10% with hydration or hematocrit <30%, BUN rise >5 mg/dL, serum calcium <8 mg/dL, arterial Po$_2$ <60 mm Hg, and base deficit >4 mEq/L

Parkinson's disease

Definition: Progressive neurologic disorder affecting 1% of population >60 years old; characterized pathologically by cytoplasmic eosinophilic inclusions (Lewy bodies) in neurons of the substantia nigra and locus caeruleus and by depigmentation of the brainstem nuclei

DIAGNOSIS
- Clinical presentation:
  - The disease often begins insidiously and can manifest as a slight loss of motor dexterity, generalized slowness, or a decrease in overall motor activity.
  - The classic manifestations of Parkinson's disease are as follows:
    - **Rigidity:** increased muscle tone. It involves agonist and antagonist muscle groups. The resistance to passive movement is widespread and more prominent at large joints ("cogwheeling" rigidity is noted).
    - **Tremor:** resting tremor, with a frequency of four to seven movements per second. It often begins unilaterally and distally and spreads proximally and to the other side over months or years. The tremor usually is noted in the hands and often involves the thumb and forefinger ("pill-rolling" tremor).
    - **Akinesia:** inability to initiate or execute a movement. The patient often sits immobile because even the simple task of getting up from a chair becomes impossible. The face shows a marked absence of movement (masked facies); the mouth is usually open, and the patient drools.

- **Gait disturbance:** The patient assumes a stooped posture (head bowed, trunk bent forward, shoulders dropped; knees and arms flexed, "soccer goalie stand"). There is difficulty initiating the first step, and this is followed by small shuffling steps that increase in speed (festinating gait) as if the patient is chasing his or her center of gravity (the patient's steps become progressively faster and shorter while the trunk inclines further forward).

- **Abnormal reflexes** Stroking the palm of the hand near the base of the thumb results in contraction of the ipsilateral mentalis muscle, causing wrinkling of the skin of the chin (palmomental reflex). Repeated gentle tapping on the glabella evokes blinking of both eyes (glabellar reflex).

- **Dementia:** occurs in approximately 25% to 50% of patients

- **Others:** orthostatic hypotension, micrographia, diminished blinking, inaudible speech, difficulty opening a jar, turning in bed

TREATMENT

- Treatment is directed toward relieving the symptoms of tremor and rigidity and slowing the disease.

- Drug therapy should generally be delayed until symptoms significantly limit the patient's daily activities because tolerance and side effects to antiparkinsonian agents are common.

- Levodopa generally should be avoided early in the course of Parkinson's disease. Selegiline (Eldepryl) or second-generation dopamine agonists (ropinirole [Requip], pramipexole [Mirapex]) carry a smaller risk of dyskinesia and are preferred for early treatment.

- **Commonly used agents in Parkinson's disease:**

- Selegiline, an inhibitor of monoamine oxidase B, is favored by some as initial treatment for younger patients with early disease because of its possible neuroprotective effect.

- Dopamine receptor agonists, including ropinirole and pramipexole, are not as potent as levodopa, but often are used as initial treatment in younger patients to attempt to delay the tolerance and onset of complications (dyskinesias, motor fluctuations [on/off effect]) associated with levodopa therapy.

- Levodopa therapy the cornerstone of symptomatic therapy, commonly is used with a peripheral dopa decarboxylase inhibitor (carbidopa) to minimize side effects (nausea, mood changes, cardiac arrhythmias, postural hypotension). The combination of the two drugs is marketed under the trade name Sinemet.

- Amantadine (Symmetrel) is an antiviral agent that may increase dopamine in the brain and improve rigidity and bradykinesia.

- Anticholinergic agents, including trihexyphenidyl (Artane) and ⬛⬛⬛ (Cogentin) are helpful in treating the tremor and

alone or in combination with levodopa.
- Implantation of electrodes to stimulate precise locations in the brain (*deep brain stimulation*) is a newer treatment modality. Thalamic stimulation and thalamotomy are equally effective for the suppression of drug-resistant tremor, but thalamic stimulation has fewer adverse effects and results in a greater improvement in function.
- Transplantation of fetal tissue, ventrolateral thalamotomy (for control of tremor, rigidity, and dystonia), and medial pallidotomy (to control akinesia or on/off effects) are available only in selected centers.

Paroxysmal atrial tachycardia

Definition: Group of arrhythmias that generally originate as reentrant rhythm from the atrioventricular node and are characterized by sudden onset and abrupt termination

DIAGNOSIS
- ECG reveals absolutely regular rhythm at rate of 150 to 220 beats/min (Fig. 13).
- P waves may or may not be seen (the presence of P waves depends on the relationship of atrial to ventricular depolarization).
- Wide QRS complex (>0.12 second) with initial slurring (delta wave) during sinus rhythm and short P-R interval (≤0.12 second) is characteristic of Wolff-Parkinson-White (WPW) syndrome;

ETIOLOGY
- Preexcitation syndromes (WPW syndrome)
- Atrial septal defect
- Acute myocardial infarction

TREATMENT
- Valsalva maneuver in the supine position is the most effective way to terminate supraventricular tachycardia (SVT); carotid sinus massage (after excluding occlusive carotid disease) also is commonly used to elicit vagal efferent impulses.
- Synchronized DC shock is used if patient shows signs of cardiogenic shock, angina, or congestive heart failure.
- Adenosine (Adenocard) is effective for treatment of SVT. Dose is 6 mg given as a rapid intravenous bolus; tachycardia usually is terminated within a few seconds; if necessary, adenosine may be repeated with 12-mg IV bolus.

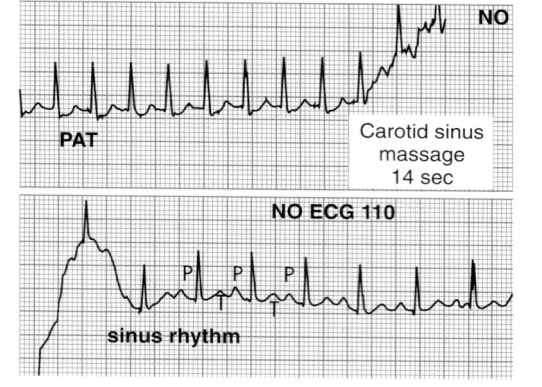

FIGURE 13. Paroxysmal atrial tachycardia. The upper and lower rows are part of one continuous strip. In the upper row, no definite P waves are visible. The diagnosis of this electrocardiogram is supraventricular tachyarrhythmia. The ventricular rate is approximately 185 beats/min. In the lower strip, taken at the end of the carotid sinus massage, sinus rhythm has appeared. The heart rate is still rapid (approximately 135 beats/min). (From Goldberger E: Treatment of Cardiac Emergencies, 5th ed. St Louis, Mosby, 1990.)

- Verapamil 5-10 mg IV is given over 5 minutes; if no effect, dose may be repeated in 30 minutes. Repeat carotid massage after intravenous verapamil if SVT persists.
- Metoprolol (5 mg/2 min IV up to 15 mg) or esmolol (500 µg/kg IV bolus, then 50 µg/kg/min) may be effective in the treatment of SVT.

Definition: Lice infestation. Humans can be infested with three kinds of lice: *Pediculus capitis* (head louse), *Pediculus corporis* (body louse), and *Phthirus pubis* (pubic, or crab, louse). Lice feed on human blood and deposit their eggs (nits) on the hair shafts (head lice and pubic lice) and along the seams of clothing (body lice). Nits generally hatch within 7 to 10 days. Lice are obligate human parasites and cannot survive away from their hosts for >7 to 10 days.

DIAGNOSIS
- Pruritus with excoriation may be caused by hypersensitivity reaction, inflammation from saliva, and fecal material from the lice.
- Nits can be identified by examining hair shafts.
- The presence of nits on clothes indicates body lice.
- Lymphadenopathy may be present (cervical adenopathy with head lice, inguinal lymphadenopathy with pubic lice).
- Head lice most frequently are found in the back of the head and neck, behind the ears.
- Scratching can result in pustules and crusting.
- Pubic lice may affect the hair around the anus.
- Wood's light examination is useful to screen a large number of children; live nits fluoresce, empty nits have a gray fluorescence, and nits with unborn louse have a white fluorescence.

DIFFERENTIAL DIAGNOSIS
- Seborrheic dermatitis
- Scabies
- Eczema
- **Other:** pilar casts, trichonodosis (knotted hair), monilethrix

TREATMENT
- The following products are available for treatment of lice:
  - Permethrin is available over the counter (1% permethrin [Nix]) or by prescription (5% permethrin [Elimite]); it should be applied to the hair and scalp and rinsed out after 10 minutes. A repeat application generally is not necessary in patients with head lice.
  - Lindane 1% (Kwell) and pyrethrin S (RID) are available as shampoos or lotions; they are applied to the affected area and washed off in 5 minutes; treatment should be repeated in 7 to 10 days to destroy hatching nits.
  - Malathion (Ovide) or organophosphate is effective in head lice. It is available by prescription. Use should be avoided in children ≤2 years old.

- In patients who previously have failed treatment or in whom resistance with 1% permethrin cream rinse occurs, a 10-day course of trimethoprim-sulfamethoxazole (8 mg/kg/day of trimethoprin in divided doses) is an effective treatment for head lice infestation.
- Ivermectin (Mectizan), an antiparasitic drug, given in a single oral dose of 200 µg/kg is effective for head lice resistant to other treatments (currently not approved by the Food and Drug Administration for pediculosis).

CLINICAL PEARLS
- Patients with body lice should discard infested clothes and improve their hygiene.
- Combing out nits is a widely recommended but unproven adjunctive therapy.
- Personal items such as combs and brushes should be soaked in hot water for 15 to 30 minutes.
- Close contacts and household members also should be examined for the presence of lice.

Pelvic inflammatory disease (PID)

Definition: Spectrum of inflammatory disorders of the upper genital tract among women, which may include any combination of endometritis, salpingitis, tuboovarian abscess, and pelvic peritonitis

DIAGNOSIS
- No single historical, physical, or laboratory finding is sensitive and specific for the diagnosis of acute PID.
- **Minimal criteria for the diagnosis of PID:**
  - Uterine/adnexal tenderness *or*
  - Cervical motion tenderness
- **Additional criteria:**
  - Oral temperature >38.3°C (101°F)
  - Abnormal cervical or vaginal mucopurulent discharge
  - Presence of white blood cells on saline microscopy of vaginal secretions
  - Elevated erythrocyte sedimentation rate
  - Elevated C-reactive protein level
  - Laboratory documentation of cervical infection with *Neisseria gonorrhoeae* or *Chlamydia trachomatis*.
- The most specific criteria for diagnosing PID include the following:
  - Histopathologic evidence of endometritis on endometrial biopsy

cned fluid-filled tubes with or without free pelvic fluid or tuboovarian complex
  - Laparoscopic abnormalities consistent with PID

ETIOLOGY

- Sexually transmitted organisms, especially *N. gonorrhoeae* and
  C. trachomatis, are implicated in most cases.
- Microorganisms that can be part of the vaginal flora, such as anaerobes, *Gardnerella vaginalis, Haemophilus influenzae,* enteric gram-
  negative rods, and *Streptococcus agalactiae,* also can cause PID.
- Some experts also believe that *Mycoplasma hominis* and *Ureaplasma
  urealyticum* are causative agents of PID.

TREATMENT

- Parenteral regimen A:
  - Cefotetan 2 g IV q12h *or* cefoxitin 2 g IV q6h *plus*
  - Doxycycline 100 mg IV or PO q12h
  - *Note:* Parenteral therapy may be discontinued 24 hours after the
    patient improves clinically; oral therapy with doxycycline 100 mg
    bid should be continued for 14 days.
- Parenteral regimen B:
  - Clindamycin 900 mg IV q8h *plus*
  - Gentamicin, loading dose 2 mg/kg body weight IV or IM followed
    by a maintenance dose 1.5 mg/kg q8h. Single daily doses may be
    substituted.
  - *Note:* Parenteral therapy may be discontinued 24 hours after a patient
    improves clinically. Continuing oral therapy should consist of doxycy-
    cline 100 mg PO bid or clindamycin 450 mg PO qid to complete 14
    days of therapy.
- **Alternative parenteral regimens:**
  - Ofloxacin 400 mg IV q12h *or* levofloxacin 500 mg IV qd *with or
    without* metronidazole 500 mg IV q8h *or*
  - Ampicillin-sulbactam (Unasyn) 3 g IV q6h *plus* doxycycline 100 mg
    IV or PO q12h
- **Outpatient oral treatment regimens:**
  - **Regimen A:**
    - Ofloxacin 400 mg PO bid for 14 days *or* levofloxacin 500 mg PO
      qd for 14 days *with or without* metronidazole 500 mg PO bid for
      14 days
  - **Regimen B:**
    - Ceftriaxone 250 mg IM once *plus* doxycycline 100 mg PO bid for
      14 days *with or without* metronidazole 500 mg PO bid for 14 days
      or

- Cefoxitin 2 g IM plus probenecid 1 g PO in a single concurrent dose *plus* doxycycline 100 mg PO bid for 14 days *with or without* metronidazole 500 mg PO bid for 14 days

CLINICAL PEARLS

- Outpatient management of PID is appropriate for most patients; however, follow-up within 72 hours is recommended to assess the patient's response to antimicrobial therapy.
- Hospitalization is recommended when the following criteria are met:
  - Surgical emergencies, such as appendicitis, cannot be excluded.
  - The patient is pregnant.
  - The patient has a tuboovarian abscess.
  - The patient has severe illness, nausea and vomiting, or high fever.
  - The patient is unable to follow or tolerate an outpatient oral regimen.
  - The patient does not respond clinically to oral antimicrobial therapy.

Peptic ulcer disease (PUD)

Définition: Ulceration in the stomach or duodenum resulting from an imbalance between mucosal protective factors and various mucosal damaging mechanisms

DIAGNOSIS

- Physical examination is often unremarkable. Patient may have epigastric tenderness, tachycardia, pallor, hypotension (from acute or chronic blood loss), nausea and vomiting (if pyloric channel is obstructed), boardlike abdomen and rebound tenderness (if perforated), and hematemesis or melena (with a bleeding ulcer).
- Diagnostic modalities include endoscopy or upper gastrointestinal series. Endoscopy is preferred.
- Routine laboratory studies are usually unremarkable. Anemia may be present in patients with significant gastrointestinal bleeding. *Helicobacter pylori* testing via endoscopic biopsy, urea breath test, stool antigen test (*H. pylori* stool antigen), or specific antibody test is recommended. Histologic evaluation of endoscopic biopsy samples is currently the gold standard for accurate diagnosis of *H. pylori* infection. Stool antigen tests are as accurate as the urea breath test for follow-up evaluation of patients treated for *H. pylori*. This test detects the presence of infection by measuring the fecal excretion of *H. pylori* antigens. A positive result on the stool antigen test 8 weeks after

pylori was unsuccessful.

ETIOLOGY

- PUD is often multifactorial; the following are common mucosal damaging factors:
  - *Helicobacter pylori* infection
  - Medications (nonsteroidal antiinflammatory drugs [NSAIDs], glucocorticoids)
  - Incompetent pylorus or lower esophageal sphincter
  - Bile acids
  - Impaired proximal duodenal bicarbonate secretion
  - Decreased blood flow to gastric mucosa
  - Acid secreted by parietal cells and pepsin secreted as pepsinogen by chief cells
  - Cigarette smoking
  - Alcohol

TREATMENT

- Eradication of *H. pylori,* when present, can be accomplished with various regimens:
  - Proton-pump inhibitor (PPI) bid (e.g., omeprazole 20 mg bid or lansoprazole 30 mg bid) *plus* clarithromycin 500 mg bid *and* amoxicillin 1000 mg bid for 7 to 10 days
  - PPI bid *plus* amoxicillin 500 mg bid *plus* metronidazole 500 mg for 7 to 10 days
  - PPI bid *plus* clarithromycin 500 mg bid *and* metronidazole 500 mg bid for 7 days
  - Trials indicate that a 1-day quadruple-therapy regimen may be as effective as a 7-day triple-therapy regimen. The 1-day quadruple therapy regimen consists of 2 tablets of 262 mg of bismuth subsalicylate qid, 1 500-mg metronidazole tablet qid, 2 g of amoxicillin suspension qid, and 2 capsules of 30 mg of lansoprazole.
  - Bismouth compound qid *plus* tetracycline 500 mg qid *and* metronidazole 500 mg qid for 14 days
  - A 5-day treatment with three antibiotics (amoxicillin 1 g bid, clarithromycin 250 mg bid, and metronidazole 400 mg bid) *plus* either lansoprazole 30 mg bid or ranitidine 300 mg bid is an efficacious cost-saving option for patients >55 years old with no history of PUD.
- PUD patients testing negative for *H. pylori* should be treated with antisecretory agents.
  - Histamine-2 receptor antagonists, including cimetidine, ranitidine, famotidine, and nizatidine, are effective; they usually are given in a split dose or at nighttime.

- PPIs also can induce rapid healing; they usually are given 30 minutes before meals.
- Antacids and sucralfate are effective agents for the treatment and prevention of PUD.
- Advise the patient to stop cigarette smoking; cigarette smoking increases the risk of PUD, decreases the healing rate, and increases the frequency of recurrence.
- Avoid NSAIDs and alcohol.
- Special diets have been proved *unrelated* to ulcer development and healing; however, foods that cause symptoms should be avoided.

Pericarditis

Definition: Inflammation (or infiltration) of the pericardium associated with a wide variety of causes

DIAGNOSIS

Clinical presentation:
- Severe constant pain localizes over the anterior chest and may radiate to arms and back; it can be differentiated from myocardial ischemia because the pain intensifies with inspiration and is relieved by sitting up and leaning forward (the pain of myocardial ischemia is not pleuritic).
- Pericardial friction rub is best heard with the patient upright and leaning forward and by pressing the stethoscope firmly against the chest; it consists of three short, scratchy sounds:
  - Systolic component
  - Diastolic component
  - Late diastolic component (associated with atrial contraction)
- Cardiac tamponade may be occurring if the following are observed:
  - Tachycardia
  - Low blood pressure and pulse pressure
  - Distended neck veins
  - Paradoxical pulse
- **Laboratory tests:** The following tests may be useful in absence of an obvious cause:
  - Complete blood count with differential
  - Viral titers (acute and convalescent)
  - Erythrocyte sedimentation rate
  - Antinuclear antibody, rheumatoid factor
  - b. ...d streptococcal derivative, antistreptolysin O titers

····ou cultures

- Cardiac isoenzymes (usually normal, but mild elevations of CK-MB may occur because of associated epicarditis)
- **Imaging:**
  - Echocardiogram detects and determines amount of pericardial effusion; absence of effusion does not rule out the diagnosis of pericarditis. Divergence of right and left ventricular systolic pressures is present in cardiac tamponade and constrictive pericarditis.
  - On chest radiograph, cardiac silhouette appears enlarged if >250 mL of fluid has accumulated. Calcifications around the heart may be seen with constrictive pericarditis.
- **ECG:**
  - ECG varies with the evolutionary stage of pericarditis.
  - **Acute phase:** diffuse ST segment elevations (particularly evident in the precordial leads), which can be distinguished from acute myocardial infarction (MI) by absence of reciprocal ST segment depression in oppositely oriented leads (reciprocal ST segment depression may be seen in aV_R and VI), elevated ST segments concave upward, and absence of Q waves
  - **Intermediate phase:** return of ST segment to baseline and T wave inversion in leads previously showing ST segment elevation
  - **Late phase:** resolution of T wave changes

ETIOLOGY

- Idiopathic (possibly postviral)
- Infectious (viral, bacterial, tuberculous, fungal, amebic, toxoplasmosis)
- Collagen vascular disease (systemic lupus erythematosus, rheumatoid arthritis, scleroderma, vasculitis, dermatomyositis)
- Drug-induced lupus syndrome (procainamide, hydralazine, phenytoin, isoniazid, rifampin, doxarubicin, mesalamine)
- Acute MI
- Trauma or posttraumatic
- Post-MI (Dressler's syndrome)
- After pericardiotomy
- After mediastinal radiation (e.g., patients with Hodgkin's disease)
- Uremia
- Sarcoidosis
- Neoplasm (primary or metastatic)
- Leakage of aortic aneurysm in pericardial sac
- Familial Mediterranean fever
- Rheumatic fever
- Leukemic infiltration

• **Other:** anticoagulants, amyloidosis, immune thrombocytopenic purpura

TREATMENT

• Antiinflammatory therapy (nonsteroidal antiinflammatory drugs [NSAIDS] [e.g., naproxen 500 mg bid, indomethacin 25-50 mg tid])
• Prednisone 30 mg bid for severe forms of acute pericarditis (before use of prednisone, tuberculous pericarditis must be excluded)
• Colchicine 0.6 mg bid may be used as an alternative in patients intolerant to NSAIDs and corticosteroids
• Consider ventricular rate control with verapamil or diltiazem because of the propensity for atrial fibrillation in these patients.
• Observe patients closely for signs of cardiac tamponade.
• Avoid anticoagulants (increased risk of hemopericardium).
• Treat underlying cause of pericarditis.

Peripheral nerve dysfunction

Definitions:
• *Peripheral neuropathy*—any disorder involving the peripheral nerves
• *Polyneuropathy (symmetric polyneuropathy)*—generalized process resulting in widespread and symmetric effects on the peripheral nervous system
• *Focal or multifocal neuropathy (mononeuropathy, mononeuropathy multiplex)*—local involvement of one or more individual peripheral nerves
• *Paresthesia*—spontaneous aberrant sensation (e.g., pins and needles)

DIAGNOSIS

History:
• Family history of neuropathies—rule out hereditary neuropathies
• Current and past employment—rule out exposure to toxic agents
• Current or recent medications—rule out neuropathy secondary to drugs
• Any systemic disease, such as diabetes, renal failure, or hypothyroidism
• Ethanol abuse—rule out alcoholic neuropathy; diabetes and alcoholism are the most common causes of peripheral neuropathy in the United States
• Any special diets (e.g., food faddists)—rule out nutritional deficiencies
• History of trauma—to rule out compression entrapment

Risk factors for AIDS

  • History of tick bite or erythema chronicum migrans (Lyme disease)
• **Physical examination:**
  • Define type of neuropathy present
  • Sensory versus motor versus mixed
  • Number of nerves involved (e.g., mononeuropathy, polyneuropathy, mononeuropathy multiplex)
  • Determine the territory of neurologic deficit
  • Evaluate deep tendon reflexes (decreased in root and peripheral nerve disease)
• **Initial laboratory evaluation:**
  • Complete blood count, electrolytes, blood urea nitrogen, creatinine, glucose, liver function tests, creatine phosphokinase, calcium, magnesium, phosphate; HIV in patients with risk factors; Lyme titer in patients with a suggestive history. Erythrocyte sedimentation rate is obtained in most patients but rarely helpful.
  • If toxic neuropathy is suspected, heavy metal screening should be ordered; in suspected lead poisoning, blood lead concentration, urinary tests for coproporphyrin and δ-aminolevulinic acid, and bone marrow aspirates (to evaluate the presence of basophilic stippling in normoblasts)
  • Thyroid-stimulating hormone level in suspected hypothyroidism
  • Vitamin B_{12} and red blood cell folate levels in suspected nutritional deficiencies
  • Antinuclear antibody, serum angiotensin-converting enzyme level, Venereal Disease Research Laboratory, serum and urine protein immunoelectrophoresis in selected patients
• Chest x-ray to rule out sarcoidosis and lung carcinoma
• Lumbar puncture in suspected Guillain-Barré syndrome
• X-ray of involved limb in suspected trauma or peripheral nerve compression
• Electromyography—in neurogenic lesions, there are spontaneous fibrillation potentials and positive sharp waves at rest
• Nerve conduction studies
• Nerve biopsy (usually sural nerve)

ETIOLOGY
• **Hereditary neuropathies:**
  • Charcot-Marie-Tooth syndrome
  • **Others:** Dejerine-Sottas disease, Refsum's disease, Riley-Day syndrome

- **Acquired neuropathies:**
  - Diabetes mellitus
  - Myxedema
  - Uremia
  - Sarcoidosis
  - Alcohol
  - Neoplasms
  - Nutritional deficiencies (thiamine, folic acid, vitamin B_{12})
  - **Others:** collagen vascular diseases, amyloidosis, multiple myeloma
- Guillain-Barré neuropathy
- **Toxic neuropathies:**
  - Drugs (chloramphenicol, lithium, isoniazid, pyridoxine, nitrofurantoin, disulfiram, dapsone, ethionamide, cisplatin, vincristine, metronidazole, gold, hydralazine, amiodarone, phenytoin, penicillamine, indomethacin, amphotericin B, amitriptyline, sulfonamides, colchicine, antiretrovirals [didanosine, stavudine, zalcitabine, interferon alfa], cimetidine)
  - Toxic chemicals (lead, arsenic, cyanide, thallium, carbon disulfide, mercury, organophosphates, trichloroethylene)
- Neuropathies associated with infection (leprosy, herpes zoster, diphtheria, Lyme disease, HIV)
- Entrapment neuropathy (e.g., carpal tunnel) syndrome

TREATMENT
- Stop offending agent(s).
- **Initiate specific treatment** dimercaprol and edetate calcium sodium in patients with lead poisoning, plasmapheresis followed by low-dose prednisone in patients with inflammatory demyelinating neuropathy, oral pyridoxine 50 mg bid to prevent isoniazid neuropathy, vitamin B_{12} supplementation in vitamin B_{12} deficiency
- Consider immunoglobulin therapy if neurotherapy is immune mediated.

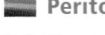 **Peritonitis, secondary**

Definition: Acute onset of severe abdominal pain secondary to peritoneal inflammation

DIAGNOSIS
- Acute peritonitis is mainly a clinical diagnosis based on patient history and physical examination. Laboratory and imaging studies assist in determining the need for and type of intervention.
- Clinical presentation includes acute abdominal pain; abdominal dis-
  ... .inal rigidity rebound, and guarding; fever;

... and tachycardia; tachypnea, and dysphea.

- If patient is hemodynamically unstable, immediate diagnostic laparotomy should be performed in lieu of adjuvant diagnostic studies.
- **Laboratory tests:**
  - Complete blood count—rule out leukocytosis, left shift, anemia
  - SMA7—rule out electrolyte imbalances, kidney dysfunction
  - Liver function tests—rule out ascites secondary to liver disease, cholelithiasis
  - Amylase—rule out pancreatitis
  - Blood cultures—rule out bacteremia, sepsis
  - Peritoneal cultures—rule out infectious etiology
  - Blood gas—rule out respiratory versus metabolic acidosis
  - Ascitic fluid analysis—rule out exudate versus transudate
  - Urinalysis and culture—rule out urinary tract infection
  - Cervical cultures for gonorrhea and *Chlamydia*
  - Urine and serum human chorionic gonadotropin
- **Diagnostic imaging:**
  - Abdominal series—free air secondary to perforation, small or large bowel dilation secondary to obstruction, identification of fecalith
  - Chest x-ray—elevated diaphragm, pneumonia
  - Pelvic/abdominal ultrasound—abscess formation, abdominal mass, intrauterine versus ectopic pregnancy, identify free fluid suggesting hemorrhage or ascites
  - CT—mass, ascites

ETIOLOGY

- Although acute peritonitis can be caused by a wide variety of problems, similar clinical presentation is a result of stimulation of pain receptors within the peritoneum by purulent exudates; bleeding; inflammation; or the release of caustic materials, such as pancreatic juice, bile, and gastric secretions.

TREATMENT

- **Surgery:** to correct underlying pathology, such as controlling hemorrhage, correct perforation, and drain abscess
- **Broad-spectrum antibiotics:**
  - **Single agent:** ceftriaxone 1-2 g IV q24h, cefotaxime 1-2 g IV q4-6h
  - **Multiple agents:**
    - Ampicillin 2 g IV q4-6h, gentamicin 1.5 mg/kg/day, clindamycin 600-900 mg IV q8h
    - Ampicillin 2 g IV q4-6h, gentamicin 1.5 mg/kg/day, metronidazole 500 mg IV q6-8h
- **Pain control:** morphine or meperidine as needed (hold until diagnosis confirmed)

Pheochromocytoma

Definition: Catecholamine-producing tumor that originates from chromaffin cells of the adrenergic system. Pheochromocytomas generally secrete norepinephrine and epinephrine, but norepinephrine is usually the predominant amine.

DIAGNOSIS

- **Clinical presentation:**
  - Hypertension can be sustained (55%) or paroxysmal (45%).
  - Headache (80%) usually is paroxysmal in nature and described as "pounding" and severe.
  - Palpitations (70%) can be present with or without tachycardia.
  - Hyperhidrosis (60%) is most evident during paroxysmal attacks of hypertension.
  - Physical examination may be normal if done in a symptom-free interval; during a paroxysm, the patient may show a marked increase in systolic and diastolic blood pressure, profuse sweating, visual disturbances (caused by hypertensive retinopathy), dilated pupils (secondary to catecholamine excess), paresthesias in the lower extremities (caused by severe vasoconstriction), tremor, or tachycardia.
- **Laboratory tests:**
  - Plasma-free metanephrines is the best test for excluding or confirming pheochromocytoma and should be the test of first choice for diagnosis of the tumor. Plasma concentrations of normetanephrines >2.5 pmol/mL or metanephrine levels >1.4 pmol/mL indicate a pheochromocytoma with 100% specificity.
  - Twenty-four-hour urine collection for metanephrines (100% sensitive) also show increased metanephrines; the accuracy of the 24-hour urinary levels for metanephrines can be improved by indexing urinary metanephrine levels by urine creatinine levels.
  - The clonidine suppression test is useful for distinguishing between high levels of plasma norepinephrine caused by release from sympathetic nerves and high levels caused by release from a pheochromocytoma. A decrease <50% in plasma norepinephrine levels after clonidine administration is normal, whereas persistent elevations indicate pheochromocytoma.
- **Imaging:**
  - Abdominal CT scan (88% sensitivity) is useful in locating pheochromocytomas >0.5 inch in diameter (90-95% accurate).

- sensitivity); MRI may become the diagnostic imaging modality of choice.
- Scintigraphy with ^{131}I-MIBG (100% sensitivity) is particularly useful in locating extraadrenal pheochromocytomas. ^{131}I-MIBG is a norepinephrine analogue that localizes in adrenergic tissue.
- 6-Fluorodopamine F 18 positron emission tomography is reserved for cases in which clinical symptoms and signs suggest pheochromocytoma and results of biochemical tests are positive, but conventional imaging studies cannot locate the tumor. An alternative approach is to use vena caval sampling for plasma catecholamines and metanephrines.

ETIOLOGY

- Catecholamine-producing tumors that usually are located in the adrenal medulla
- Specific mutations of the *RET* protooncogene cause familial predisposition to pheochromocytoma in multiple endocrine neoplasia II.
- Mutations in the von Hippel–Landau tumor suppressor gene (*VHL* gene) cause familial disposition to pheochromocytoma in von Hippel–Landau disease.
- More recently identified genes for succinate dehydrogenase subunit D (*SDHD*) and succinate dehydrogenase subunit B (*SDHB*) predispose carriers to pheochromocytoma and globus tumors.

TREATMENT

- Laparoscopic removal of the tumor (surgical resection for benign and malignant disease):
  - Preoperative stabilization with combination of phenoxybenzamine, β-blocker, metyrosine, and liberal fluid and salt intake starting 10 to 14 days before surgery
  - Volume expansion to prevent postoperative hypotension
  - α-Blockade to control hypertension—phenoxybenzamine (Dibenzyline) 5 mg PO bid initially, gradually increased to 10 mg q3d to 50-100 mg bid; prazosin may be used when phenoxybenzamine therapy alone is not effective or not well tolerated
  - β-Blockade with propranolol 20-40 mg PO q6h (to be used only after α-blockade) is useful to prevent catecholamine-induced arrhythmias and tachycardia.
  - Metyrosine reduces tumor stores of catecholamines, decreases need for intraoperative medication to control blood pressure, and lowers intraoperative fluid requirements.
  - Hypertensive crisis preoperatively and intraoperatively should be controlled with phentolamine (Regitine) 2-5 mg IV q1-2h as

needed or nitroprusside used in combination with β-adrenergic blockers.
- Combination chemotherapy with cyclophosphamide, vincristine, and dacarbazine is useful for symptomatic advanced malignant pheochromocytoma.

CLINICAL PEARLS
- Obtaining a detailed family history is important because 10% of pheochromocytomas are familial.
- Screening for pheochromocytoma should be considered in patients with malignant hypertension, poor response to antihypertensive therapy, and paradoxical hypertensive response.

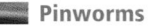 **Pinworms**

Definition: Noninvasive infestation of the intestinal tract by *Enterobius vermicularis,* a helminth of the nematode family

DIAGNOSIS
- Identification of adult worms or eggs on transparent tape placed on the perianal skin on awakening. (*Note:* Five consecutive negative tests rule out the diagnosis.)
- Most infested persons are asymptomatic.
- Perianal itching is the most common reported symptom, with scratching leading to excoriation and sometimes secondary infection.

ETIOLOGY
- Humans are the only host for this worm. Infestation is by fecal-oral route; ingested eggs hatch in the stomach and the larvae migrate to the colon, where they mature. Gravid female worms migrate to the perianal skin at night, lay their eggs there, and die. The eggs cause itching; scratching causes egg deposition under fingernails, from which they can contaminate food or lead to autoreinfection.

TREATMENT
- Single dose of mebendazole or pyrantel pamoate repeated after 2 to 3 weeks

Definition: A common self-limiting skin eruption of unknown etiology

DIAGNOSIS
- Initial lesion (herald patch) precedes the eruption by approximately 1 to 2 weeks; it typically measures 3 to 6 cm; it is round to oval in appearance and most frequently located on the trunk.
- Eruptive phase follows within 2 weeks and peaks after 7 to 14 days.
- Lesions are located most frequently in the lower abdominal area. They have a salmon-pink appearance in whites and a hyperpigmented appearance in blacks.
- Most lesions are 4 to 5 mm in diameter; the center has a "cigarette paper" appearance; the border has a characteristic ring of scale (collarette).
- Lesions occur in a symmetric distribution and follow the cleavage lines of the trunk (Christmas tree pattern).
- The number of lesions varies from a few to hundreds.
- Most patients are asymptomatic; pruritus is the most common symptom.
- History of recent fatigue, headache, sore throat, and low-grade fever is present in approximately 25% of cases.

DIFFERENTIAL DIAGNOSIS
- Tinea corporis (can be ruled out by potassium hydroxide examination)
- Secondary syphilis (absence of herald patch, positive serologic test for syphilis)
- Psoriasis
- Nummular eczema
- Drug eruption
- Viral exanthem
- Eczema
- Lichen planus
- Tinea versicolor (the lesions are more brown and the borders are not as ovoid)

TREATMENT
- Use calamine lotion or oral antihistamines in patients with significant pruritus.
- Use prednisone tapered over 2 weeks in patients with severe pruritus.
- Direct sun exposure or use of ultraviolet light within the first week of eruption is beneficial in decreasing the severity of disease.

CLINICAL PEARLS
- Spontaneous complete resolution of the rash occurs within 4 to 8 weeks.
- Recurrence is rare (<2% of cases).

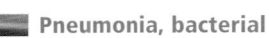

Pneumonia, bacterial

Definition: Infection involving the lung parenchyma

DIAGNOSIS
- **Clinical presentation:**
  - Fever, tachypnea, chills, tachycardia, cough
  - Presentation varies with the cause of pneumonia, the patient's age, and the clinical situation, as follows:
    - Patients with streptococcal pneumonia usually present with high fever, shaking chills, pleuritic chest pain, cough, and copious production of purulent sputum.
    - Elderly or immunocompromised hosts initially may present with only minimal symptoms (e.g., low-grade fever, confusion); respiratory and nonrespiratory symptoms are reported less commonly by older patients with pneumonia.
    - Generally, auscultation reveals crackles and diminished breath sounds.
    - Percussion dullness is present if the patient has pleural effusion.
- **Imaging:**
  - Classically, pneumococcal pneumonia presents with a segmental lobe infiltrate.
  - Diffuse infiltrates on chest x-ray can be seen with *Legionella pneumophila, Mycobacterium pneumoniae,* viral pneumonias, *Pneumocystis carinii,* miliary tuberculosis, aspiration pneumonia, and aspergillosis.

TREATMENT
- Macrolides (azithromycin or clarithromycin) or levofloxacin is recommended for empiric outpatient treatment of community-acquired pneumonia; cefotaxime or a β-lactam/β-lactamase inhibitor can be added in patients with more severe presentation who insist on outpatient therapy. Duration of treatment is 7 to 14 days.
- In the hospital setting, patients admitted to the general ward can be treated empirically with a second-generation or third-generation cephalosporin (ceftriaxone, ceftizoxime, cefotaxime, or cefuroxime) plus a macrolide (azithromycin or clarithromycin) or doxycycline.
  - ... oral quinolone (levofloxaxin, moxifloxacin, or

doxycycline.
- In hospitalized patients at risk for *Pseudomonas aeruginosa* infection, empiric treatment should consist of an antipseudomonal β-lactam (cefepime or piperacillin-tazobactam) *plus* an aminoglycoside *plus* an antipseudomonal quinolone or macrolide.

CLINICAL PEARLS

- Causes of slowly resolving or nonresolving pneumonia include the following:
  - Difficult-to-treat infections—viral pneumonia, *Legionella*, pneumococci, or staphylococci with impaired host response, tuberculosis, fungi
  - Neoplasm—lung, lymphoma, metastasis
  - Congestive heart failure
  - Pulmonary embolism
  - Immunologic or idiopathic—Wegener's granulomatosis, pulmonary eosinophilic syndromes, systemic lupus erythematosus
  - Drug toxicity (e.g., amiodarone)

Pneumonia, mycoplasmal

Definition: Infection of the lung parenchyma caused by *Mycoplasma pneumoniae*

DIAGNOSIS

- **Chest x-ray:** predilection for lower lobe involvement (upper lobes involved in less than a fourth), with radiographic abnormalities frequently out of proportion to abnormalities on physical examination; small pleural effusions in about 30% of patients
- **Clinical presentation:** nonexudative pharyngitis (common), rhonchi or rales, without evidence of consolidation (common) in lower lung zones. Associated with bullous myringitis (perhaps no more frequently than in other pneumonias)

TREATMENT

- Therapy (10-14 days) with erythromycin (500 mg qid), azithromycin (500 mg daily), or clarithromycin (500 mg bid) is preferred to tetracycline, especially in young children or women of childbearing age.

Pneumonia, Pneumocystis carinii

Definition: Serious respiratory infection caused by the fungal or protozoal organism *Pneumocystis carinii*

DIAGNOSIS

- Fever, cough, and shortness of breath are present in almost all cases.
- Lungs frequently are clear to auscultation, although rales occasionally are present.
- Chest x-ray should be performed.
- Arterial blood gases should be obtained.
- Perform sputum examination for cysts of *Pneumocystis*
- Perform bronchoscopy with bronchoalveolar lavage or lung biopsy if sputum examination is negative or equivocal.
- Diffuse uptake on gallium scanning of the lungs is suggestive but not diagnostic.
- Perform HIV antibody test if cause of underlying immune deficiency state is unclear.

TREATMENT

- For confirmed or suspected *Pneumocystis* pneumonia:
  - Trimethoprim-sulfamethoxazole (TMP-SMZ) 20 mg/kg trimethoprim and 100 mg/kg sulfamethoxazole PO or IV qd
  - Either regimen with prednisone 40 mg PO bid
  - Pentamidine 4 mg/kg IV qd
  - If arterial oxygen pressure <70 mm Hg
  - If arterial-alveolar oxygen pressure difference >35 mm Hg
  - Dose tapered to 20 mg bid after 5 days and 20 mg qd after 10 days
  - Therapy is continued for 3 weeks.
- Alternative therapies are available for patients unable to tolerate conventional therapy.
  - Dapsone-trimethoprim
  - Clindamycin-primaquine
  - Atovaquone
- After completion of therapy, lifelong prophylaxis should be maintained with TMP-SMZ (1 single-strength tablet PO qd or double-strength three times weekly).
- Patients intolerant of this therapy should be treated with dapsone 50 mg qd *plus* pyrimethamine 50 mg PO weekly *plus* leucovorin 25 mg PO weekly.

less effective and is reserved for patients intolerant to other forms of prophylaxis.

▰ Polyarteritis nodosa

Definition: Vasculitic syndrome involving medium-size to small arteries, characterized histologically by necrotizing inflammation of the arterial media and inflammatory cell infiltration

DIAGNOSIS

- The presence of any 3 of the following 10 items allows the diagnosis of polyarteritis nodosa with a sensitivity of 82% and a specificity of 86%:
  - Weight loss >4 kg
  - Livedo reticularis
  - Testicular pain or tenderness
  - Myalgias, weakness, or leg tenderness
  - Neuropathy
  - Diastolic blood pressure >90 mm Hg
  - Elevated blood urea nitrogen or creatinine
  - Positive test for hepatitis B virus
  - Arteriography revealing small or large aneurysms and focal constrictions between dilated segments
  - Biopsy of small or medium-size artery containing white blood cells

TREATMENT

- Prednisone 1-2 mg/kg/day; cyclophosphamide in refractory cases

CLINICAL PEARL

- The 5-year survival is <20% in untreated patients. Treatment with corticosteroids increases survival to approximately 50%. Use of corticosteroids and immunosuppressive drugs may increase 5-year survival to >80%. Poor prognostic signs are severe renal or gastrointestinal involvement.

Polycythemia vera (PCV)

Definition: Chronic myeloproliferative disorder characterized mainly by erythrocytosis (increase in red blood cell [RBC] mass)

DIAGNOSIS

- The diagnosis of PCV generally requires the following three major criteria or the first two major criteria plus two minor criteria:
- **Major criteria:**
  - Increased RBC mass (>36 mL/kg in men, >32 mL/kg in women)
  - Normal arterial oxygen saturation (>92%)
  - Splenomegaly
- **Minor criteria:**
  - Thrombocytosis (>400,000/mm³)
  - Leukocytosis (>12,000/mm³)
  - Elevated leukocyte alkaline phosphatase (>100 U/L)
  - Elevated serum vitamin B_{12} (>900 pg/mL) or vitamin B_{12} binding protein (>2200 pg/mL)
- Serum erythropoietin level is the best initial test for the diagnosis of PCV. A low serum erythropoietin level is highly suggestive of PCV. A normal level does not exclude the diagnosis. If the erythropoietin level is elevated, obtain abdominal and pelvic CT scans to rule out renal cercal carcinoma and other causes of polycythemia.
- Bone marrow aspiration reveals RBC hyperplasia and absent iron stores.

DIFFERENTIAL DIAGNOSIS

- Smoking—polycythemia secondary to increased carboxyhemoglobin, resulting in left shift in the hemoglobin dissociation curve
- Hypoxemia (secondary polycythemia)—living for prolonged periods at high altitudes, pulmonary fibrosis, congenital cardiac lesions with right-to-left shunts
- Erythropoietin-producing states—renal cell carcinoma, hepatoma, cerebral hemangioma, uterine fibroids, polycystic kidneys
- Stress polycythemia (secondary polycythemia)—laboratory evaluation shows normal RBC mass, arterial oxygen saturation, and erythropoietin level; plasma volume decreased
- Hemoglobinopathies associated with high oxygen affinity—an abnormal oxyhemoglobin-dissociation curve (P50) is present.

TREATMENT

- Phlebotomy keeps hematocrit <45% in men and <42% in women and is the mainstay of therapy.

decrease the incidence of thrombotic events.

- Interferon alfa-2b also is effective in controlling RBC values without significant side effects.
- Myelosuppressive therapy with chlorambucil is effective but not routinely used because of its leukemogenic potential.
- **Adjunctive therapy:** Treat pruritus with antihistamines, control significant hyperuricemia with allopurinol, reduce gastric hyperacidity with antacids or H_2 blockers, and administer low-dose aspirin to treat vasomotor symptoms in patients without bleeding diathesis. Low-dose aspirin also may prevent thrombotic complications.

▰ Polymyalgia rheumatica (PMR)

Definition: Clinical syndrome predominantly involving individuals >50 years old and characterized by pain and stiffness involving mainly the shoulders, pelvic girdle musculature, and torso

DIAGNOSIS

- Diagnosis is based on clinical presentation and elevated erythrocyte sedimentation rate (ESR) (≥40 mm/hr), although the latter is not essential for the diagnosis (>20% of patients with PMR have a normal ESR at time of diagnosis).
- Symmetric polymyalgias and arthralgias involve back, shoulder, neck, and pelvic girdle muscles; duration is generally >1 month.
- Constitutional symptoms include fever, malaise, and weight loss.
- Headache occurs in patients with coexisting temporal arteritis.
- Symptoms are worse in the morning (difficulty getting out of bed) and at night.
- Muscle strength is usually normal.
- Crescendo of symptoms occurs over several weeks or months.
- Depression or weight loss may be present.
- Laboratory tests show elevated ESR and mild anemia.

TREATMENT

- Low-dose corticosteroids (e.g., prednisone 10-20 mg/day) generally produce dramatic relief of symptoms within 48 hours and confirm the diagnosis; failure to improve within 1 week suggests other diagnoses (e.g., fibromyalgia, polymyositis, viral myalgias, hypothyroidism, depression, rheumatoid arthritis, occult neoplasm, or infection).
- The corticosteroid dosage is gradually tapered over several months on the basis of repeated clinical observation and serial measurements of ESR. When symptoms have resolved and the ESR has

decreased, the dose of prednisone can be gradually decreased. If the initial prednisone dose is 20 mg/day, reduce it by 2.5 mg every week until 10 mg/day, then reduce it by 1 mg every month.
- In patients with minimal symptoms, nonsteroidal antiinflammatory drugs may be used instead of corticosteroids.

CLINICAL PEARLS
- In general, temporal artery biopsy is not indicated in patients with pure PMR (i.e., in the absence of giant cell arteritis signs and symptoms). The clinician should monitor patients with PMR carefully and give higher doses of corticosteroids and arrange for biopsy if symptoms of giant cell arteritis appear.
- A baseline bone-density study in female patients is recommended.

Prolactinoma

Definition: Monoclonal tumor that secretes prolactin

DIAGNOSIS
- The diagnosis of prolactinoma is established by demonstration of an elevated serum prolactin level (after exclusion of other causes of hyperprolactinemia) and radiographic evidence of a pituitary adenoma.
- Prolactin levels can vary with time of day, stress, sleep cycle, and meals. More accurate measurements can be obtained 2 to 3 hours after awakening, prandially, and when patient is not distressed. Levels >300 ng/mL are virtually diagnostic of prolactinomas. Serial measurements are recommended in patients with mild prolactin elevations.
- MRI with gadolinium enhancement is the preferred imaging procedure. In absence of MRI, a radiographic diagnosis is best accomplished with high-resolution CT and special coronal cuts through the pituitary region.
- Thyrotropin-releasing hormone (TRH) stimulation test may be useful in equivocal cases. The normal response is an increase in serum prolactin levels by 100% within 1 hour of TRH infusion; failure to show an increase in prolactin level suggests pituitary lesion.

ETIOLOGY
- Hyperprolactinemia may be caused by the following:
  - Drugs (phenothiazines, methyldopa, reserpine, monoamine oxidase inhibitors, androgens, progesterone, cimetidine, tricyclic antidepressants, haloperidol, meprobamate, chlordiazepoxide, estrogens, nar-

contraceptives)

- Hepatic cirrhosis, renal failure, primary hypothyroidism
- Ectopic prolactin-secreting tumors (hypernephroma, bronchogenic carcinoma)
- Infiltrating diseases of the pituitary (sarcoidosis, histiocytosis)
- Head trauma, chest wall injury, spinal cord injury
- Polycystic ovary disease, pregnancy, nipple stimulation
- Idiopathic hyperprolactinemia, stress, exercise

TREATMENT

- Management of prolactinomas depends on their size and encroachment on the optic chiasm and other vital structures, the presence or absence of gonadal dysfunction, and the patient's desires with respect to fertility.
- Medical therapy is preferred when fertility is an important consideration. Bromocriptine (Parlodel) and cabergoline (Dostinex) are commonly used.
- Transsphenoidal resection is option in an infertile patient who cannot tolerate bromocriptine or cabergoline or when medical therapy is ineffective. It results in a cure in 50% to 75% of patients with microadenomas and 10% to 20% of patients with macroadenomas.
- Pituitary irradiation is useful as adjunctive therapy of macroadenomas (>10 mm in diameter) and in patients with persistent hypersecretion after surgery.
- Stereotactic radiosurgery (gamma knife) has become popular as a modality in the treatment of prolactinomas.

 Prostatitis

Definition: Inflammation of the prostate gland. There are four major categories:

- Acute bacterial prostatitis
- Chronic bacterial prostatitis
- Nonbacterial prostatitis
- Prostatodynia

DIAGNOSIS

- **Acute bacterial prostatitis:**
  - Sudden or rapidly progressive onset of dysuria, frequency, urgency, and nocturia occurs.
  - Perineal pain may radiate to the back, rectum, or penis.

- Hematuria or a purulent urethral discharge may occur.
- Occasionally, urinary retention complicates the course.
- Fever, chills, and signs of sepsis also can be part of the clinical picture.
- On rectal examination, the prostate is typically tender.

- **Chronic bacterial prostatitis:**
  - Prostatitis may be asymptomatic when the infection is confined to the prostate.
  - Prostatitis may present as an increase in severity of baseline symptoms of benign prostatic hypertrophy.
  - When cystitis also is present, urinary frequency, urgency, and burning may be reported.
  - Hematuria may be a presenting complaint.
  - In elderly men, new onset of urinary incontinence may be noted.

- **Nonbacterial prostatitis and prostatodynia:**
  - These present similarly with symptoms of bladder irritation (urinary frequency, urgency, dysuria, increase in nocturia episodes) and perineal discomfort.
  - The symptoms can be of variable severity, but tend to be more bothersome in prostatodynia.

- **Laboratory tests:**
  - Perform urinalysis.
  - Perform urine culture and sensitivity.
  - Bacterial localization studies can be performed, but are cumbersome and impractical in most clinical settings.
  - Cell count and culture of expressed prostatic secretions should be performed.
  - The yield of a urine culture may be increased if the specimen is obtained after a prostatic massage.
  - Prostate-specific antigen (PSA) is not used to diagnose prostatitis; however, a rapid rise over baseline should raise the possibility of prostatitis even in the absence of symptoms. In such cases, a follow-up PSA after treatment of prostatitis is appropriate.
  - Complete blood count and blood cultures should be obtained if fever, chills, or signs of sepsis exist.

ETIOLOGY

- **Acute bacterial prostatitis:**
  - Acute, usually gram-negative infection of the prostate gland
    - Generally associated with cystitis
    - Resulting from the ascent of bacteria in the urethra
  - Occasionally the route of infection is hematogenous or lymphogenous spread of rectal bacteria.
  - Most seen in young or middle-aged men.

- Often asymptomatic
  - Exacerbation of symptoms of benign prostatic hypertrophy caused by the same mechanism as in acute bacterial prostatitis
- **Nonbacterial prostatitis:**
  - Refers to symptoms of prostatic inflammation associated with the presence of white blood cells (WBCs) in prostatic secretions with no identifiable bacterial organism
  - *Chlamydia* infection may be etiologically implicated in some cases.
- **Prostatodynia:**
  - Refers to symptoms of prostatic inflammation with no or few WBCs in the prostatic secretion
  - Spasm in the bladder neck or urethra is believed to be the cause of symptoms.

TREATMENT

- **Acute bacterial prostatitis:** Culture-guided antibiotic therapy for 4 weeks (beginning with a few days of intravenous antibiotics if the infection is serious or if the patient is bacteremic).
- **Chronic bacterial prostatitis:**
  - Trimethoprim-sulfamethoxazole (TMP-SMZ) is first-line choice for 4 weeks if the organism is sensitive.
  - Second-line choice for treatment failure or organisms resistant to TMP-SMZ is a fluoroquinolone.
  - Patients with refractory infection or with multiple relapses may be offered long-term suppressive therapy.
- **Nonbacterial prostatitis and prostatodynia:**
  - No specific treatment
  - Antibiotics not effective
  - A trial of treatment with an adrenergic blocker (terazosin, doxazosin, or tamsulosin) may be considered.
  - Any underlying bladder pathology should be ruled out by cystoscopy and treated if identified.

Pseudogout

Definition: Crystal-induced synovitis resulting from the deposition of calcium pyrophosphate dehydrate (CPPD) crystals in joint hyaline and fibrocartilage. The cartilage deposition is termed *chondrocalcinosis.*

DIAGNOSIS

- The American Rheumatism Association revised diagnostic criteria for CPPD crystal deposition disease (pseudogout) are often used:

    I Demonstration of CPPD crystals (obtained by biopsy, necroscopy, or aspirated synovial fluid) by definitive means (e.g., characteristic "fingerprint" by x-ray diffraction powder pattern or by chemical analysis)

    II a Identification of monoclinic or triclinic crystals showing either no or only a weakly positive birefringence by compensated polarized light microscopy

    b Presence of typical calcifications on radiographs

    III a Acute arthritis, especially of knees or other large joints, with or without concomitant hyperuricemia

    b Chronic arthritis, especially of knees, hips, wrists, carpus, elbow, shoulder, and metacarpophalangeal joints, especially if accompanied by acute exacerbations; the following features are helpful in differentiating chronic arthritis from osteoarthritis:

    - Uncommon site (e.g., wrist, metacarpophalangeal joint, elbow, shoulder)
    - Appearance of lesion radiologically (e.g., radiocarpal or patellofemoral joint space narrowing, especially if isolated [(patella "wrapped around" the femur])
    - Subchondral cyst formation
    - Severity of degeneration—progressive, with subchondral bony collapse (microfractures), and fragmentation, with formation of intraarticular radiodense bodies
    - Osteophyte formation—variable and inconstant
    - Tendon calcifications, especially Achilles, triceps, obturators

- **Categories:**
    - Definite—criteria I or IIa plus IIb must be fulfilled.
    - Probable—criteria IIa or IIb must be fulfilled.
    - Possible—criteria IIIa or IIIb should alert the clinician to the possibility of underlying CPPD deposition.

TREATMENT

- Nonsteroidal antiinflammatory drugs (as for gout)
- Colchicine
- Aspiration/steroid injection

Pseudomembranous colitis

Definition: Occurrence of diarrhea and bowel inflammation associated with antibiotic use

DIAGNOSIS
- The clinical signs of pseudomembranous colitis generally include diarrhea, fever, and abdominal cramps after use of antibiotics.
- *Clostridium difficile* toxin can be detected by cytotoxin tissue-culture assay (gold standard for identifying *C. difficile* toxin in stool specimen) and by ELISA for *C. difficile* toxins A and B. The latter is used most widely in the clinical setting. It has a sensitivity of 85% and a specificity of 100%.
- Fecal leukocytes (assessed by microscopy or lactoferrin assay) are generally present in stool samples.
- Complete blood count usually reveals leukocytosis.

ETIOLOGY
- Cephalosporins are the most frequent offending agent in pseudomembranous colitis because of their high rates of use.
- The antibiotic with the highest incidence is clindamycin (10% incidence of pseudomembranous colitis with its use).
- *C. difficile* causes >250,000 cases of diarrhea and colitis in the United States every year.

TREATMENT
- Metronidazole 250 mg PO qid for 10 to 14 days
- Vancomycin 125 mg PO qid for 10 to 14 days in cases resistant to metronidazole
- Cholestyramine 4 g PO qid for 10 days in addition to metronidazole to control severe diarrhea (avoid use with vancomycin)
- When parenteral therapy is necessary (e.g., patient with paralytic ileus), metronidazole 500 mg IV qid can be used. It also can be supplemented with vancomycin 500 mg via nasogastric tube or enema.

Pulmonary edema, cardiogenic

Definition: Life-threatening condition caused by severe left ventricular decompensation

DIAGNOSIS
- **Clinical presentation:**
  - Dyspnea with rapid, shallow breathing

- Diaphoresis, peroral and peripheral cyanosis
- Pink, frothy sputum
- Moist, bilateral pulmonary rales
- Increased pulmonary second sound, S_3 gallop (in association with tachycardia)
- Bulging neck veins

- **Imaging studies:**
  - Chest x-ray shows pulmonary congestion with Kerley B lines, fluffy perihilar infiltrates in the early stages, and bilateral interstitial alveolar infiltrates and pleural effusions in later stages.
  - Echocardiogram is useful to evaluate valvular abnormalities and diastolic versus systolic dysfunction (can evaluate ejection fraction), it also can aid in differentiation of cardiogenic versus noncardiogenic pulmonary edema.
  - Right heart catheterization is done in selected patients. Cardiac pressures and cardiogenic pulmonary edema reveal increased pulmonary artery diastolic pressure and pulmonary capillary wedge pressure (PCWP) 225 mm Hg.

ETIOLOGY

- Increased pulmonary capillary pressure secondary to:
  - Acute myocardial infarction
  - Exacerbation of congestive heart failure
  - Valvular regurgitation
  - Ventricular septal defect
  - Severe myocardial ischemia
  - Mitral stenosis
- **Other:** cardiac tamponade, endocarditis, myocarditis, arrhythmias, cardiomyopathy, hypertensive crisis

TREATMENT

All the following steps can be performed concomitantly:

- Give 100% oxygen by facemask. Continuous positive airway pressure and biphasic positive airway pressure systems can improve oxygenation and lower carbon dioxide tension. Check arterial blood gases; if marked hypoxemia or severe respiratory acidosis, intubate the patient and place on a ventilator.
- Furosemide 1 mg/kg IV bolus (typically 40-100 mg) rapidly establishes diuresis and decreases venous return through its vasodilator action; the dose may be doubled in 30 minutes if no effect. Institute vasodilator therapy. Nitrates are particularly useful if the patient has concomitant chest pain.
- Give nitroglycerin.
  - Nitroglycerin 150-600 µg sublingually or nitroglycerin spray can be given immediately on arrival

and blood pressure remains stable.

- Apply 2% nitroglycerin ointment, 1-3 inches out of the tube applied continuously; absorption may be erratic.
- Give intravenous nitroglycerin 100 mg in 500 mL of 5% dextrose in water solution; start at 6 µg/min (2 mL/hr).
- Nitroprusside is useful for afterload reduction in hypertensive patients with decreased cardiac index.
- Vasodilator and diuretic therapy should be tailored to achieve PCWP ≤18 mm Hg, renal artery pressure ≤8 mm Hg, systolic blood pressure >90 mm Hg, and systemic vascular resistance (SVR) >1200 dynes · sec · cm^{-5}.
- Nesiritide (Natrecor), a B-type natriuretic peptide, has venous, arterial, and coronary vasodilatory properties that decrease preload and afterload and increase cardiac output without direct inotropic effects. It is effective in cardiogenic pulmonary edema.
- Morphine 2-4 mg IV/SC/IM (may repeat q15min as needed) decreases venous return, anxiety, and SVR (naloxone should be available at bedside to reverse the effects of morphine if respiratory depression occurs). Morphine may induce hypotension in volume-depleted patients.
- Reduce afterload with angiotensin-converting enzyme (ACE) inhibitors. Captopril 25 mg PO tablet can be used for sublingual administration (placing a drop or two of water on the tablet and placing it under the tongue helps dissolve it). Onset of action is <10 minutes, and peak effect can be reached in 30 minutes. ACE inhibitors also can be given intravenously (e.g., enalaprilat 1 mg IV q2h as needed).
- Dobutamine 2.5-10 µg/kg/min IV is the parenteral inotropic agent of choice in severe cases of cardiogenic pulmonary edema. Intravenous phosphodiesterase inhibitors (amrinone, milrinone) may be useful in refractory cases.
- Aminophylline is useful *only* if the patient has concomitant severe bronchospasm.
- Digitalis has limited use in acute pulmonary edema caused by myocardial infarction. It may be useful in pulmonary edema resulting from atrial fibrillation or flutter with a fast ventricular response.

CLINICAL PEARL

- Acute cardiogenic pulmonary edema caused by idiopathic hypertrophic subaortic stenosis must be treated with intravenous normal saline solution and negative inotropic agents, such as verapamil and β-blockers.

![] Pulmonary embolism (PE)

Definition: Lodging of a thrombus or other embolic material from a distant site in the pulmonary circulation

DIAGNOSIS

- Chest x-ray may be normal; suggestive findings include elevated diaphragm, pleural effusion, dilation of pulmonary artery, infiltrate or consolidation, abrupt vessel cutoff, or atelectasis. A wedge-shaped consolidation in the middle and lower lobes suggests a pulmonary infarction and is called *Hampton's hump.*
- Perform lung scan in patients with normal chest x-ray. A ventilation-perfusion mismatch suggests PE, and a lung scan interpretation of high probability is confirmatory.
- Spiral CT is an excellent modality for diagnosing PE. It may be used in place of lung scan and is favored in patients with baseline lung abnormalities on initial chest x-ray. It has the added advantage of detecting other pulmonary pathology that can mimic PE.
- Pulmonary angiography is the gold standard; however, it is invasive, expensive, and not readily available in some clinical settings.
- Arterial blood gases generally reveal decreased PaO_2 and $PaCO_2$ and increased pH; normal results do not rule out PE.
- Alveolar-arteriolar (A-a) oxygen gradient, a measure of the difference in oxygen concentration between alveoli and arterial blood, is a more sensitive indicator of the alteration in oxygenation than PaO_2; it can be calculated easily using the information from arterial blood gases; a normal A-a gradient among patients without history of PE or deep vein thrombosis (DVT) makes the diagnosis of PE unlikely.
- Measure plasma D dimer by ELISA. A normal plasma D dimer level is useful to exclude PE in patients with a nondiagnostic lung scan and a low pretest probability of PE. It cannot be used to "rule in" the diagnosis, however, because it increases with many other disorders (e.g., metastatic cancer, trauma, sepsis, postoperative state). Plasma D dimer also can be used in conjunction with lower extremity compression ultrasound in patients with indeterminate ventilation-perfusion and spiral CT scans. Absence of DVT and presence of a normal D dimer level in these settings generally rules out clinically significant PE.
- ECG is abnormal in 85% of patients with acute PE. Frequent abnormalities are sinus tachycardia; nonspecific ST segment or T wave changes; S-I, Q-III, T-III pattern (10% of patients); S-I, S-II, S-III pattern; T wave inversion in V_1 to V_6; acute right bundle branch block; new-onset atrial fibrillation; ST segment depression in lead II; and right

- **Risk factors for PE:**
  - Prolonged immobilization
  - Postoperative state
  - Trauma to lower extremities
  - Estrogen-containing birth control pills
  - Prior history of DVT or PE
  - Congestive heart failure
  - Pregnancy and early puerperium
  - Visceral cancer (lung, pancreas, alimentary and genitourinary tracts)
  - Trauma, burns
  - Advanced age
  - Obesity
  - Hematologic disease (e.g., antithrombin III deficiency, protein C deficiency, protein S deficiency, lupus anticoagulant, polycythemia vera, dysfibrinogenemia, paroxysmal nocturnal hemoglobinuria, factor V Leiden mutation, G20210A prothrombin mutation)
  - Chronic obstructive pulmonary disease, diabetes mellitus
  - Prolonged air travel

TREATMENT

- Heparin by continuous infusion for at least 5 days has been the traditional treatment of PE. In hemodynamically stable patients with PE, initial treatment with once-daily subcutaneous administration of the synthetic antithrombotic agent fondaparinux without monitoring has been reported to be at least as safe and as effective as adjusted-dose intravenous unfractionated heparin. Several other trials also have shown fixed-dose low-molecular-weight heparin to be as effective and safe as dose-adjusted intravenous unfractionated heparin for the initial treatment of nonmassive PE.
- Thrombolytic agents (urokinase, tissue plasminogen activator, streptokinase) provide rapid resolution of clots; thrombolytic agents are the treatment of choice in patients with massive PE who are hemodynamically unstable and with no contraindication to their use.
- Long-term treatment generally is carried out with warfarin therapy started on day 1 or 2 and given in a dose to maintain the international normalized ratio at 2 to 3. The duration of oral anticoagulant treatment is 6 months in patients with reversible risk factors and indefinitely in patients with persistence of risk factors that caused the initial PE.
- If thrombolytics and anticoagulants are contraindicated (e.g., gastrointestinal bleeding, recent central nervous system surgery, recent trauma), or if the patient continues to have recurrent PE despite

anticoagulation therapy, vena caval interruption is indicated by transvenous placement of a Greenfield vena caval filter.
- Acute pulmonary artery embolectomy may be indicated in a patient with massive PE and refractory hypotension.

Pyelonephritis

Definition: Infection, usually bacterial in origin, of the upper urinary tract

DIAGNOSIS
- Clinical presentation includes fever, flank pain, dysuria, and hematuria.
- Laboratory tests include complete blood count with differential, blood cultures, urinalysis, urine cultures, blood urea nitrogen, creatinine, and Gram stain of urine.
- Urgent renal sonography is indicated if obstruction or closed space infection is suspected.
- CT scans may better define the extent of collections of pus.
- Helical CT scans excellent to detect calculi.

ETIOLOGY
- Gram-negative bacilli, such as *Escherichia coli* and *Klebsiella*, in >95% of cases
- Other, more unusual gram-negative organisms, especially if instrumentation of the urinary system has occurred
- Resistant gram-negative organisms or even fungi in hospitalized patients with indwelling catheters
- Gram-positive organisms, such as enterococci
- *Staphylococcus aureus*—presence in urine indicates hematogenous origin
- Viruses—rarely, but these usually are limited to the lower tract

TREATMENT
- Antibiotic therapy should be initiated after cultures are obtained and guided by the results of culture and sensitivity testing.
- Oral trimethoprim-sulfamethoxazole (TMP-SMZ) double-strength bid for 10 days or ciprofloxacin 500 mg orally bid for 10 days—adequate for stable patients who can tolerate oral medications with sensitive pathogens
- Intravenous TMP-SMZ or ciprofloxacin for more toxic patients
- Ceftazidime 1 g IV q6-8h

- g $\cdots$ q... adjusted for renal function, but nephrotoxic especially in diabetics with azotemia
- Vancomycin 1 g IV q12h to cover gram-positive cocci, such as enterococci or staphylococci
- Ampicillin 1-2 g IV q4-6h to cover enterococci, but an aminoglycoside is needed for synergy
- Oral ampicillin or amoxicillin—no longer adequate for therapy of gram-negative infections because of resistance
- Prompt drainage with nephrostomy tube placement for obstruction
- Surgical drainage of large collections of pus to control infection
- Diabetic patients and patients with indwelling catheters especially prone to complicated infections and abscess formation

▆▆ Raynaud's phenomenon

Definition: Vasospastic disorder generally involving arterioles of the hands; however, it can involve toes, ears, and other body appendages

DIAGNOSIS
- Raynaud's phenomenon classically manifests in three stages:
  - **Pallor phase:** The initial spasm causes decreased cutaneous blood flow, resulting in pallor, numbness, paresthesias, and pain in the affected digits.
  - **Cutaneous cyanosis phase:** The digits develop a blue-purple color caused by deoxygenated blood in the capillary bed.
  - **Hyperemic phase:** Increased blood flow to the affected digits resulting from the reopening of the digital artery results in blushing of the skin.

TREATMENT
- Avoid triggering factors (cold ambient temperatures, emotional stress, drugs [tobacco, caffeine, antihistamines, amphetamines, cocaine, β-blockers, estrogen replacement without progesterone]).
- Behavioral therapy can decrease emotional stress.
- Institute drug therapy when lifestyle changes fail to control symptoms.
  - Calcium channel blockers (nifedipine, amlodipine, diltiazem)
  - α-Adrenergic blockers (prazosin)
  - Others (pentoxifylline, captopril, ketanserin, prostacyclin)

CLINICAL PEARL
• Raynaud's phenomenon can be primary or secondary. The most common cause of secondary Raynaud's phenomenon is connective tissue diseases (scleroderma, systemic lupus erythematosus).

Renal failure, acute (ARF)

Definition: Rapid impairment in renal function resulting in retention of products in the blood that normally are excreted by the kidneys

DIAGNOSIS
• Identify contributing factors (e.g., nephrotoxin exposure, hypertension, diabetes mellitus).
• Laboratory evaluation can quantify degree of abnormality; radiographic studies exclude prerenal and postrenal factors.
• Categorization of renal failure into oliguric (urinary output <400 mL/day) or nonoliguric is important. The physical examination should focus on volume status.

Laboratory tests:
• Elevated serum creatinine: The rate of rise of creatinine is approximately 1 mg/dL/day in complete renal failure.
• Elevated blood urea nitrogen (BUN): BUN/creatinine ratio is >20:1 in prerenal azotemia, postrenal azotemia, and acute glomerulonephritis; it is <20:1 in acute interstitial nephritis (AIN) and acute tubular necrosis (ATN).
• Electrolytes (potassium, phosphorus) are elevated; bicarbonate level and calcium are decreased.
• Complete blood count may reveal anemia because of decreased erythropoietin production, hemoconcentration, or hemolysis.
• Urinalysis may reveal the presence of hematuria (glomerular nephritis), proteinuria (nephrotic syndrome); casts (e.g., granular casts in ATN, red blood cell casts in acute glomerular nephritis, white blood cell casts in AIN, or eosinophiluria (AIN).
• Urinary sodium and urinary creatinine also should be obtained to calculate the fractional excretion of sodium (FE_{Na}) (FE_{Na} = urine sodium/plasma sodium × plasma creatinine/urine creatinine × 100). FE_{Na} is <1 in prerenal failure and >1 in intrinsic renal failure in patients with urine output <400 mL/day.
• Urinary osmolarity is 250 to 300 mOsm/kg in ATN, >400 mOsm/kg in postrenal azotemia, and <500 mOsm/kg in prerenal azotemia and acute glomerulonephritis.

...have sepsis, liver function tests, immunoglobulins, and protein electrophoresis in patients suspected to have myeloma; and creatinine kinase in patients suspected to have rhabdomyolysis.

- Renal biopsy may be indicated in patients with intrinsic renal failure when considering specific therapy; major uses of renal biopsy are differential diagnosis of nephrotic syndrome, separation of lupus vasculitis from other vasculitis and lupus membranous from idiopathic membranous, confirmation of hereditary nephropathies on the basis of the ultrastructure, diagnosis of rapidly progressing glomerulonephritis, separation of allergic interstitial nephritis from ATN, and separation of primary glomerulonephritis syndromes. The biopsy may be performed percutaneously or by open method. The percutaneous approach is favored and generally yields adequate tissue in >90% of cases. Open biopsy generally is reserved for uncooperative patients, patients with solitary kidney, and patients at risk for uncontrolled bleeding.

- **Imaging:**
  - Chest x-ray is useful to evaluate for congestive heart failure (CHF) and for pulmonary renal syndromes (Goodpasture's syndrome, Wegener's granulomatosis).
  - Ultrasound of kidneys is used to evaluate for kidney size (useful to distinguish ARF from chronic renal failure), to evaluate for the presence of obstruction, and to evaluate renal vascular status (with Doppler evaluation).

- **Clinical presentation:**
  - Variable clinical presentation depending on the duration and rapidity of onset of renal failure
  - Peripheral edema
  - Skin pallor, ecchymoses
  - Oliguria (however, patients can have nonoliguric renal failure), anuria
  - Delirium, lethargy, myoclonus, seizures
  - Back pain, fasciculations, muscle cramps
  - Tachypnea, tachycardia
  - Weakness, anorexia, generalized malaise, nausea

ETIOLOGY

- **Prenal:** inadequate perfusion caused by hypovolemia, CHF, cirrhosis, or sepsis. Sixty percent of community-acquired cases of ARF are due to prerenal conditions.

- **Postrenal:** outlet obstruction from prostatic enlargement, ureteral obstruction (stones), bilateral renal vein occlusion. Postrenal causes account for 5% to 15% of community-acquired ARF.
- **Intrinsic renal:** glomerulonephritis, ATN, drug toxicity, contrast nephropathy

TREATMENT

- Stop all nephrotoxic medications.
- Implement dietary modification to supply adequate calories while minimizing accumulation of toxins; control fluid balance appropriately. Physicians should recommend a nutrition program with an energy prescription of 120–150 kJ/kg/day and restriction of potassium (60 mEq/day), sodium (90 mEq/day), and phosphorus (800 mg/day).
- Ideal protein supplementation ranges from 0.6 to 1.4 g/kg depending on whether dialysis is required.
- Daily weight
- Modifications of dosage of renally excreted drugs
- Specific treatment varies with etiology of ARF.
- **Prerenal:** intravenous volume expansion in hypovolemic patients
- **Intrinsic renal:** discontinuation of any potential toxins and treatment of condition causing the renal failure
- **Postrenal:** removal of obstruction
- General indications for initiation of dialysis are:
  - Floor symptoms of uremia (encephalopathy, pericarditis)
  - Severe volume overload
  - Severe acid-base imbalance
  - Significant derangement in electrolyte concentrations (e.g., hyperkalemia, hyponatremia)

CLINICAL PEARLS

- Anuria is common in obstructive uropathy and acute cortical necrosis.
- Hydration with sodium bicarbonate (addition of 154 mL of 1000 mEq/L sodium bicarbonate to 846 mL of 5% dextrose in water) before contrast exposure is more effective than hydration with sodium chloride for prophylaxis of contrast-induced renal failure.

Definition: Progressive decrease in renal function (CFR <60 mL/min for ≥3 months) with subsequent accumulation of waste products in the blood, electrolyte abnormalities, and anemia

DIAGNOSIS

- Laboratory evaluation and imaging studies should be aimed at identifying reversible causes of acute decrements in glomerular filtration rate (GFR) (e.g., volume depletion, urinary tract obstruction, congestive heart failure [CHF]) superimposed on chronic renal disease.
- The clinical presentation varies with the degree of renal failure and its underlying etiology. Common symptoms are generalized fatigue, nausea, anorexia, pruritus, insomnia, and taste disturbances.
- **Laboratory tests:**
  - Blood urea nitrogen (BUN), creatinine, and creatinine clearance are elevated.
  - Urinalysis may reveal proteinuria and red blood cell casts.
  - Serum chemistry shows elevated BUN and creatinine, hyperkalemia, hyperuricemia, hypocalcemia, hyperphosphatemia, hyperglycemia, and decreased bicarbonate.
  - Measure urinary protein excretion. The finding of a ratio of protein to creatinine of >1000 mg/g suggests the presence of glomerular disease.
  - Special studies include serum and urine immunoelectrophoresis (in suspected multiple myeloma) and antinuclear antibody (in suspected systemic lupus erythematosus).
- **Imaging:** ultrasound of kidneys to measure kidney size and to rule out obstruction

ETIOLOGY

- Diabetes (37%), hypertension (30%), chronic glomerulonephritis (12%)
- Polycystic kidney disease
- Tubular interstitial nephritis (e.g., drug hypersensitivity, analgesic nephropathy), obstructive nephropathies (e.g., nephrolithiasis, prostatic disease)
- Vascular diseases (renal artery stenosis, hypertensive nephrosclerosis)

TREATMENT

- Provide adequate nutrition and calories (147-168 kJ/kg/day in energy intake, chiefly from carbohydrate and polyunsaturated fats). Referral to a dietitian for nutritional therapy for patients wtih GFR <50 mL/1.73 m^2 is recommended and is now a covered service by Medicare.

- Restrict sodium (approximately 100 mmol/day), potassium (≤60 mmol/day), and phosphate (<800 mg/day).
- Adjust daily doses or correct for prolonged half-lives.
- Restrict fluid if significant edema is present.
- Protein restriction (≤0.8 g/kg/day) may slow deterioration of renal function; however, studies have not confirmed this benefit. There is insufficient evidence to recommend or advise against routine restriction of protein intake to <0.8 g/kg/day.
- Resistance exercise training can preserve lean body mass, nutritional status, and muscle function in patients with moderate chronic kidney disease.
- Avoid radiocontrast agents.
- Angiotensin-converting enzyme (ACE) inhibitors, angiotensin receptor blockers (ARBs), and nondihydropyridine calcium channel blockers (diltiazem or verapamil) are useful in reducing proteinuria and slowing the progression of CRF especially in hypertensive diabetic patients. A systolic blood pressure between 129 mm Hg and <1 g/day Systolic blood pressure <110 mm Hg may be associated with a higher risk for kidney disease progression.
- **Initiate dialysis:**
  - **Urgent Indications:** uremic pericarditis, neuropathy, neuromuscular abnormalities, CHF, hyperkalemia, seizures
  - **Judgmental Indications:** creatinine clearance 10 to 15 mL/min, progressive anorexia, weight loss, reversal of sleep pattern, pruritus, uncontrolled fluid gain with hypertension and signs of CHF
- Give erythropoietin for anemia—2000-3000 IU/SC three times a week to maintain hematocrit 30% to 33%.
- Reduce significant fluid overload with diuretics (loop diuretics are preferred).
- Correct hypertension to at least 130/85 mm Hg with ACE inhibitors (avoid in patients with significant hyperkalemia). ARBs or nondihydropyridine calcium channel blockers (verapamil, diltiazem) can be used in patients intolerant to ACE inhibitors or when other drugs are needed to control blood pressure.
- Correct electrolyte abnormalities (e.g., calcium chloride, glucose, sodium polystyrene sulfonate for hyperkalemia); use sodium bicarbonate in patients with severe metabolic acidosis.
- Prescribe lipid-lowering agents in patients with dyslipidemia; target low-density lipoprotein cholesterol of <100 mg/dL.
- Control renal osteodystrophy with calcium supplementation and vitamin D. Starting dose of calcium carbonate is 0.5 g with each meal.

...if the phosphorus concentration is normalized

increasing serum calcium concentration. Paracalcitol, a new vitamin D analogue, has been reported as more effective than calcitriol in lessening the elevations in serum calcium and phosphorus levels.
- Sevelamer (Renagel) is a useful phosphate binder to reduce serum phosphate levels.
- Kidney transplantation is indicated in selected patients.

CLINICAL PEARLS

- Kidney biopsy is generally not performed in patients with small kidneys or with advanced disease.
- The GFR is the best overall indicator of kidney function. It can be estimated using prediction equations that take into account the serum creatinine level and some or all of specific variables (body size, age, sex, race). GFR calculators are available on the National Kidney Foundation Web site (http://www.kidney.org/kls/professionals/gfr_calculator.cfm).

Renal tubular acidosis (RTA)

Definition: Disorder characterized by inability to excrete H^+ or inadequate generation of new HCO_3^-. There are four types of RTA:

- Type I (classic, distal RTA)—abnormality in distal hydrogen secretion resulting in hypokalemic hyperchloremic metabolic acidosis
- Type II (proximal RTA)—decreased proximal bicarbonate reabsorption resulting in hypokalemic hyperchloremic metabolic acidosis
- Type III (RTA of glomerular insufficiency)—normokalemic hyperchloremic metabolic acidosis as a result of impaired ability to generate sufficient NH_3 in the setting of decreased glomerular filtration rate (<30 mL/min). This type of RTA is described in older textbooks and is considered by many not to be a distinct entity.
- Type IV (hyporeninemic hypoaldosteronemic RTA)—aldosterone deficiency or antagonism resulting in decreased distal acidification and decreased distal sodium reabsorption with subsequent hyperkalemic hyperchloremic acidosis.

DIAGNOSIS

- Arterial blood gases reveal metabolic acidosis; serum potassium is low in RTA types I and II, normal in type III, and high in type IV.
- Minimal urine pH is >5.5 in RTA type I and <5.5 in types II, III, and IV.
- Urinary anion gap is 0 or positive in all types of RTA.

- Additional useful studies include serum calcium level and urine calcium.
- Anion gap is normal.
- Parathyroid hormone measurement is useful in patients suspected to have primary hyperparathyroidism (may be associated with type II RTA).
- Renal sonogram or noncontrast helical CT of abdomen can be used to evaluate renal size or presence of stones.

ETIOLOGY

- **Type I RTA:** primary biliary cirrhosis and other liver diseases, medications (amphotericin, nonsteroidals), systemic lupus erythematosus, Sjögren's syndrome
- **Type II RTA:** Fanconi's syndrome, primary hyperparathyroidism, multiple myeloma, medications (acetazolamide)
- **Type IV RTA:** diabetes mellitus, sickle cell disease, Addison's disease, urinary obstruction

TREATMENT

- Types I and II RTA are treated with oral sodium bicarbonate (1-2 mEq/kg/day in RTA type I, 2-4 mEq/kg/day in RTA type II) titrated to correct acidosis.
- Potassium supplementation is needed in hypokalemic patients.
- Type IV RTA can be treated with furosemide to lower elevated potassium levels and sodium bicarbonate to correct significant acidosis. Fludrocortisone 100-300 µg/day can be used to correct mineralocorticoid deficiency.
- Monitor potassium levels frequently in RTA type IV.
- Monitor for bone disease in RTA type II.
- Monitor for nephrocalcinosis and nephrolithiasis in RTA type I.

CLINICAL PEARLS

- Untreated distal RTA may result in hypercalcemia, hyperphosphaturia, nephrolithiasis, and nephrocalcinosis.

▓ Renal vein thrombosis

Definition: Thrombotic occlusion of one or both renal veins

DIAGNOSIS

- Abdominal ultrasound
- Abdominal MRI
- Renal arteriography (delayed films during venous phase)

clots, if present, could be dislodged)
- **Clinical presentation:** flank pain, renal failure, hematuria, edema, deep vein thrombosis of lower extremities, dilated abdominal pain, back pain

ETIOLOGY
- Extrinsic compression by a tumor or retroperitoneal mass
- Invasion of the renal vein or inferior vena cava by tumor (almost always renal cell cancer)
- Trauma
- Hypercoagulable states
- Dehydration
- Glomerulopathies (membranous glomerulonephritis, crescenting glomerulonephritis, systemic lupus erythematosus, amyloidosis), especially in the presence of nephrotic syndrome when the serum albumin is <2 g/dL

TREATMENT
- Institute anticoagulation therapy in acute renal vein thrombosis to prevent pulmonary emboli and in an attempt to improve renal function and decrease proteinuria.
- Thrombolytic therapy or surgical thrombectomy also has been reported to be effective.
- The value of anticoagulation in chronic renal vein thrombosis is dubious except in nephrotic patients with membranous glomerulonephritis with profound hypoalbuminemia, in which prolonged prophylactic anticoagulation may be of benefit even if renal vein thrombosis has not been documented.

Rhabdomyolysis

Definition: Acute or subacute event resulting in damage or necrosis of striated muscle

DIAGNOSIS
- **Creatine kinase (CK):** Elevations may be >100,000 U/L in fulminant rhabdomyolysis; the development of renal failure is not directly related to the threshold level of CK; isoenzyme fractionation is useful: if CK-MB is >5% of the total CK, involvement of the myocardium is likely.
- **Serum creatinine:** This is usually elevated; the etiology of the renal failure is uncertain and probably multifactorial (renal tubular

obstruction by precipitated myoglobin, direct myoglobin toxicity, hypotension, dehydration, decreased glomerular filtration rate, intravascular coagulation).

- **Serum potassium:** Preexisting hyperkalemia is a contributing factor to rhabdomyolysis; fulminant rhabdomyolysis can result in life-threatening hyperkalemia secondary to increased K^+ release from damaged muscle and impaired renal excretion.
- **Calcium and phosphate:** Initially there is hyperphosphatemia from muscle necrosis, secondary hypocalcemia from Ca^{2+} deposition in the injured muscle, and decreased 1,25-dihydroxycholecalciferol; later (in the diuretic phase of renal failure); hypercalcemia is present as a result of remobilization of the deposited Ca^{2+} and secondary hyperparathyroidism.
- **Myoglobin:** Myoglobin is present in the serum and urine; the urine is brownish. This method detects granular casts, and is orthotoluidine-positive. A quick visual method to separate myoglobinuria from hemoglobinuria is to examine the urine and serum simultaneously: Reddish brown urine and pink serum indicate hemoglobinuria, whereas brown urine and clear serum suggest myoglobinuria. A rise in serum myoglobin precedes the rise in CK level and is useful to estimate the risk of renal failure (serum myoglobin levels <2000 μg/L may be associated with renal insufficiency.)

ETIOLOGY

- Trauma (e.g. crush syndrome, burns, electrical shock)
- Muscle ischemia (e.g. thrombosis, embolism, vasculitis, sickle cell disease, pressure necrosis, tourniquet shock)
- **Drugs:** Drug-induced rhabdomyolysis can occur via several mechanisms.
  - Primary toxin-induced (e.g. ethanol, methadone, ethylene glycol, isopropyl alcohol, carbon monoxide poisoning)
  - Caused by chronic intake of drugs associated with hypokalemia (e.g. thiazides)
  - Caused by overdose of certain drugs (e.g. barbiturates, heroin, cocaine)
  - Malignant hyperthermia (usually seen in genetically predisposed individuals after exposure to halothane, succinylcholine, or pancuronium)
  - Neuroleptic malignant syndrome (associated with use of phenothiazines, butyrophenones, antipsychotics, cocaine, or diphenhydramine usually in patients with dehydration and electrolyte imbalance)
  - Use of certain lipid-lowering agents (e.g. combination of statins and fenofibrate)

- **Infections:**
  - Bacterial (e.g., *Streptococcus, Salmonella, Clostridium, Legionella, Leptospira, Shigella*)
  - Viral (e.g., echovirus, coxsackievirus, influenza, cytomegalovirus, herpesvirus, Epstein-Barr virus, hepatitis)
  - Parasites (trichinosis)
- Excessive muscular stress (e.g., marathon runners, status epilepticus, delirium tremens)
- Genetic defects (carnitine deficiency, phosphorylase deficiency, glucosidase deficiency, cytochrome disturbances)
- **Miscellaneous:** brown recluse spider bite, snake bite, hornet sting, polymyositis, dermatomyositis, heatstroke, diabetic ketoacidosis, hyponatremia, hypophosphatemia, myxedema, thyroid storm, Rocky Mountain spotted fever, hypothermia, carbon monoxide, cyclic antidepressants, phenylpropanolamine, codeine, phencyclidine, amphetamines, LSD, Reye's syndrome

TREATMENT

- Vigorous fluid replacement to maintain a good urinary output, at least until myoglobin disappears from the urine. Initially, normal saline should be given at a rate of 1.5 L/hr with close monitoring of cardiac, pulmonary, and electrolyte status. Maintain a high rate of intravenous fluids at least until creatine phosphokinase is <1,000 U/L. Patients may require >15 L of fluid in the initial 24 hours to achieve urine flow rates of 200 to 300 mL/hr.
- Administration of a single dose of mannitol (100 mL of a 25% solution IV over 15 minutes) is controversial. Mannitol acts as an osmotic diuretic, renal vasodilator, and intravascular volume expander and may convert oliguric renal failure to nonoliguric renal failure.
- Alkalinization of the urine with addition of 44 mEq/L of sodium bicarbonate is advocated by some experts. The goal is to maintain urine pH >6.5. Sodium bicarbonate may increase solubility of uric acid and myoglobulin; however, it may promote calcium deposition.
- Hyperkalemia caused by rhabdomyolysis is most severe 10 to 40 hours after injury; initial treatment with sodium polystyrene sulfonate may be indicated; hyperkalemia caused by rhabdomyolysis responds poorly to treatment with glucose and insulin; attempts to correct hyperkalemia and initial hypocalcemia with calcium infusion may result in metastatic calcifications and severe hypercalcemia in the recovery period; hemodialysis may be necessary in patients with severe hyperkalemia, volume overload, uremic pericarditis, or uremic encephalopathy.

▦ Rheumatoid arthritis (RA)

Definition: Inflammatory disease that affects primarily synovial-lined joints, but also can affect the cardiac, nervous, pulmonary, reticuloendothelial, and integumentary systems

DIAGNOSIS

- RA is a clinical diagnosis. The seven criteria of the American College of Rheumatology are:
  - Morning stiffness in or around joints lasting at least 1 hour before improvement
  - Arthritis of three or more joint areas
  - Arthritis of hand joints with at least one swollen area in a wrist, metacarpophalangeal, or proximal interphalangeal joint
  - Symmetric arthritis
  - Presence of rheumatoid nodules (subcutaneous nodules over bony prominences or extensor surfaces or juxtaarticular regions)
  - Positive serum rheumatoid factor
  - Typical radiographic changes (erosions or bony decalcifications localized in or most marked adjacent to involved joints)
- Existence of four or more of these criteria denotes RA.
- **Laboratory tests:** There is no single laboratory test that can exclude or prove the diagnosis of RA. Any of the following laboratory abnormalities may be present:
  - **Rheumatoid factor (RF):** Latex positivity may be initially absent, but over the course of the disease, approximately 85% of patients become latex positive. RF is not specific for RA and may be found in other conditions (e.g. osteomyelitis, infective endocarditis, liver disease, and nonspecific elevation in the elderly).
  - Erythrocyte sedimentation rate is generally elevated during exacerbations.
  - Antinuclear antibody is detected in approximately 15% of patients.
  - Decreased hemoglobin or hematocrit and granulocytopenia are other laboratory findings.

TREATMENT

- Drug therapy of RA generally consists of a stepwise approach based on the severity of disease and clinical response.
- There are two major categories of drugs:
  - **Rapid acting:** indicated for initial rapid relief of painful joint symptoms; examples are salicylates, other nonsteroidal anti-inflammatory drugs (NSAIDs), and systemic corticosteroids

are hydroxychloroquinine, gold, penicillamine, and immunosuppressive agents (methotrexate, azathioprine)
- Current recommendations favor early aggressive treatment with DMARDs to minimize long-term joint damage. Most clinicians begin therapy with a DMARD (hydroxychloroquine or sulfasalazine for mild forms of RA or methotrexate in more severe disease) in addition to an NSAID or corticosteroid. Combination DMARD therapy (e.g., methotrexate and leflunomide) can be used in moderate-to-severe disease. Appropriate liver enzyme and hematologic monitoring is mandatory.

Sarcoidosis

Definition: Chronic systemic granulomatous disease of unknown cause, characterized histologically by the presence of nonspecific, noncaseating granulomas

DIAGNOSIS
- Clinical manifestations often vary with the stage of the disease and degree of organ involvement; patients may be asymptomatic, but a chest x-ray may show findings consistent with sarcoidosis. Nearly 50% of patients with sarcoidosis are diagnosed by incidental findings on chest x-ray.
- **Frequent manifestations:**
  - Pulmonary manifestations—dry, nonproductive cough; dyspnea; chest discomfort
  - Constitutional symptoms—fatigue, weight loss, anorexia, malaise
  - Visual disturbances—blurred vision, ocular discomfort, conjunctivitis, iritis, uveitis
  - Dermatologic manifestations—erythema nodosum, macules, papules, subcutaneous nodules, hyperpigmentation, lupus pernio
  - Myocardial disturbances—arrhythmias, cardiomyopathy
  - Splenomegaly; hepatomegaly
  - Rheumatologic manifestations—arthralgias reported in 40% of patients
  - Neurologic and other manifestations—cranial nerve palsies, diabetes insipidus, meningeal involvement, parotid enlargement, hypothalamic and pituitary lesions, peripheral adenopathy
- Initial laboratory evaluation should include complete blood count, serum chemistries, urinalysis, and tuberculin test. Common laboratory abnormalities are:

- Hypergammaglobulinemia, anemia, leukopenia
- Liver function test abnormalities
- Hypercalcemia, hypercalciuria (secondary to increased gastro-intestinal absorption, abnormal vitamin D metabolism, and increased calcitriol production by sarcoid granuloma)
- Cutaneous anergy to *Trichophyton*, *Candida*, mumps, and tuberculin
- Angiotensin-converting enzyme is elevated in approximately 60% of patients with sarcoidosis; this is nonspecific and generally not useful in following the course of the disease.
- Biopsy should be done on accessible tissues suspected of sarcoid involvement (conjunctiva, skin, lymph nodes); bronchoscopy with transbronchial biopsy is the procedure of choice in patients without any readily accessible site.
- Chest x-ray shows adenopathy of the hilar and paratracheal nodes; parenchymal changes also may be present, depending on the stage of the disease:
  - Stage 0—normal x-ray
  - Stage I—bilateral hilar adenopathy
  - Stage II—stage I plus pulmonary infiltrate
  - Stage III—pulmonary infiltrate without adenopathy
  - Stage IV—advanced fibrosis with evidence of honeycombing, hilar retraction, bullae, cysts, and emphysema
- Pulmonary function tests (PFTs), including spirometry and diffusing capacity of the lung for carbon dioxide, may be normal or may reveal a restrictive pattern or obstructive pattern or both.
- ECG should be obtained in all patients with sarcoidosis.

TREATMENT

- Corticosteroids remain the mainstay of therapy when treatment is required (e.g., prednisone 40 mg qd for 8 to 12 weeks with gradual tapering of the dose to 10 mg qod over 8 to 12 months). Corticosteroids should be considered in patients with severe symptoms (e.g., dyspnea, chest pain); hypercalcemia; ocular, central nervous system, or cardiac involvement; and progressive pulmonary disease. Patients with interstitial lung disease benefit from oral steroid therapy for 6 to 24 months.
- Patients with progressive disease refractory to corticosteroids may be treated with methotrexate 7.5-15 mg once/week or azathioprine.
- Hydroxychloroquine is effective for chronic disfiguring skin lesions.
- Nonsteroidal antiinflammatory drugs are useful for musculoskeletal symptoms and erythema nodosum.
- Pulmonary rehabilitation is indicated in patients with significant respiratory insufficiency.

most patients with sarcoidosis have spontaneous remission within 2 years and do not require treatment. Their course can be followed by periodic clinical evaluation, chest x-ray, and PFTs.

Scabies

Definition: Contagious disease caused by the mite *Sarcoptes scabiei*

DIAGNOSIS
- Diagnosis is made based on the clinical presentation and on the demonstration of mites, eggs, or mite feces.
- Primary lesions are caused when the female mite burrows within the stratum corneum, laying eggs within the tract she leaves behind; burrows (linear or serpiginous tracts) end with a minute papule or vesicle.
- Primary lesions are found most commonly in the web spaces of the hands, wrists, buttocks, scrotum, penis, breasts, axillae, and knees.
- Secondary lesions result from scratching or infection.
- Intense pruritus, especially nocturnal, is common; it is caused by an acquired sensitivity to the mite or fecal pellets and usually is noted 1 to 4 weeks after the primary infestation.
- Examination of the skin may reveal burrows, tiny vesicles, excoriations, or inflammatory papules.
- For microscopic demonstration of the organism, feces, or eggs, a drop of mineral oil may be placed over the suspected lesion before removal; the scrapings are transferred directly to a glass slide; a drop of potassium hydroxide is added, and a coverslip is applied.

TREATMENT
- After a warm bath or shower, lindane (Kwell, Scabene) lotion should be applied to all skin surfaces below the neck (can be applied to the face if area is infested); it should be washed off 8 to 12 hours after application. Repeat application 1 week later is usually sufficient to eradicate infestation.
- Pruritus generally abates 24 to 48 hours after treatment, but it can last 2 weeks; oral antihistamines are effective in decreasing postscabietic pruritus.
- Topical corticosteroid creams may hasten the resolution of secondary eczematous dermatitis.
- If the patient is a resident of an extended care facility, it is important to educate the patients, staff, family, and frequent visitors about scabies and the need to have full cooperation in treatment. Scabicide

should be applied to all patients, staff, and frequent visitors, whether symptomatic or not; symptomatic family members of staff and visitors also receive treatment.

- Permethrin 5% cream (Elimite) also is effective with usually one treatment; it should be massaged into the skin from the head to the soles of the feet. Remove cream 8 to 14 hours later by washing. If living mites are present after 14 days, treat again.
- A single dose (150-200 mg/kg in 6-mg tablets) of ivermectin, an anti-helminthic agent, is as effective as topical lindane for the treatment of scabies.

CLINICAL PEARLS

- Scabies generally is acquired by sleeping with or in the bedding of infected individuals.
- Widespread and crusted lesions (Norwegian or crusted scabies) may be seen in elderly and immunocompromised patients.

Seizure disorder, absence

Definition: A type of generalized nonconvulsive seizure characterized by episodes of loss of awareness (typically ≤10 seconds) associated with a 3-Hz generalized spike and slow-wave electroencephalogram (EEG) pattern, followed by abrupt return to full consciousness

DIAGNOSIS

- Findings are normal between seizures in children with typical absence epilepsy.
- During seizure, the patient typically appears awake, but abruptly ceases ongoing activity and does not respond to or recall stimuli.
- More prolonged episodes may be associated with automatisms and mistaken for complex partial seizures.
- Tonic-clonic seizures can occur in approximately 40% of patients.
- EEG is the most powerful tool for identification of this seizure type.
- In most untreated individuals, vigorous hyperventilation for 3 to 5 minutes provokes characteristic EEG finding.

ETIOLOGY

- Idiopathic with a presumed genetic cause
- Absence seizures also can be seen with some types of generalized epilepsy syndromes, such as juvenile absence epilepsy or juvenile myoclonic epilepsy.
- **Experimental data:** Seizures arise from impaired regulation of rhyth-

- Drug of choice is ethosuximide or sodium valproate.
- Ethosuximide does not suppress tonic-clonic seizures. Sodium valproate is the drug of choice for patients with absence and tonic clonic seizures.
- The initial dose of ethosuximide in children is 10-15 mg/kg/day with maintenance dose of 15-40 mg/kg/day divided into a bid or tid dosing schedule. Gastrointestinal side effects can occur, so ethosuximide is best taken with meals.
- Common pediatric doses for valproic acid are 15-60 mg/kg/day (bid-qid). Hepatotoxicity and blood dyscrasias can occur.
- Lamotrigine also is effective but is not approved by the Food and Drug Administration for the treatment of absence epilepsy.

CLINICAL PEARLS
- Because most patients have spontaneous resolution of seizures, one can consider withdrawing anticonvulsant therapy typically when the patient has been seizure-free for at least 2 years.
- Absence seizures may be mistakenly diagnosed as complex partial seizures based on clinical descriptions. The EEG is essential for making this distinction.
- Administering other anticonvulsants (particularly carbamazepine or phenytoin) to patients with typical absence epilepsy may exacerbate seizures.

Seizure disorder, partial

Definition: In partial seizures, the onset of abnormal electrical activity originates in a focal region or lobe of the brain. Clinical manifestations may involve sensory, motor, autonomic, or psychic symptoms. Consciousness may be preserved (*simple partial seizures*) or impaired (*complex partial seizures*).

DIAGNOSIS
- Clinical presentation varies and depends on the site of origin of the abnormal electrical discharges.
- Symptoms of simple partial seizures include focal motor or sensory symptoms; language disturbance; olfactory, visual or auditory hallucinations; and visceral sensations, or fear or panic.
- With complex partial seizures, there is a loss or reduction of awareness. This may be preceded by an aura (simple partial seizure). There may be associated automatisms or alterations in behavior.

- There may be a relatively quick "march" or progression of symptoms over seconds to minutes as the ictal focus spreads along the cortex.
- Electroencephalogram is the most powerful tool for localization of the seizure focus.
- MRI with contrast is the modality of choice because of its high sensitivity for stroke, tumor, abscess, atrophy, and vascular malformations.

ETIOLOGY

- Seizures are a symptom of an underlying abnormality affecting the central nervous system, not a disease.
- Partial-onset seizures may be caused by underlying disorders, including stroke, tumor, infection, trauma, vascular malformations, or genetic factors.

TREATMENT

- Carbamazepine and phenytoin are common first-line therapeutic agents.
- Sodium valproate also may be effective.
- Newer agents, such as lamotrigine, oxcarbazepine, levetiracetam, and topiramate, may be better tolerated.

CLINICAL PEARL

- Individual seizures lasting <5 minutes generally require no acute pharmacologic intervention.

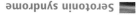 **Serotonin syndrome**

Definition: Syndrome that is characterized by a change in mental status and alteration in neuromuscular activity and autonomic dysfunction. The constellation of signs and symptoms results from increased activity of serotonin (5-hydroxytryptamine) in the central nervous system.

DIAGNOSIS

- Onset of symptoms is usually within minutes to hours after starting a new pharmacologic agent.
- Neuromuscular manifestations include confusion, agitation, hypomania, myoclonus, rigidity, tremor, hyperreflexia, ataxia, and shivering.
- Cardiovascular manifestations include tachycardia, hypertension, hypotension, and cutaneous flushing.
- Gastrointestinal manifestations include abdominal pain, diarrhea, vomiting, nausea, and salivation.

adding a serotoninergic agent to the patient's established regimen
- Drugs that increase serotonin release—amphetamines, cocaine, codeine, dextromethorphan, levodopa, fenfluramine, pentazocine, risperidone
- Drugs that decrease serotonin reuptake—SSRIs, carbamazepine, cyclic antidepressants, trazodone, venlafaxine, meperidine, methadone
- Direct or indirect serotonin receptor agonists—buspirone, lithium, sumatriptan, mescaline and other phenylalkylamines

TREATMENT
- No specific antidote exists for SSRI overdose.
- Useful medications to antagonize certain serotonin receptors are the following:
  - Cyproheptadine 4-8 mg PO q1-4h until a therapeutic dose is achieved (maximum adult dose is 32 mg). It also can be administered in liquid form via nasogastric tube (0.25 mg/kg/day divided into three equal doses).
  - Lorazepam 1 mg IV q30min can be used to treat muscle rigidity, myoclonus, and seizure complications.
  - Propranolol also has some serotonin blocking activity.
- Ventricular dysrhythmias should be treated with standard antidysrhythmic agents.

 Sialoadenitis

Definition: Inflammation of the salivary glands

DIAGNOSIS
- Pain and swelling of affected salivary gland
- Increased pain with meals
- Erythema, tenderness at the duct opening
- Purulent discharge from duct orifice
- Induration and pitting of the skin with involvement of the masseteric and submandibular spatial planes in severe cases
- Laboratory tests—complete blood count with differential possibly to reveal leukocytosis with left shift
- Ultrasound or CT scan useful in patients not responding to medical therapy

ETIOLOGY

- Ductal obstruction is generally secondary to a mucus plug caused by stasis of saliva with increased viscosity with subsequent stasis and infection.
- Most frequent infecting organisms are *Staphylococcus aureus*, *Pseudomonas*, *Enterobacter*, *Klebsiella*, *Enterococcus*, *Proteus*, and *Candida*.
- Sjögren's syndrome, trauma, radiation therapy, chemotherapy, dehydration, and chronic illness are predisposing factors.

TREATMENT

- Amoxicillin-clavulanate 500-875 mg or cefuroxime 250 mg bid should be given for 10 days. Clindamycin is an alternative choice in penicillin-allergic patients.
- Intravenous antibiotics (e.g., cefoxitin, nafcillin) can be given in severe cases.
- Massage of the gland may express pus and relieve some of the pressure.
- Rehydration
- Warm compresses
- Oral cavity irrigations

Sick sinus syndrome

Definition: Group of cardiac rhythm disturbances characterized by abnormalities of the sinus node, including (1) sinus bradycardia, (2) sinus arrest or exit block, (3) combinations of sinoatrial or atrioventricular conduction defects, and (4) supraventricular tachyarrhythmias. These abnormalities may coexist in a single patient so that a patient may have episodes of bradycardia and episodes of tachycardia.

DIAGNOSIS

- ECG
- Ambulatory cardiac rhythm monitoring
- Twenty-four-hour ambulatory ECG (Holter)
- Event recorder
- **Clinical presentation:** lightheadedness, dizziness, syncope, palpitation

ETIOLOGY

- Fibrosis or fatty infiltration involves the sinus node, atrioventricular node, or its branches.

...nding the sinus nodes and other sclerodegenerative changes may be found.

TREATMENT
- A permanent pacemaker is placed if symptoms are present.
- Drug treatment of the tachycardia (e.g., with digitalis or calcium channel blockers) may worsen or bring out the bradycardia and become the reason for pacemaker requirement.

▨ Sjögren's syndrome

Definition: Autoimmune disorder characterized by lymphocytic and plasma cell infiltration and destruction of salivary and lacrimal glands with subsequent diminished lacrimal and salivary gland secretions

- *Primary*—dry mouth (xerostomia) and dry eyes (xerophthalmia) develop as isolated entities
- *Secondary*—associated with other disorders

DIAGNOSIS
- Workup involves the demonstration of the following criteria for diagnosis of primary and secondary Sjögren's syndrome.
- **Primary:**
  - **Symptoms and objective signs of ocular dryness:**
    - Schirmer's test—<8 mm wetting per 5 minutes
    - Positive rose bengal or fluorescein staining of cornea and conjunctiva to show keratoconjunctivitis sicca
  - **Symptoms and objective signs of dry mouth:**
    - Decreased parotid flow using Lashley cups or other methods
    - Abnormal biopsy result of minor salivary gland (focus score >2 based on average of four assessable lobules)
  - **Evidence of systemic autoimmune disorder:**
    - Elevated titer of rhematoid factor (RF) >1 : 320
    - Elevated titer of antinuclear antibody (ANA) >1 : 320
    - Presence of anti-SSA (Ro) or anti-SSB (La) antibodies
- **Secondary:**
  - **Characteristic signs and symptoms:**
    - Dry mouth with dry lips (cheilosis), erythema of tongue and other mucosal surfaces, carious teeth
    - Dry eyes (conjunctival injection, decreased luster, and irregularity of the corneal light reflex)

- Possible salivary gland enlargement and dysfunction with subsequent difficulty in chewing and swallowing food and in speaking without frequent water intake
- Purpura (nonthrombocytopenic, hyperglobulinemic, vasculitic)
- Evidence of associated conditions (e.g., rheumatoid arthritis [RA] or other connective disease, lymphoma, hypothyroidism, chronic obstructive pulmonary disease, trigeminal neuropathy, chronic liver disease, polymyopathy)
- Clinical features sufficient to allow a diagnosis of RA, systemic lupus erythematosus, polymyositis, or scleroderma
- Laboratory tests: positive ANA (>60% of patients) with autoantibodies anti-SSA and anti-SSB may be present. Additional laboratory abnormalities may include elevated erythrocyte sedimentation rate, anemia (normochromic, normocytic), abnormal liver function studies, elevated serum β_2-microglobulin levels, RF.
- A definite diagnosis of Sjögren's syndrome can be made with a salivary gland biopsy.

TREATMENT

- Provide adequate fluid replacement.
- Proper oral hygiene reduces the incidence of caries.
- Use artificial tears frequently.
- Pilocarpine 5 mg PO qid is useful to improve dryness. A cyclosporine 0.05% ophthalmic emulsion (Restasis) also may be useful for dry eyes. Recommended dose is 1 drop bid in both eyes.
- Cevimeline (Evoxac), a cholinergic agent with muscarinic agonist activity, 30 mg PO tid is effective for the treatment of dry mouth in patients.

Spontaneous bacterial peritonitis (SBP)

Definition: Bacterial peritonitis without an evident source of infection in a patient with ascites

DIAGNOSIS

- **Ascitic fluid analysis:**
  - Polymorphonuclear neutrophil (PMN) cell count >250/mm³ in ascitic fluid; this is the most sensitive and specific test for SBP if >500/mm³.
  - Presence of bacteria on initial Gram stain of ascitic fluid
  - Lactic acid (lactate) >32 mg/dL

Glucose 500 mg/dL

- Lactate dehydrogenase (LDH) <225 mU/mL
- Positive culture of peritoneal fluid
- Major distinguishing factors between SBP and secondary peritonitis (perforation of bowel wall):
  - Presence of free air on abdominal x-ray films in secondary peritonitis
  - Common presence of multiple organisms and anaerobes in ascitic fluid in secondary peritonitis
  - Analysis of ascitic fluid in secondary peritonitis generally reveals leukocyte count >10,000/mm^3, LDH >225 mU/mL, protein >1 g/dL, and glucose <50 mg/dL.
  - Repeat paracentesis after 48 hours of appropriate antibiotic therapy reveals a significant decrease in ascitic fluid PMN count in patients with SBP and no decrease in patients with a secondary bacterial peritonitis.

ETIOLOGY

- SBP usually occurs as a complication of hepatic ascites. The following mechanisms may account for bacterial seeding of the ascitic fluid:
  - Hematogenous transmission
  - Direct transmural passage after mucosal drainage (ischemia, edema)
  - Bowel perforation after paracentesis (uncommon)
- **Infecting organisms:** *Escherichia coli,* group D streptococci, *Streptococcus pneumoniae, Streptococcus viridans, Enterobacter, Pseudomonas, Klebsiella*

TREATMENT

- Cefotaxime 2 g IV q8h or ceftriaxone 2 g IV q24h in patients with normal renal function; treatment duration is generally 7 to 10 days. Oral quinolone therapy (ofloxacin 100-800 mg/day) may be an acceptable alternative in selected patients.

CLINICAL PEARLS

- Renal failure is a major cause of morbidity in patients with SBP.
- SBP is associated with hepatic ascites in 8% to 25% of cases of ascites. Trimethoprim-sulfamethoxazole (Bactrim DS, Septra DS) 1 tablet five times per week and ciprofloxacin 750 mg PO every week are effective for the prevention of SBP in patients with cirrhosis.

Status asthmaticus

Definition: Severe continuous bronchospasm

DIAGNOSIS

- Physical examination during status asthmaticus may reveal:
  - Tachycardia and tachypnea
  - Use of accessory respiratory muscles
  - Pulsus paradoxus (inspiratory decline in systolic blood pressure >10 mm Hg)
  - Wheezing
  - Mental status changes generally secondary to hypoxia and hypercapnia, which constitute an indication for urgent intubation
  - Paradoxical abdominal and diaphragmatic movement on inspiration (detected by palpation over the upper part of the abdomen in a semirecumbent position); this is an important sign of impending respiratory crisis, indicating diaphragmatic fatigue
  - The following abnormalities in vital signs indicate severe asthma:
    - Pulsus paradoxus >18 mm Hg
    - Respiratory rate >30 breaths/min
    - Tachycardia with heart rate >120 beats/min
- **Pulmonary function studies:** During acute severe bronchospasm, forced expiratory volume in 1 second is <1 L, and peak expiratory flow rate is <80 L/min.
- Arterial blood gases can be used in staging the severity of an asthmatic attack.
  - Mild—decreased PaO_2 and $PaCO_2$, increased pH
  - Moderate—decreased PaO_2, normal $PaCO_2$ and pH
  - Severe—marked decreased PaO_2, increased $PaCO_2$, decreased pH
- Complete blood count shows leukocytosis with left shift, which may indicate the existence of bacterial infection.
- Chest x-ray usually is normal; it may show evidence of thoracic hyperinflation (e.g., flattening of the diaphragm, increased volume over the retrosternal air space).
- ECG shows tachycardia, and nonspecific ST-T wave changes; it also may show cor pulmonale, right bundle branch block, right axial deviation, and counterclockwise rotation.

ETIOLOGY

- **Intrinsic asthma:** occurs in patients who have no history of allergies; may be triggered by upper respiratory infections or psychological stress
- **Extrinsic asthma (allergic asthma):** brought on by exposure to allergens, industrial chemicals)

...matitis with bronchospasm after initiation of exercise and improves with discontinuation of exercise
- **Drug-induced asthma:** often associated with use of nonsteroidal antiinflammatory drugs, β-blockers, sulfites, certain foods and beverages

TREATMENT
- Oxygen generally is started at 2-4 L/min via nasal cannula or Venti-Mask at 40% fraction of inspired oxygen; further adjustments are made according to arterial blood gases.
- **Bronchodilators:**
  - Various agents and modalities are available. Inhaled bronchodilators are preferred when they can be administered quickly. Parenteral administration of sympathomimetics (e.g., subcutaneous epinephrine) when necessary should be accompanied by ECG monitoring.
  - Albuterol 0.5-1 mL (2.5-5 mg) in 3 mL of saline solution tid or qid via nebulizer is effective.
- **Corticosteroids:**
  - Early administration is advised, particularly in patients using steroids at home.
  - Patients may be started on hydrocortisone 2.5-4 mg/kg or methylprednisolone 0.5-1 mg/kg IV loading dose, then q6h as needed; higher doses may be necessary in selected patients (particularly patients receiving steroids at home). Steroids given by inhalation also are useful for controlling bronchospasm and tapering oral steroids and should be used in all patients with severe asthma.
  - Rapid but judicious tapering of corticosteroids eliminates serious steroid toxicity; long-term low-dose methotrexate may be an effective means of reducing the systemic corticosteroid requirement in some patients with severe refractory asthma.
- Judicious use of intravenous hydration is necessary to avoid congestive heart failure in elderly patients.
- Intravenous antibiotics are indicated when there is suspicion of bacterial infection (e.g., infiltrate on chest x-ray, fever, or leukocytosis).
- Intubation and mechanical ventilation are indicated when the above-listed measures fail to produce significant improvement.
- General anesthesia with halothane may reverse bronchospasm in a severe asthmatic who cannot be ventilated adequately by mechanical means.
- Intravenous magnesium sulfate supplementation (20-minute infusion of 40 mg/kg to a maximum of 2 g of magnesium sulfate) in children

with low or borderline-low magnesium levels may improve acute bronchospasm.

CLINICAL PEARLS

- The most common errors regarding steroid therapy in acute bronchospasm are the use of "too little, too late" and too-rapid tapering with return of bronchospasm.
- Absence of wheezing (silent chest) or decreased wheezing can indicate worsening obstruction in status asthmaticus.

Status epilepticus

Definition: Seizure activity continuing for 30 minutes or intermittently over a 30-minute period without the patient's regaining consciousness

TREATMENT

- Insert oral airway.
- Start intravenous line with normal saline solution.
- Draw samples to evaluate arterial blood gases, electrolyte, glucose, blood urea nitrogen, creatinine, calcium, magnesium, toxicology screen, and anticonvulsant levels (in patients receiving anticonvulsants).
- Institute ECG, respiratory, and blood pressure monitoring.
- Give thiamine 100 mg IM.
- Give 50-mL bolus injection of a 50% glucose solution if hypoglycemia is present.
- Give lorazepam 0.1 mg/kg IV at 2 mg/min (maximum 8 mg) or diazepam 0.2 mg/kg IV at 5 mg/min (maximum 20 mg).
- Monitor closely for respiratory depression and hypotension.
- Emergency intubation may be required.
- Increase saline solution infusion if the patient becomes hypotensive.
- Give fosphenytoin simultaneously 15-20 mg /kg infused at a rate of 100-150 mg /min with ECG monitoring.
- The preceding measures control seizures in 90% of all patients within 30 to 40 minutes; if seizures continue, *intubate patients,* and proceed with the following measures.
  - Give phenobarbital 100 mg/min IV to a maximum of 20 mg/kg *or*
  - Give diazepam 100 mg in 500 mL of dextrose in water infused at 40 mL/hr; this results in diazepam serum levels of 0.2 to 0.8 μg/mL.
- If seizure activity persists >60 minutes, consider instituting general anesthesia with isoflurane and neuromuscular blockade. Continuous seizures at this point are often due to metabolic disturbances (e.g., _____) or serious intracranial lesions (e.g.,

Stevens-Johnson syndrome

Definition: Severe vesiculobullous form of erythema multiforme affecting skin, mouth, eyes, and genitalia

DIAGNOSIS
- Diagnosis generally is based on clinical presentation and characteristic appearance of the lesions.
- The cutaneous eruption generally is preceded by vague, nonspecific symptoms of low-grade fever and fatigue occurring 1 to 14 days before the skin lesions. Cough is often present. Fever may be high during the active stages.
- Bullae generally occur on the conjunctiva and mucous membranes of the mouth, nares, and genital regions.
- Ulcerative stomatitis results in hemorrhagic crusting.
- Flat, atypical target lesions or purpuric maculae may be distributed on the trunk or be widespread.
- Skin biopsy generally is reserved for when classic lesions are absent and diagnosis is uncertain.

DIFFERENTIAL DIAGNOSIS
- Toxic erythema (drugs or infection)
- Pemphigus
- Pemphigoid
- Urticaria
- Hemorrhagic fevers
- Serum sickness
- *Staphylococcus* scalded-skin syndrome
- Behçet's syndrome

ETIOLOGY
- Drugs (e.g., phenytoin, penicillins, phenobarbital, sulfonamides) are the most common cause.
- Upper respiratory tract infections (e.g., *Mycoplasma pneumoniae*) and herpes simplex viral infections also have been implicated.

TREATMENT
- Withdrawal of any potential drug precipitants
- Treatment of associated conditions (e.g., acyclovir for herpes simplex virus infection, erythromycin for *Mycoplasma* infection)
- Antihistamines for pruritus

- Treatment of cutaneous blisters with cool, wet Burow's compresses
- Relief of oral symptoms by frequent rinsing with lidocaine (Xylocaine Viscous)
- Liquid or soft diet with plenty of fluids to ensure proper hydration
- Treatment of secondary infections with antibiotics
- **Corticosteroids:** use remains controversial; when used, prednisone 20-30 mg bid until new lesions no longer appear, then rapidly tapered
- **Topical steroids:** may use to treat papules and plaques; however, should not be applied to eroded areas
- **Vitamin A:** may be used for lacrimal hyposecretion

CLINICAL PEARLS

- Prognosis varies with severity of disease. It is generally good in patients with limited disease; however, mortality may approach 10% in patients with extensive involvement.
- Oral lesions may continue for several months.
- Scarring and corneal abnormalities may occur in 20% of patients.

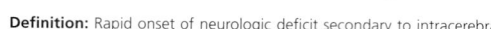

Stroke, intracerebral hemorrhage

Definition: Rapid onset of neurologic deficit secondary to intracerebral hemorrhage

DIAGNOSIS

- On CT scan of the head, area of hemorrhagic infarct appears as a zone of increased density; shifts of intracranial contents and compression of the ventricles may be present.
- The hemorrhage usually occurs during periods of activity, often manifesting with headache, vomiting, and sudden onset of neurologic deficits that can progress rapidly to coma and death; the neurologic deficits vary with the area involved.
- In addition to the focal deficits, the patient may show signs of increased intracranial pressure (ICP) (e.g., bradycardia, decreased respiratory rate, third nerve palsy).

ETIOLOGY

- Hypertension (50-60% of cases), cerebral amyloid angiopathy (10%), hemorrhagic infarcts (10%), use of anticoagulants and fibrinolytic agents (10%), brain tumors (5%), vascular malformations (5%)

TREATMENT

- Patients with intracranial hemorrhage should be admitted to the ICU. Hourly neurologic checks for at least the initial 12 hours are recom-
- ~~mended. Place on bed rest with head of the bed ele-~~

...are necessary to prevent deep vein thrombosis.

- All fluids should be given in normal saline if possible to maintain serum sodium and osmolarity. Hypotonic fluids may worsen cerebral edema. Total intravenous fluid intake generally should be limited to 1.5 L/day.
- Supportive measures include urinary catheter insertion, arterial line placement (if blood pressure management is needed), intubation of patients with depressed level of consciousness and inability to protect airway from aspiration, and rotation schedule to prevent decubitus ulcers.
- **Control of severe hypertension:** Lower blood pressure may reduce cerebral edema, but risks promoting border zone ischemia. As a rough guide, blood pressure reduction should be considered if systolic blood pressure is >180 mm Hg or diastolic blood pressure is >100 mm Hg. If the prehemorrhage blood pressure is known, the mean arterial pressure (MAP) should not be lowered >25% from baseline (MAP = diastolic blood pressure + pulse pressure/3). Intravenous nitroprusside is a good agent for blood pressure control because it is effective, has rapid onset of action, and can be titrated easily.
- **Management of increased ICP:**
  - Increased ICP can be managed with mannitol.
  - Intubation and ventilation of patients with increased ICP are recommended to prevent hypoxia and hypercapnia (both powerful stimuli for cerebral vasodilation).
  - Use of benzodiazepines or short-acting barbiturates is helpful to prevent increased intracranial and intrathoracic pressure from agitation and fighting the ventilator in intubated patients.
- Correction of coagulation disturbances includes platelet transfusions to increase platelet count >50,000/mm³ in thrombocytopenic patients and use of fresh frozen plasma in patients with abnormal coagulation secondary to liver disease or warfarin.
- **Surgical evacuation of hematomas:** Surgery is indicated in the following situations:
  - Noncomatose patients with cerebellar hemorrhage
  - Patients with surgically accessible cerebral hematomas that produce progressive signs of temporal lobe herniation
  - Size of the hematoma and level of consciousness are of prognostic significance; awake patients with a small hematoma (<3 cm) often recover without surgery, whereas comatose patients with hemorrhages >6 cm do poorly regardless of medical or surgical management.

Stroke, ischemic

Definition: Rapid onset of neurologic deficit involving a certain vascular territory secondary to thrombosis or embolism

DIAGNOSIS

- Clinical presentation varies with the cerebral vessel involved.
- CT scan of the head shows cerebral infarction as an area of decreased density. Initial CT scan may be negative, and infarct may not be evident for 2 to 3 days after the infarction.

TREATMENT

- **Thrombolysis:** Patients who present within 3 hours of ischemic stroke onset and who meet specific inclusion and exclusion criteria should be considered for intravenous thrombolytic therapy.
- Acute anticoagulation with heparin, low-molecular-weight heparin, and heparinoids provides no benefit, while increasing hemorrhagic complications in patients with cardioembolic stroke, lacunar stroke, or stroke of unknown etiology. It may be reasonable, however, to give intravenous heparin to selected patients who present within 24 hours of symptom onset and who have signs of unstable or progressing atherothrombotic stroke of large intracranial or extracranial arteries. When given, intravenous heparin generally is maintained for 3 to 7 days while a decision is made about long-term prophylaxis therapy with either antiplatelet drugs or warfarin. CT scan should be performed initially (before anticoagulation is started) and may be repeated after 48 hours to show no hemorrhagic transformation.
- Antiplatelet agents for secondary prevention of atherothrombotic strokes include aspirin, clopidogrel, and combination of aspirin and dipyridamole.
- Lowering systemic blood pressure in patients with acute cerebral infarction is contraindicated because it may produce clinical deterioration (secondary to spontaneous fluctuation in blood pressure and impaired cerebral autoregulation), unless one of the following conditions is present:
  - Diastolic pressure is ≥120 mm Hg or systolic pressure is >230 mm Hg.
  - Hypertensive encephalopathy is present.
  - Vital organs (heart, kidney) are compromised.
  - There is cerebral ischemia secondary to aortic dissection.
  - Most patients with acute cerebral infarction have elevated blood pressure, which generally returns to baseline within 48 hours without additional treatment.

- Carotid endarterectomy may be indicated for patients after atherothrombotic stroke whose surgery can be delayed at least 1 month and who have minor residual deficits associated with high-grade ipsilateral stenosis or large ulcerative lesions and have a low-to-medium surgical risk.

Subarachnoid hemorrhage (SAH)

Definition: Presence of active bleeding into the subarachnoid space

DIAGNOSIS

- CT scan of head confirms the presence of subarachnoid blood localized to the basal cisterns or extending intracerebrally or in the ventricles (Fig. 14); a fresh hemorrhage produces an area of increased density; the scan may be normal if done >48 hours after the SAH or if the hemorrhage is small. Very thin cuts (3 mm in thickness) through the base of the brain are recommended because thicker cuts (10 mm) may miss small collections of blood. MRI has a lower index of accuracy than CT in SAH.
- **Clinical manifestations:**
  - Abrupt onset of severe occipital or generalized headache that radiates into the posterior neck region and is worsened by neck and head movements; often described as "the worst headache" of the patient's life
  - Restlessness, vomiting, diminished level of consciousness, syncope
- **Physical examination:**
  - Focal neurologic signs usually are absent.
  - Level of consciousness varies from normal to deeply comatose.
  - Fever and nuchal rigidity are present or usually develop within 24 hours.
  - Fundi may show papilledema or retinal hemorrhage.
  - Cranial nerve abnormalities may be noted (e.g., pupillary dilation secondary to oculomotor nerve dysfunction).
  - Hypertension may be present and can lead to an incorrect diagnosis of primary hypertensive emergency.
  - Tachycardia and irregular heartbeat may be present (91% of patients with SAH have cardiac arrhythmias).

ETIOLOGY

- Ruptured congenital aneurysm or arteriovenous malformation (AVM)

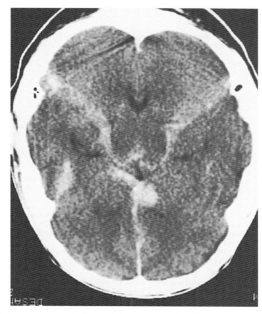

FIGURE 14. Noncontrast CT scan shows diffuse subarachnoid hemorrhage. The rounded area of hyperdensity anterior to the suprasellar cistern represents an aneurysm of the anterior communicating artery. (From Specht N [ed]: Practical Guide to Diagnostic Imaging, St Louis, Mosby, 1998.)

- Management of SAH varies with the patient's clinical status and the location and surgical accessibility of the aneurysm.
- **Medical management:**
  - Implement strict bed rest in a quiet, darkened private room with cardiac monitoring (frequent arrhythmias).
  - Control headache with acetaminophen and codeine.
  - Have the patient avoid all forms of straining (stool softeners and mild laxatives are indicated to prevent constipation).
  - Stress ulcer prophylaxis (e.g., intravenous H_2 blockers, proton-pump inhibitors, or sucralfate 1 g in 20 mL H_2O via nasogastric tube tid) is indicated in patients on mechanical ventilation or with prior history of gastric ulcers.
  - Reduce cerebral edema with mannitol.
  - Nimodipine, a calcium channel blocker, is useful in the treatment of cerebral blood vessel spasm after SAH from ruptured congenital intracranial aneurysms in patients who are in good neurologic condition postevent; it decreases the incidence of permanent neurologic damage and death. Therapy should be initiated within 96 hours of the onset of hemorrhage; dosage is 60 mg q4h for 21 days; it may be administered via nasogastric tube. Dosage reduction is necessary in patients with liver disease.
- **Surgical management (clipping versus coiling):** The indications for surgery and the patient's prognosis depend on the size of the aneurysm, the patient's age and clinical condition, and the experience of the neurosurgeon. Endovascular coiling with a platinum coil device also is effective in enabling endovascular occlusion of intracranial aneurysms and reducing risk for further rupture without craniotomy.

CLINICAL PEARL

- **Prognosis of cerebral AVMs:** The rate of rebleeding for cerebral AVMs in patients with hemorrhage is approximately 6% in the first 6 months after the hemorrhage; thereafter, it is approximately 4% per year, a rate identical to the yearly risk of a first hemorrhage in patients with AVMs that have never bled; surgery or endovascular coiling to prevent rebleeding or the initial bleed is much more desirable in a younger patient.

Subclavian steal syndrome

Definition: Occlusion or severe stenosis of the proximal subclavian artery leading to decreased antegrade flow or retrograde flow in the ipsilateral vertebral artery and neurologic symptoms referable to the posterior circulation

DIAGNOSIS

- Upper extremity ischemic symptoms include fatigue, exercise-related aching, coolness, and numbness of the involved upper extremity.
- Neurologic symptoms, including brief spells of vertigo, diplopia, and unsteady gait, are reported by 25% of patients with known unilateral subclavian steal. Exercising the ischemic upper extremity occasionally provokes these spells (classic subclavian steal). Left subclavian steal is more common than right, but the latter is more serious.
- Physical findings include delayed and smaller volume pulse (wrist or antecubital) in the affected upper extremity, lower blood pressure in the affected upper extremity, and supraclavicular bruit.
  - *Note:* Inflating a blood pressure cuff increases the bruit if it originates from a vertebral artery stenosis and decreases the bruit if it originates from a subclavian artery stenosis.
- Doppler sonography of the vertebral, subclavian, and innominate arteries
- Arteriography

ETIOLOGY

- Atherosclerosis
- Arteritis (Takayasu's disease and temporal arteritis)
- Embolism to the subclavian or innominate artery
- Cervical rib
- Chronic use of a crutch
- Occupational (baseball pitchers and cricket bowlers)

TREATMENT

- In most patients, the disease is benign and requires no treatment other than atherosclerosis risk factor modification and aspirin. Symptoms tend to improve over time as collateral circulation develops.
- Vascular surgical reconstruction requires a thoracotomy; it may be indicated in innominate artery stenosis or when upper extremity ischemia is incapacitating.

Definition: Set of symptoms that results when a mediastinal mass compresses the SVC or the veins that drain into it

DIAGNOSIS
- **Clinical presentation:** shortness of breath, chest pain, cough, dyspnea, dysphagia, syncope
- **Physical examination:** chest wall vein distention, neck vein distention, facial edema, upper extremity swelling, cyanosis
- Chest x-ray
- Venography
- Chest CT scan or MRI
- Although invasive procedures, such as mediastinoscopy or thoracotomy, are associated with higher than usual risk of bleeding, a tissue diagnosis usually is needed before starting therapy.

ETIOLOGY
- Lung cancer (80% of all cases, of which half are small cell lung cancer)
- Lymphoma (15%)
- Tuberculosis
- Goiter
- Aortic aneurysm (arteriosclerotic or syphilitic)
- SVC thrombosis
  - **Primary:** associated with a central venous catheter
  - **Secondary:** as a complication of SVC syndrome associated with one of the above-mentioned causes

TREATMENT
- Emergency empiric radiation is indicated in critical situations, such as respiratory failure or central nervous system signs associated with increased intracranial pressure.
- Treat the underlying malignancy.
- Anticoagulant or fibrinolytic therapy is indicated in patients who do not respond to cancer treatment within 1 week or if an obstructing thrombus has been documented.

Syncope

Definition: Temporary loss of consciousness resulting from an acute global reduction in cerebral blood flow

DIAGNOSIS

- **History:**
  - **Sudden loss of consciousness:** Consider cardiac arrhythmias or vertebrobasilar transient ischemic attack.
  - **Gradual loss of consciousness:** Consider orthostatic hypotension, vasodepressor syncope, or hypoglycemia.
  - **Patient's activity at the time of syncope:**
    - **Micturition, coughing, defecation:** Consider syncope caused by decreased venous return.
    - **Turning head while shaving:** Consider carotid sinus syndrome.
    - **Physical exertion in a patient with murmur:** Consider aortic stenosis.
    - **Arm exercise:** Consider subclavian steal syndrome.
    - **Assuming an upright position:** Consider orthostatic hypotension.
  - **Associated events:**
    - **Chest pain:** Consider myocardial infarction or pulmonary embolism.
    - **Palpitations:** Consider dysrhythmias.
    - **History of aura, incontinence during episode, and transient confusion after "syncope":** Consider seizure disorder.
    - **Psychic stress:** Consider vasovagal syncope.
    - Consider current medications, particularly antihypertensive drugs.
- **Physical examination:**
  - **Blood pressure:** If low, consider orthostatic hypotension. If unequal in both arms (difference >20 mm Hg), consider subclavian steal or dissecting aneurysm. Blood pressure and heart rate should be recorded in the supine, sitting, and standing positions.
  - **Pulse:** If patient has tachycardia, bradycardia, or irregular rhythm, consider dysrhythmia.
  - **Mental status:** If patient is confused after the syncopal episode, consider postictal state.
  - **Heart:** If murmurs are present, suggestive of aortic stenosis or idiopathic hypertrophic subaortic stenosis (IHSS), consider syncope secondary to left ventricular outflow obstruction; if jugular venous

- **Carotid sinus pressure:** This can be diagnostic if it reproduces symptoms and other causes are excluded. A pause ≥3 seconds or a systolic blood pressure drop >50 mm Hg without symptoms or <30 mm Hg with symptoms when sinus pressure is applied separately on each side for ≤5 seconds is considered abnormal; this test should be avoided in patients with carotid bruits or cerebrovascular disease. ECG monitoring, intravenous access, and bedside atropine should be available when carotid sinus pressure is applied.
- **Initial diagnostic tests:**
  - Routine blood tests rarely yield diagnostically useful information and should be done only when they are suggested specifically by the results of the history and physical examination. The following tests should be considered:
    - Complete blood count—rule out anemia, infection
    - Electrolytes, blood urea nitrogen, creatinine, magnesium, and calcium—rule out electrolyte abnormalities, hypomagnesemia, hypocalcemia; evaluate fluid status
    - ECG—rule out arrhythmias; may be diagnostic in 5% to 10% of patients
    - Chest x-ray—evaluate cardiac size, lung fields
    - Arterial blood gases—rule out pulmonary embolus, hyperventilation
    - Pregnancy test in women of child-bearing age
  - Tilt-table testing.
    - This test is useful to support the diagnosis of neurocardiogenic syncope. It also is useful to identify patients with prominent bradycardic response who may benefit from a permanent pacemaker.
    - It is indicated in patients with recurrent episodes of unexplained syncope. Patients >50 years old should have stress testing before undergoing tilt-table testing.
  - Additional diagnostic tests may be indicated depending on the patient's history and physical examination.
    - If arrhythmias are suspected, a 24-hour Holter monitor and admission to a telemetry unit are appropriate; in general, Holter monitoring is rarely useful, revealing a cause for syncope in <3% of cases. Loop recorders that can be activated after a syncopal event and retrieve information about the cardiac rhythm during the preceding 4 minutes have added considerable diagnostic yield in patients with unexplained syncope.

- An echocardiogram is indicated in patients with a heart murmur to rule out aortic stenosis, IHSS, or atrial myxoma.
- If a seizure is suspected, a CT scan of the head and an electroencephalogram are indicated.
- If pulmonary embolism is suspected, a ventilation-perfusion scan or a spiral CT scan should be done.
- Cardiac isoenzymes or troponin levels or both should be obtained if the patient gives a history of chest pain before the syncopal episode.
- Check drug and alcohol levels when suspecting toxicity.

ETIOLOGY

- **Vasovagal (vasodepressor):**
  - Psychophysiologic (panic disorders, hysteria)
  - Visceral reflex
  - Carotid sinus
  - Glossopharyngeal neuralgia
  - Reduction of venous return resulting from Valsalva maneuver, cough, defecation, or micturition
- **Orthostatic hypotension:**
  - Hypovolemia
  - Hypotensive drugs
  - Neurogenic, idiopathic
  - Pheochromocytoma
  - Systemic mastocytosis
- **Cardiac:**
  - Reduced cardiac output
    - Left ventricular outflow obstruction (aortic stenosis, hypertrophic cardiomyopathy)
    - Obstruction to pulmonary flow (pulmonary embolism, pulmonic stenosis, primary pulmonary hypertension)
    - Myocardial infarction with pump failure
    - Cardiac tamponade
    - Mitral stenosis
  - Dysrhythmias or asystole
    - Extreme tachycardia (>160-180 beats/min)
    - Severe bradycardia (<30-40 beats/min)
    - Sick sinus syndrome
    - Atrioventricular block (second or third degree)
    - Ventricular tachycardia or fibrillation
    - Long Q-T syndrome
    - Pacemaker malfunction
- **Cerebrovascular:**

- basilar migraine
- Colloid cyst of the third ventricle
- **Other causes:**
  - Mechanical reduction of venous return (atrial myxoma, ball-valve thrombus)
  - Not related to decreased blood flow—hypoxia, hypoglycemia, anemia, hyperventilation, seizure disorder, drug or alcohol abuse

TREATMENT
- Varies with etiology of syncope

PROGNOSIS
- Varies with the age of the patient and the etiology of the syncope
  - **Benign prognosis (low 1-year morbidity and mortality):**
    - Patients ≤30 years old and having noncardiac syncope
    - Patients ≤70 years old and having vasovagal or psychogenic syncope
  - **Poor prognosis (high morbidity and mortality):** Patients with cardiac syncope. Patients with syncope of unknown cause also are at increased risk for death from any cause.
- Patients with three or more of the following risk factors have a >30% 1-year mortality risk: abnormal ECG, history of ventricular arrhythmias, history of congestive heart failure, age >45 years.

Syndrome of inappropriate antidiuretic hormone secretion (SIADH)

Definition: Syndrome characterized by excessive secretion of antidiuretic hormone (ADH) in absence of normal osmotic or physiologic stimuli (increased serum osmolarity, decreased plasma volume, hypotension)

DIAGNOSIS
- Demonstration through laboratory evaluation of excessive secretion of ADH in absence of appropriate osmotic or physiologic stimuli. Laboratory tests reveal:
  - Hyponatremia
  - Urinary osmolarity > serum osmolarity
  - Urinary sodium usually >30 mEq/L
  - Normal blood urea nitrogen, creatinine (indicates normal renal function and absence of dehydration)

- Decreased uric acid
- For diagnostic purposes, patient should have normal thyroid, adrenal, and cardiac function and no recent or concurrent use of diuretics.
- Chest x-ray should be obtained to rule out neoplasm or infectious process.

ETIOLOGY

- **Neoplasm:** lung, duodenum, pancreas, brain, thymus, bladder, prostate, mesothelioma, lymphoma, Ewing's sarcoma
- **Pulmonary disorders:** pneumonia, tuberculosis, bronchiectasis, emphysema, status asthmaticus
- **Intracranial pathology:** trauma, neoplasms, infections (meningitis, encephalitis, brain abscess), hemorrhage, hydrocephalus
- **Postoperative period:** surgical stress, ventilators with positive pressure, anesthetic agents
- **Drugs:** chlorpropamide, thiazide diuretics, vasopressin, desmopressin, oxytocin, chemotherapeutic agents (vincristine, vinblastine, cyclophosphamide), carbamazepine, phenothiazines, monoamine oxidase inhibitors, tricyclic antidepressants, narcotics, nicotine, clofibrate, haloperidol, selective serotonin reuptake inhibitors
- **Other:** acute intermittent porphyria, Guillain-Barré syndrome, myxedema, psychosis, delirium tremens, adrenocorticotropic hormone deficiency (hypopituitarism)

TREATMENT

- In emergency situations (seizures, coma), SIADH can be treated with combination of hypertonic saline solution (slow infusion of 250 mL of 3% sodium chloride) and furosemide; this increases the serum sodium by causing diuresis of urine that is more dilute than plasma; the rapidity of correction varies depending on the degree of hyponatremia and if the hyponatremia is acute or chronic; generally the serum sodium should be corrected only halfway to normal in the initial 24 hours, and serum sodium should be increased by <0.5 mEq/L/hr.
- Depending on the underlying etiology, fluid restriction may be needed indefinitely. Monthly monitoring of electrolytes is recommended in patients with chronic SIADH.
- Demeclocycline (Declomycin) 300-600 mg PO bid may be useful in patients with chronic SIADH (e.g., secondary to neoplasm), but use with caution in patients with hepatic disease; side effects include nephrogenic diabetes insipidus, and photosensitivity. This medication is very expensive

Use of hypertonic (3%) saline is contraindicated in patients with congestive heart failure, nephrotic syndrome, or cirrhosis.
- Too-rapid correction of hyponatremia can cause demyelination and permanent central nervous system damage.

▰ Syphilis

Definition: Systemic infectious disease caused by *Treponema pallidum*. *Latent syphilis* is defined as syphilis characterized by seroreactivity without other evidence of disease. *Tertiary syphilis* refers to gummatous and cardiovascular syphilis, but not to neurosyphilis.

DIAGNOSIS

- Dark-field examinations and direct fluorescent antibody tests of lesion exudate or tissue are the definitive methods for diagnosing early syphilis.
- Presumptive diagnosis is possible with the use of two types of serologic tests for syphilis: (1) nontreponemal (e.g., Venereal Disease Research Laboratory and rapid plasma reagin) and (2) treponemal (e.g., fluorescent treponemal antibody absorbed and microhemagglutination assay for antibody to *T. pallidum*). The use of one type of test alone is not sufficient for diagnosis.
- Patients with syphilis may seek treatment for signs or symptoms of primary infection (ulcer or chancre at site of infection), secondary infection (manifestations that include rash, mucocutaneous lesions, and adenopathy), or tertiary infection (cardiac, neurologic, ophthalmic, auditory, or gummatous lesions).
- Patients can be diagnosed as having early latent syphilis if, within the year preceding the evaluation, they had the following:
  - A documented seroconversion
  - Unequivocal symptoms of primary or secondary syphilis
  - A sex partner who had primary, secondary, or early latent syphilis

TREATMENT

- **Primary and secondary syphilis:**
  - Nonallergic patients with primary or secondary syphilis should be treated with the following regimen: benzathine penicillin G 2.4 million U IM in a single dose.
  - **Penicillin allergy:** Nonpregnant penicillin-allergic patients who have primary or secondary syphilis should be treated with the following regimen:
    - Doxycycline 100 mg orally bid for 2 weeks *or*

- Tetracycline 500 mg orally qid for 2 weeks
  - **Pregnancy:** Pregnant patients allergic to penicillin should be treated with penicillin, after desensitization if necessary.
- **Latent syphilis:**
  - Treatment of early latent syphilis is with benzathine penicillin G 2.4 million U IM in a single dose. Late latent syphilis or latent syphilis of unknown duration is treated with benzathine penicillin G 7.2 million U total, administered as three doses of 2.4 million U IM each at 1-week intervals.
  - Nonpregnant patients who have latent syphilis and who are allergic to penicillin should be treated with doxycycline 100 mg PO bid or tetracycline 500 mg PO qid for 2 weeks if the duration of infection is known to have been <1 year; otherwise, these agents should be administered for 4 weeks.
- **Tertiary syphilis:**
  - Recommended treatment regimen is benzathine penicillin G 7.2 million U total, administered as three doses of 2.4 million U IM at 1-week intervals.
  - Penicillin-allergic patients should be treated according to the recommended regimens for late latent syphilis.
- **Neurosyphilis:**
  - Recommended treatment regimen is aqueous crystalline penicillin G 18-24 million U a day administered as 3-4 million U q4h for 10 to 14 days.
  - Alternative treatment regimen is with procaine penicillin 2.4 million U IM a day *plus* probenecid 500 mg PO qid, both for 10 to 14 days.

Systemic lupus erythematosus (SLE)

Definition: Chronic multisystemic disease characterized by production of autoantibodies and protean clinical manifestations

DIAGNOSIS
- The diagnosis of SLE can be made by showing the presence of any four or more of the following criteria of the American Rheumatism Association:
  - Butterfly rash
  - Discoid rash
  - Photosensitivity (particularly leg ulcerations)
  - Oral ulcers

tion not performed, cellular casts)
* Neurologic disorder (seizures, psychosis [in absence of offending drugs or metabolic derangement])
* Hematologic disorder:
  * Hemolytic anemia with reticulocytosis
  * Leukopenia (<4000/mm^3 total on two or more occasions)
  * Lymphopenia (<1500/mm^3 on two or more occasions)
  * Thrombocytopenia (<100,000/mm^3 in the absence of offending drugs)
* Immunologic disorder:
  * Positive SLE cell preparation
  * Anti-DNA (presence of antibody to native DNA in abnormal titer)
  * Anti-Sm (presence of antibody to Smith nuclear antigen)
  * False-positive serologic test for syphilis known to be positive for at least 6 months and confirmed by negative treponemal immobilization or fluorescent treponemal antibody tests
* Antinuclear antibody (ANA)—an abnormal titer of ANA by immunofluorescence or equivalent assay at any time in the absence of drugs known to be associated with "drug-induced lupus" syndrome
* **Laboratory tests:** Suggested initial laboratory evaluation of suspected SLE:
  * **Immunologic evaluation:** ANA, anti-DNA antibody, anti-Sm antibody
  * **Other laboratory tests:** complete blood count with differential, platelet count (Coombs' test if anemia detected), urinalysis (24-hour urine collection for protein if proteinuria is detected), partial thromboplastin time and anticardiolipin antibodies in patients with thrombotic events, blood urea nitrogen, creatinine to evaluate renal function
* **Clinical presentation:**
  * **Skin:** erythematous rash over the malar eminences, generally with sparing of the nasolabial folds (butterfly rash); alopecia; raised erythematous patches with subsequent edematous plaques and adherent scales (discoid lupus); leg, nasal, or oropharyngeal ulcerations; livedo reticularis; pallor (from anemia); petechiae (from thrombocytopenia)
  * **Joints:** tenderness, swelling, or effusion generally involving peripheral joints

- **Cardiac:** pericardial rub (in patients with pericarditis), heart murmurs (if endocarditis or valvular thickening and dysfunction)
- **Other:** fever, conjunctivitis, dry eyes, dry mouth (sicca syndrome), oral ulcers, abdominal tenderness, decreased breath sounds (pleural effusions)
- **Imaging:**
  - Chest x-ray for evaluation of pulmonary involvement (e.g., pleural effusions, pulmonary infiltrates)
  - Echocardiogram to screen for significant valvular heart disease (present in 18% of patients with SLE); echocardiography can identify a subset of lesions (valvular thickening and dysfunction) other than verrucous (Libman-Sacks) endocarditis that are prone to hemodynamic deterioration

TREATMENT

- Joint pain and mild serositis generally are well controlled with nonsteroidal antiinflammatory drugs; antimalarials also are effective (e.g., hydroxychloroquine [Plaquenil]).
- **Cutaneous manifestations:**
  - Topical corticosteroids; intradermal corticosteroids are helpful for individual discoid lesions, especially in the scalp
  - Antimalarials (e.g., hydroxychloroquinine and quinacrine)
  - Sunscreens that block UVA and UVB radiation
  - Immunosuppressive drugs (methotrexate or azathioprine) used as steroid-sparing drugs
- **Renal disease:**
  - The use of high-pulsed doses of cyclophosphamide given at monthly intervals is more effective in preserving renal function than treatment with glucocorticoids alone. The combination of methylprednisolone and cyclophosphamide is superior to bolus therapy with methylprednisolone or cyclophosphamide alone in patients with lupus nephritis. For patients with proliferative lupus nephritis, short-term therapy with intravenous cyclophosphamide followed by maintenance therapy with mycophenolate mofetil or azathioprine seems to be more efficacious and safer than long-term therapy with intravenous cyclophosphamide.
  - Use of plasmapheresis combined with immunosuppressive agents (to prevent the rebound phenomenon of antibody levels after plasmapheresis) generally is reserved for rapidly progressive renal failure or life-threatening systemic vasculitis.
- **Central nervous system involvement:** Treatment generally consists of corticosteroid therapy; however, its efficacy is uncertain, and it is generally reserved for organic brain syndrome. Anticonvulsants and antipsychotics also are indicated in selected cases; headaches are

anemia consists of high doses of corticosteroids; nonhemolytic anemia (secondary to chronic disease) does not require specific therapy.

- **Thrombocytopenia:**
  - Initial treatment consists of corticosteroids.
  - In patients with poor response to steroids, encouraging results have been reported with the use of danazol, vincristine, and immunoglobulins. Combination chemotherapy with cyclophosphamide and prednisone combined with vincristine, vincristine and procarbazine, or etoposide may be useful in patients with severe refractory idiopathic thrombocytopenic purpura.
  - Splenectomy generally does not cure the thrombocytopenia of SLE, but it may be necessary as an adjunct in managing selected cases.
- Infections are common because of compromised immune function secondary to SLE and the use of corticosteroid, cytotoxic, and antimetabolite drugs; pneumococcal bacteremia is associated with high mortality rate.
- Close monitoring for exacerbation of the disease and for potential side effects from medications (corticosteroids, cytotoxic agents) with frequent laboratory evaluation and office visits is necessary in all patients with SLE.

CLINICAL PEARL
- Valvular heart disease is present in 18% of patients with SLE. The prevalence of infective endocarditis is approximately 1% (similar to the prevalence after prosthetic valve surgery, but greater than the prevalence after rheumatic valvulitis). Valvular heart disease in patients with SLE frequently changes over time (e.g., vegetations can appear unexpectedly for the first time, resolve, or change in size or appearance). These frequent changes are temporarily unrelated to other clinical features of SLE and can be associated with substantial morbidity and mortality.

▰ Thrombocytopenia

Definition: Platelet count <150,000/mm^3

DIAGNOSIS
  - Obtain a thorough history (particularly drug history).
- Physical examination should look for presence of splenomegaly (hypersplenism, leukemia, lymphoma).

- Examine peripheral blood smear; note platelet size and other abnormalities (e.g., fragmented red blood cells may indicate thrombotic thrombocytopenic purpura [TTP] or disseminated intravascular coagulation [DIC]; increased platelet size suggests accelerated destruction and release of large young platelets into the circulation).
- Check international normalized ratio, partial thromboplastin time, bleeding time, and Coombs test.
- On bone marrow examination, increased megakaryocytes indicate thrombocytopenia resulting from accelerated destruction.

ETIOLOGY

- ### Increased destruction:
  - #### Immunologic:
    - Drugs (quinine, quinidine, digitalis, procainamide, thiazide diuretics, sulfonamides, phenytoin, aspirin, penicillin, heparin, gold, meprobamate, sulfa drugs, phenylbutazone, nonsteroidal anti-inflammatory drugs, methyldopa, cimetidine, furosemide, isoniazid, cephalosporins, chlorpropamide, organic arsenicals, chloroquine, platelet glycoprotein IIb/IIIa receptor inhibitors, ranitidine, indomethacin, carboplatin, ticlopidine, clopidogrel)
    - Idiopathic thrombocytopenic purpura
    - Transfusion reaction—transfusion of platelets with plasminogen activator (PLA) in recipients without PLA-1
    - Fetal/maternal incompatibility
    - Collagen vascular diseases (e.g., systemic lupus erythematosus)
    - Autoimmune hemolytic anemia
    - Lymphoproliferative disorders (e.g., chronic lymphocytic leukemia)
  - #### Nonimmunologic:
    - Prosthetic heart valves
    - TTP
    - Sepsis
    - DIC
    - Hemolytic-uremic syndrome
    - Giant cavernous hemangioma
- ### Decreased production:
  - Abnormal marrow
  - Marrow infiltration (e.g., leukemia, lymphoma, fibrosis)
  - Marrow suppression (e.g., chemotherapy, alcohol, radiation)
  - Vitamin deficiencies (Vitamin B_{12}, folate)
- ### Hereditary disorders:
  - Wiskott-Aldrich syndrome—X-linked disorder characterized by thrombocytopenia, eczema, and repeated infections
  - May-Hegglin anomaly—increased megakaryocytes but ineffec-

- Dilutional (massive transfusion)

TREATMENT
- Varies with cause of thrombocytopenia

▰ Thrombophlebitis, superficial

Definition: Inflammatory thrombosis in subcutaneous veins

DIAGNOSIS
- **Clinical presentation:**
  - Subcutaneous vein is palpable, tender; tender cord is present with erythema and edema of the overlying skin and subcutaneous tissue.
  - Induration, redness, and tenderness are localized along the course of the vein. This linear appearance rather than circular appearance is useful to distinguish thrombophlebitis from other conditions (e.g., cellulitis, erythema nodosum).
  - There is no significant swelling of the limb (superficial thrombophlebitis generally does not produce swelling of the limb).
  - Low-grade fever may be present. High fever and chills suggest septic phlebitis.
- **Laboratory tests:** complete blood count with differential, blood cultures, culture of intravenous catheter tip (when secondary to intravenous cannulation)
- **Imaging:**
  - Serial ultrasound or venography in patients with suspected deep vein thrombosis (DVT)
  - CT scan of abdomen in patients with suspected malignancy (Trousseau's syndrome—recurrent migratory thrombophlebitis)

ETIOLOGY
- Trauma to preexisting varices
- Intravenous cannulation of veins (most common cause)
- Abdominal cancer (e.g., carcinoma of pancreas)
- Infection (*Staphylococcus* most common pathogen)
- Hypercoagulable state
- DVT

TREATMENT

- Apply warm, moist compresses.
- It is not necessary to restrict activity; however, if there is extensive thrombophlebitis, bed rest with the leg elevated limits the thrombosis and improves symptoms.
- Give nonsteroidal antiinflammatory drugs to relieve symptoms.
- Treat septic thrombophlebitis with antibiotics with adequate coverage of *Staphylococcus*.
- Ligation and division of the superficial vein at the junction avoids propagation of the clot in the deep venous system when the thrombophlebitis progresses toward the junction of the involved superficial vein with deep veins.

Thrombotic thrombocytopenic purpura (TTP)

Definition: Rare disorder characterized by thrombocytopenia (often accompanied by purpura) and microangiopathic hemolytic anemia; neurologic impairment, renal dysfunction, and fever also may be present

DIAGNOSIS

- Severe anemia and thrombocytopenia are present.
- Evidence of hemolysis includes elevated reticulocyte count, indirect bilirubin, and lactate dehydrogenase and decreased haptoglobin.
- Urinalysis shows hematuria (red blood cells [RBCs] and RBC casts in urine sediment) and proteinuria.
- Peripheral smear shows severely fragmented RBCs (schistocytes).
- There is no laboratory evidence of disseminated intravascular coagulation (normal fibrin degradation product, fibrinogen).
- Blood urea nitrogen and creatinine are elevated.

ETIOLOGY

- The exact cause of TTP is unknown. Studies reveal that there is platelet aggregation as a result of abnormalities in circulating von Willebrand factor caused by endothelial injury.
- Many drugs, including clopidogrel, penicillin, antineoplastic agents, oral contraceptives, quinine, and ticlopidine, have been associated with TTP Other precipitating causes include infectious agents, pregnancy, malignancies, allogeneic bone marrow transplantation, and neurologic disorders.

- continue potential offending agents.
- Institute plasmapheresis with fresh frozen plasma (FFP) replacement; cryosupernatant may be substituted for FFP in patients who fail to respond to this treatment. Daily plasma exchange generally is performed until hemolysis has ceased, and the platelet count has normalized.
- Corticosteroids (prednisone 1-2 mg/kg/day) may be effective alone in patients with mild disease or may be administered concomitantly with plasmapheresis plus plasma exchange with FFP.
- Vincristine has been used in patients refractory to plasmapheresis.
- Use of antiplatelet agents (acetylsalicylic acid, dipyridamole) is controversial.
- Platelet transfusions are contraindicated except in severely thrombocytopenic patients with documented bleeding.
- Splenectomy is performed in refractory cases.
- Relapsing TTP may be treated with plasma exchange.
- Remission of chronic TTP that is unresponsive to conventional therapy has been reported after treatment with cyclophosphamide and the monoclonal antibody rituximab.

Thyroid nodule

Definition: Abnormal growth of the thyroid gland found on physical examination; nodules can be benign (70%) or malignant

DIAGNOSIS
- Palpable, firm, and nontender nodule in the thyroid area should prompt suspicion of carcinoma. Signs of metastasis are regional lymphadenopathy and inspiratory stridor.
- Signs and symptoms of thyrotoxicosis can be found in functioning nodules.
- Fine-needle aspiration (FNA) biopsy is the best diagnostic study; the accuracy can be >90%, but it is directly related to the level of experience of the physician and the cytopathologist interpreting the aspirate.
- FNA biopsy is less reliable with thyroid cystic lesions; surgical excision should be considered for most thyroid cysts not abolished by aspiration.
- **Laboratory tests:**
  - Thyroid-stimulating hormone (TSH), thyroxine, and serum thyroglobulin levels should be obtained before thyroidectomy in patients with confirmed thyroid carcinoma on FNA biopsy.

- Serum calcitonin at random or after pentagastrin stimulation is useful when medullary carcinoma of the thyroid is suspected and in anyone with a family history of medullary thyroid carcinoma.
- Serum thyroid autoantibodies are useful when thyroiditis is suspected.

Imaging:
- Thyroid ultrasound is done in some patients to evaluate the size of the thyroid and the number, composition (solid versus cystic), and dimensions of the thyroid nodule; solid thyroid nodules have a higher incidence of malignancy, but cystic nodules also can be malignant.
- Perform thyroid scan with technetium-99m pertechnetate.
  - Scan classifies nodules as hyperfunctioning ("hot"), normally functioning ("warm"), or nonfunctioning ("cold"); cold nodules have a higher incidence of malignancy.
  - Scan has difficulty evaluating nodules near the thyroid isthmus or at the periphery of the gland.
  - Normal tissue over a nonfunctioning nodule might mask the nodule as warm or normally functioning.

TREATMENT
- Evaluate results of FNA.
  - Normal cells: may repeat biopsy during present evaluation or reevaluate patient after 3 to 6 months of suppressive therapy (levothyroxine, prescribed in doses to suppress the TSH level to 0.1–0.5). Failure to regress indicates increased likelihood of malignancy. Reliance on repeat needle biopsy is preferable to routine surgery for nodules not responding to levothyroxine.
  - Malignant cells: surgery
  - Hypercellularity: thyroid scan
    - Hot nodule: radioactive iodine therapy if the patient is hyperthyroid
    - Warm or cold nodule: surgery (rule out follicular adenoma versus carcinoma)

CLINICAL PEARLS
- *Thyroid scan and ultrasound provide information about the risk of malignant neoplasia based on the characteristics of the thyroid nodule, but their value in the initial evaluation of a thyroid nodule is limited because neither one provides a definite tissue diagnosis.
- Increased likelihood that nodule is malignant: nodule increasing in size or >2 cm, regional lymphadenopathy fixation to adjacent tissues, age <40 years, symptoms of local invasion (dysphagia, hoarseness, neck pain), male sex, family history of thyroid cancer or polyposis

Definition: An inflammatory disease of the thyroid. It is a multifaceted disease with varying etiology, different clinical characteristics (depending on the stage), and distinct histopathology. Thyroiditis can be subdivided into three common types (*Hashimoto's, painful, painless*) and two rare forms (*suppurative, Riedel's*). To add to the confusion, there are various synonyms for each form, and there is no internationally accepted classification of autoimmune thyroid disease.

DIAGNOSIS
- **Clinical presentation:**
  - **Hashimoto's:** Patients may have signs of hyperthyroidism (tachycardia, diaphoresis, palpitations, weight loss) or hypothyroidism (fatigue, weight gain, delayed reflexes) depending on the stage of the disease. Usually there is diffuse, firm enlargement of the thyroid gland; thyroid gland also may be of normal size (atrophic form with clinically manifested hypothyroidism).
  - **Painful subacute:** Exquisitely tender, enlarged thyroid; fever; and signs of hyperthyroidism are initially present. Signs of hypothyroidism subsequently may develop.
  - **Painless thyroiditis:** Clinical features are similar to subacute thyroiditis except for the absence of tenderness of the thyroid gland.
  - **Suppurative:** Patient is febrile with severe neck pain, focal tenderness of the involved portion of the thyroid, and erythema of the overlying skin.
  - **Riedel's:** Slowly enlarging hard mass is present in the anterior neck, often mistaken for thyroid cancer. Signs of hypothyroidism occur in advanced stages.
- **Laboratory tests:**
  - Thyroid-stimulating hormone (TSH) and free thyroxine may be normal or indicative of hypothyroidism or hyperthyroidism depending on the stage of the thyroiditis.
  - White blood cell (WBC) count with differential shows increased WBCs with shift to the left with subacute and suppurative thyroiditis.
  - Antimicrosomal antibodies are detected in >90% of patients with Hashimoto's thyroiditis and 50% to 80% of patients with silent thyroiditis.
  - Serum thyroglobulin levels are elevated in patients with subacute and silent thyroiditis; this test is nonspecific but may be useful in monitoring the course of subacute thyroiditis and distinguishing

silent thyroiditis from factitious hyperthyroidism (low or absent serum thyroglobulin level).

Imaging: Twenty-four-hour radioactive iodine (RAI) uptake is useful to distinguish Graves' disease (increased RAI uptake) from thyroiditis (normal or low RAI uptake).

ETIOLOGY

- **Hashimoto's:** autoimmune disorder that begins with the activation of CD4 (helper) T lymphocytes specific for thyroid antigens. The etiologic factor for the activation of these cells is unknown.
- **Painful subacute:** possibly postviral; usually from a respiratory illness. It is not considered to be a form of autoimmune thyroiditis.
- **Suppurative:** infectious etiology, generally bacterial, although fungi and parasites also have been implicated. It often occurs in immunocompromised hosts or after a penetrating neck injury.
- **Painless thyroiditis:** frequently occurs postpartum
- **Riedel's:** fibrous infiltration of the thyroid. Etiology is unknown.
- **Drug induced:** lithium, interferon alfa, amiodarone, interleukin-2

TREATMENT

- Treat hypothyroid phase with levothyroxine 25–50 µg/day initially, and monitor serum TSH initially every 6 to 8 weeks.
- Control symptoms of hyperthyroidism with β-blockers (e.g. propranolol 20–40 mg PO q6h).
- Control pain in patients with subacute thyroiditis with nonsteroidal antiinflammatory drugs (NSAIDs). Prednisone 20–40 mg qd may be used if NSAIDs are insufficient, but it should be gradually tapered off over several weeks.
- Use intravenous antibiotics and drain abscess (if present) in patients with suppurative thyroiditis.

CLINICAL PEARLS

- In Hashimoto's thyroiditis, long-term prognosis is favorable; most patients recover thyroid function.
- In painful subacute thyroiditis, permanent hypothyroidism occurs in 10% of patients.
- In painless thyroiditis, 6% of patients have permanent hypothyroidism.

Definition: Abrupt and severe exacerbation of thyrotoxicosis

DIAGNOSIS
- **Clinical presentation:**
  - Tremor, tachycardia, fever
  - Warm, moist skin
  - Lid lag, lid retraction, proptosis
  - Altered mental status (psychosis, coma, seizures)
- **Laboratory tests:**
  - Free thyroxine, thyroid-stimulating hormone
  - Complete blood count with differential
  - Blood and urine cultures
  - Glucose
  - Liver enzymes
  - Blood urea nitrogen, creatinine
  - Serum calcium
  - Creatine phosphokinase

DIFFERENTIAL DIAGNOSIS
- Psychiatric disorders
- Alcohol or other drug withdrawal
- Pheochromocytoma
- Metastatic neoplasm

TREATMENT
- **Inhibition of thyroid hormone synthesis:**
  - Administer propylthiouracil (PTU) 300-600 mg initially (PO or via nasogastric tube), then 150-300 mg q6h.
  - If the patient is allergic to PTU, use methimazole (Tapazole) 80-100 mg PO or PR followed by 30 mg PR q8h.
- **Inhibition of stored thyroid hormone:**
  - Iodide can be administered as sodium iodine 250 mg IV q6h, potassium iodide 5 gtt PO q8h, or Lugol's solution 10 gtt q8h. It is important to administer PTU or methimazole 1 hour *before* the iodide to prevent the oxidation of iodide to iodine and its incorporation in the synthesis of additional thyroid hormone.
  - **Corticosteroids:** Dexamethasone 2 mg IV q6h or hydrocortisone 100 mg IV q6h for approximately 48 hours is useful to inhibit thyroid hormone release, impair peripheral conversion of tri-iodothyronine from thyroxine, and provide additional adrenocortical hormone to correct deficiency (if present).

- **Suppression of peripheral effects of thyroid hormone:** β-Adrenergic blockers are useful. Administer propranolol 80-120 mg PO q4-6h. Propranolol also may be given 1 mg/min IV for 2 to 10 minutes under continuous ECG and blood pressure monitoring.
- Control fever with acetaminophen 325-650 mg q4h; avoid aspirin because it displaces thyroid hormone from its binding protein.
- Treat any precipitating factors (e.g., antibiotics if infection is strongly suspected).

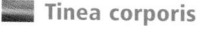 Tinea corporis

Definition: Dermatophyte fungal infection caused by *Trichophyton* or *Microsporum*

DIAGNOSIS

- Diagnosis usually is made on clinical grounds. It can be confirmed by direct visualization under the microscope of a small fragment of the scale using wet mount preparation and potassium hydroxide solution; dermatophytes appear as translucent branching filaments (hyphae) with lines of separation appearing at irregular intervals.
- Infection typically appears as single or multiple annular lesions with an advancing scaly border; the margin is slightly raised and reddened and may be pustular.
- The central area becomes hypopigmented and less scaly as the active border progresses outward.
- The trunk and legs are primarily involved.
- Pruritus is variable.

DIFFERENTIAL DIAGNOSIS

- Pityriasis rosea
- Erythema multiforme
- Psoriasis
- Systemic lupus erythematosus
- Syphilis
- Nummular eczema
- Eczema
- Granuloma annulare
- Lyme disease
- Tinea versicolor
- Contact dermatitis

TREATMENT

- Various creams are effective; the application area should include

into the affected areas and surrounding areas bid for 4 weeks
- Naftifine 1% cream (Naftin) applied qd
- Econazole 1% (Spectazole) applied qd
- Systemic therapy is reserved for severe cases and usually is given for 4 weeks; commonly used agents are ketoconazole (Nizoral) 200 mg qd, fluconazole (Diflucan) 200 mg qd, and terbinafine (Lamisil) 250 mg qd.

Tinea cruris

Definition: Dermatophyte infection of the groin. Dermatophytes are of the genera *Trichophyton, Epidermophyton,* and *Microsporum. Trichophyton rubrum* and *Epidermophyton floccosum* are the most common causes.

DIAGNOSIS
- Erythematous plaques have a half-moon shape and a scaling border.
- The acute inflammation tends to move down the inner thigh and usually spares the scrotum; in severe cases, the fungus may spread onto the buttocks.
- Itching may be severe.
- Red papules and pustules may be present.
- An important diagnostic sign is the advancing well-defined border with a tendency toward central clearing.
- Diagnosis is based on clinical presentation and demonstration of hyphae microscopically using potassium hydroxide.

TREATMENT
- Drying powders (e.g., miconazole nitrate [ZeaSorb-AF]) may be useful in patients with excessive perspiration.
- Various topical antifungal agents are available, including miconazole (Lotrimin AF), terbinafine (Lamisil AT), sulconazole nitrate (Exelderm), and betamethasone dipropionate/clotrimazole (Lotrisone).
- Oral antifungal therapy generally is reserved for cases unresponsive to topical agents. Effective medications are itraconazole (Sporanox) 100 mg/day for 2 to 4 weeks, ketoconazole (Nizoral) 200 mg qd, fluconazole (Diflucan) 200 mg qd, and terbinafine (Lamisil) 250 mg qd.

CLINICAL PEARL
- Transmission occurs from direct contact (e.g., infected persons, animals). The patient's feet should be evaluated as a source of infection because tinea cruris often is associated with tinea pedis.

Tinea pedis

Definition: Dermatophyte infection of the feet

DIAGNOSIS

- Typical presentation varies from erythematous scaling plaques and isolated blisters to interdigital maceration.
- The infection usually starts in the interdigital spaces of the foot. Most infections are found in the toe webs or in the soles.
- Fourth or fifth toes are most commonly involved.
- Pruritus is common and is most intense after removal of shoes and socks.
- Infection with *Tinea rubrum* often manifests with a moccasin distribution affecting the soles and lateral feet.
- Diagnosis usually is made by clinical observation.
- Laboratory testing, when performed, generally consists of a simple potassium hydroxide preparation with mycologic examination under a light microscope to confirm the presence of dermatophytes.

TREATMENT

- Butenafine HCl 1% (Mentax) cream applied bid for 1 week or qd for 4 weeks is effective in interdigital tinea pedis.
- Ciclopirox 0.77% (Loprox) cream applied bid for 4 weeks also is effective.
- Clotrimazole 1% (Lotrimin AF) cream is an OTC treatment. It should be applied to affected and surrounding area bid for 4 weeks.
- Naftifine 1% (Naftin) cream applied qd or gel applied bid for 4 weeks also produces a significantly high cure rate.
- Sertaconazole 2% (Ertaczo) cream is an azole antifungal effective for the topical treatment of interdigital tinea pedis.
- When using topical antifungals, the application area should include normal skin about 2 cm beyond the affected area.
- Areas of maceration can be treated with Burow's solution soaks for 10 to 20 minutes twice day followed by foot elevation.
- Oral agents (fluconazole 150 mg q1wk for 4 weeks) can be used in combination with topical agents in resistant cases.

CLINICAL PEARLS

- Keep infected area clean and dry. Aerate feet by using sandals when possible.
- Use 100% cotton socks rather than Nylon socks to reduce moisture.
- Areas likely to become infected should be dried completely before being covered with clothes.

Definition: Fungal infection of the skin caused by the yeast *Pityrosporum orbiculare*

DIAGNOSIS
- Diagnosis is based on clinical appearance; identification of hyphae and budding spores ("spaghetti and meatballs" appearance) with microscopy confirms diagnosis.
- Most lesions begin as multiple small, circular macules of various colors.
- The macules may be darker or lighter than the surrounding normal skin and scale with scraping.
- Most frequent site of distribution is trunk.
- Facial lesions are more common in children (forehead is most common facial site).
- Eruption is generally of insidious onset and asymptomatic.

TREATMENT
- Topical treatment with selenium sulfide 2.5% suspension (Selsun or Exsel) applied daily for 10 minutes for 7 consecutive days results in a cure rate of 80% to 90%.
- Antifungal topical agents (e.g., miconazole, ciclopirox, clotrimazole) also are effective but generally expensive.
- Oral treatment generally is reserved for resistant cases. Effective agents are ketoconazole (Nizoral) 200 mg qd for 5 days or single 400-mg dose (cure rate >80%), fluconazole (Diflucan) 400 mg given as a single dose (cure rate >70% at 3 weeks after treatment), or itraconazole 200 mg/day for 5 days.

CLINICAL PEARLS
- Lesions may be hyperpigmented in blacks.
- Patients should be informed that the hypopigmented areas do not disappear immediately after treatment and that several months may be necessary for the hypopigmented areas to regain their pigmentation.

Torsades de pointes

Definition: Form of ventricular tachycardia manifested by episodes of alternating electrical polarity with the amplitude of the QRS complex twisting around an isoelectric baseline resembling a spindle; rhythm usually starts with a premature ventricular contraction and is preceded by widening of the Q-T interval.

ETIOLOGY
- Torsades may be caused by electrolyte disturbances (hypokalemia, hypomagnesemia, hypocalcemia), antiarrhythmic drugs that prolong the Q-T interval (procainamide, quinidine, disopyramide), N-acetyl-procainamide, droperidol, amiodarone, phenothiazines, haloperidol, tricyclic antidepressants, terfenadine, astemizole, ketoconazole, erythromycin, trimethoprim-sulfamethoxazole, high-dose methadone, or cocaine. Torsades also is associated with hereditary long Q-T interval syndromes.

TREATMENT
- Electrical termination of the tachycardia is done with cardioversion when the ventricular tachyarrhythmia is sustained.
- Intravenous infusion of isoproterenol decreases the Q-T interval and prevents recurrences.
- Eliminate contributing factors (correction of electrolyte abnormalities, discontinuation of suspected drugs); implement early diagnosis of hereditary long Q-T syndromes and treatment of them with β_1-adrenergic receptor blocking agents. Surgical sympathectomy and use of implantable cardioverter defibrillator also should be considered in high-risk patients with hereditary long Q-T syndrome.
- Intravenous magnesium sulfate may be helpful even if magnesium levels are normal. Magnesium sulfate (10% solution) may be administered by bolus (1-2 g IV over 1-2 minutes and repeated 5-15 minutes later if no response) or by infusion (50 mg/min over 2 hours).
- Sequential overdrive pacing is indicated if the episodes of torsades are sustained and seem to be precipitated by bradycardia.

Definition: Transient neurologic dysfunction caused by focal brain or retinal ischemia with symptoms typically lasting <60 minutes but always <24 hours and followed by a full recovery of function. Acute brain ischemia is a medical emergency requiring prompt neurologic evaluation and potential intervention.

DIAGNOSIS

- During an episode, neurologic abnormalities are confined to discrete vascular territory.
- Typical carotid territory symptoms are ipsilateral monocular visual disturbance, contralateral homonymous hemianopsia, contralateral hemimotor or sensory dysfunction, and language dysfunction (dominant hemisphere) alone or in combination.
- Typical vertebrobasilar territory symptoms are binocular visual disturbance, vertigo, diplopia, dysphagia, dysarthria, and motor or sensory dysfunction involving the ipsilateral face and contralateral body.
- **Imaging studies:**
  - Head CT scan to exclude hemorrhage, including a subdural hemorrhage
  - MRI and magnetic resonance angiography (MRA). In several studies, MRI with diffusion-weighted imaging identified early ischemic brain injury in 50% of patients with TIA. MRA of the brain and neck can identify large vessel intracranial and extracranial stenoses, arteriovenous malformations, and aneurysms.
  - Carotid Doppler studies to identify carotid stenosis. Neck ultrasound also can visualize stenoses of the vertebrobasilar arteries.
  - Echocardiography if cardiac source is suspected
  - Telemetry for hospitalized patients for at least 24 hours. Consider 24-hour Holter monitoring if patient is being discharged.
  - Four-vessel cerebral angiogram if considering carotid endarterectomy or carotid stent
- **Laboratory tests:**
- Complete blood count with platelets
- Prothrombin time (international normalized ratio) and partial thromboplastin time
- Glucose
- Lipid profile
- Erythrocyte sedimentation rate (if clinical suspicion for infectious or inflammatory process)
- Urinalysis
- Chest x-ray

- ECG and consider cycling cardiac enzymes
- Other tests as dictated by suspected etiology

ETIOLOGY

- Cardioembolic
- Large vessel atherothrombotic disease
- Lacunar disease
- Hypoperfusion with fixed arterial stenosis
- Hypercoagulable states

TREATMENT

- If the time of the onset of symptoms is clear, there are significant deficits on neurologic examination, and brain hemorrhage has been ruled out, the patient may be a candidate for thrombolytic therapy.
- No data support the benefits of acute anticoagulation in the acute setting. Heparin is considered for new-onset atrial fibrillation and atherothrombotic carotid disease causing recurrent transient neurologic symptoms, especially in the setting before carotid endarterectomy or carotid stenting. Heparin also is considered for basilar artery thrombosis, given concern for progression to brainstem stroke with high morbidity and mortality.
- No data support the use of long-term anticoagulation in the management of TIA, although stroke patients with atrial fibrillation or demonstrated cardiac thrombi have been shown to benefit from long-term warfarin therapy.
- First line treatment traditionally has been aspirin. No significant benefit of high-dose aspirin (1500 mg/day) has been found conclusively over lower doses (75-325 mg/day). A baby aspirin (81 mg/day) is appropriate.
- Also consider aspirin/dipyridamole extended-release capsules (Aggrenox) 1 capsule PO bid or clopidogrel (Plavix) as a first-line therapy
- In patients with cerebrovascular disease, HMG-CoA reductase inhibitors (statins) have been shown to provide significant protection against subsequent vascular events, such as myocardial infarction and stroke even with low-density lipoprotein (LDL) values <100. Consider starting a statin agent unless LDL is <70.
- Carotid endarterectomy for carotid territory TIA associated with an ipsilateral stenosis of 70% to 99% should be done by a surgeon who is experienced with and performs this procedure regularly. Carotid stenting also is being performed in patients who are not surgical candidates. Ongoing trials are comparing stenting versus surgery for carotid disease.
- Modification of risk factors, including smoking cessation, should be

Definition: Malabsorption syndrome occurring primarily in tropical regions, including Puerto Rico, India, and South East Asia

DIAGNOSIS

- Clinical features of tropical sprue include anorexia, diarrhea, weight loss, abdominal pain, and steatorrhea; these symptoms can develop in expatriates several months after emigrating to temperate regions.
- Diagnostic workup includes a comprehensive history (especially travel history), physical examination, laboratory evidence of malabsorption, and jejunal biopsy. The biopsy results are nonspecific, with blunting, atrophy, and even disappearance of the villi and sub-epithelial lymphocytic infiltration.
- **Laboratory tests:**
  - Megaloblastic anemia (>50% of cases)
  - Vitamin B_{12} deficiency, folate deficiency
  - Steatorrhea, abnormal d-xylose absorption
- **Imaging:** Gastrointestinal series with small bowel follow-through may reveal coarsening of the jejunal folds.

DIFFERENTIAL DIAGNOSIS

- Celiac disease
- Parasitic infestation
- Inflammatory bowel disease
- Other causes of malabsorption (e.g., Whipple's disease)

TREATMENT

- Folic acid therapy (5 mg bid for 2 weeks followed by a maintenance dose of 1 mg tid) improves anemia and malabsorption in more than two thirds of patients.
- Tetracycline 250 mg qid should be given for 4 to 6 weeks in individuals who have returned to temperate zones and for 6 months in patients in endemic areas; ampicillin 500 mg bid should be given for at least 4 weeks in patients intolerant to tetracycline.
- Correct vitamin B_{12} deficiency with vitamin B_{12} 1000 μg IM weekly for 4 weeks, then monthly for 3 to 6 months.
- Correct other nutritional deficiencies (e.g., calcium, iron).

▩ Tuberculosis (TB), pulmonary

Definition: An infection of the lung and, occasionally, surrounding structures, caused by the bacterium *Mycobacterium tuberculosis*

DIAGNOSIS

- Tuberculin skin testing is used in diagnosing latent tuberculosis infection (LTBI) and includes measurement of the delayed type hypersensitivity response 48 to 72 hours after intradermal injection of purified protein derivative (PPD).
- Perform acid-fast stain and cultures of sputum.
- Perform chest x-ray.
  - Initial film may show a variety of patterns; rarely, it may be completely normal if the patient has endobronchial TB.
  - Parenchymal infiltrates most commonly involve the upper lobes (apical and posterior segments).
  - Hilar and paratracheal adenopathy, unilateral pleural effusion, and cavitary lesions also may be present.
  - A chest radiograph is indicated for all persons being considered for treatment of LTBI to exclude active pulmonary TB. If chest radiographs are normal, and no symptoms consistent with active TB are present, tuberculin-positive persons may be candidates for treatment of LTBI. If radiographic or clinical findings are consistent with pulmonary or extrapulmonary TB, further studies (e.g., medical evaluation, bacteriologic examinations, and a comparison of the current and old chest radiographs) should be done to determine if treatment for active TB is indicated.
- Baseline laboratory testing is not routinely indicated for all patients at the start of treatment for LTBI. Patients whose initial evaluation suggests a liver disorder should have baseline hepatic measurements of serum aspartate aminotransferase or alanine aminotransferase and bilirubin. Baseline testing also is indicated for patients with HIV infection, pregnant women, and women in the immediate postpartum period (i.e., within 3 months of delivery), patients with a history of chronic liver disease (e.g., hepatitis B or C, alcoholic hepatitis, or cirrhosis), persons who use alcohol regularly, and persons at risk for chronic liver disease. Baseline testing is not routinely indicated in older patients.

TREATMENT

- **Preventive treatment for PPD conversion only (infection without disease):** isoniazid 300 mg daily for 6 to 12 months (at least

600 mg plus ethambutol 30 mg/kg (maximum 2500 mg) plus pyrazinamide 2 g (50 kg), 2.5 g (51-74 kg), or 3 g (>75 kg) thrice weekly for 6 months
- **Drug-resistant TB:** A 6-month regimen of isoniazid, rifampin, pyrazinamide, and either ethambutol or streptomycin has been shown to be effective for the treatment of TB resistant only to isoniazid.

Urethritis, gonococcal

Definition: Urethral inflammation caused by *Neisseria gonorrhoeae*

DIAGNOSIS
- Typically in men there is a purulent discharge from the anterior urethra with dysuria appearing 2 to 7 days after infecting exposure. Women may experience initial urethritis and cervicitis, accompanied by purulent discharge.
- **Laboratory diagnosis:** Gram stain of discharge reveals gram-negative intracellular diplococci. Gonorrhea culture is performed on Thayer-Martin medium.

TREATMENT
- **Recommended regimens:**
  - Cefixime 400 mg PO in a single dose, *or*
  - Ceftriaxone 125 mg IM in a single dose, *or*
  - Ciprofloxacin 500 mg PO in a single dose, *or*
  - Ofloxacin 400 mg in a single dose, *or*
  - Levofloxacin 250 mg PO in a single dose
  - *plus, if chlamydial infection is not ruled out*
    - Azithromycin 1 g PO in a single dose *or* doxycycline 100 mg PO bid for 7 days

CLINICAL PEARL
- Patients infected with *N. gonorrhoeae* often are coinfected with *Chlamydia trachomatis;* this finding has led to the recommendation that patients treated for gonococcal infection also be treated routinely with a regimen effective against uncomplicated genital *C. trachomatis* infection.

Urethritis, nongonococcal

Definition: Urethral inflammation caused by any of several organisms

DIAGNOSIS
- Diagnosis requires demonstration of urethritis and exclusion of infection with *Neisseria gonorrhoeae*.
- The best specimen for culture is an endourethral swab taken from an area 2 to 4 cm inside the urethra.
- Diagnosis also can be made by ELISA and direct immunofluorescence.

ETIOLOGY
- *Chlamydia trachomatis*
- The etiology of most cases of nonchlamydial nongonococcal urethritis (NGU) is unknown. *Ureaplasma urealyticum* and possibly *Mycoplasma genitalium* are implicated in some studies.
- *Trichomonas vaginalis* and herpes simplex virus sometimes cause NGU.

TREATMENT
- **Recommended regimen:** azithromycin 1 g PO in a single dose *or* doxycycline 100 mg PO bid for 7 days.
- **Alternative regimens:**
  - Erythromycin base 500 mg PO qid for 7 days, *or*
  - Erythromycin ethylsuccinate 800 mg PO qid for 7 days, *or*
  - Ofloxacin 300 mg PO bid for 7 days, *or*
  - Levofloxacin 500 mg PO qd for 7 days
- **Management of sex partners:** Patients should be instructed to refer sex partners within the preceding 60 days for evaluation and treatment.
- Patients with recurrent/persistent urethritis can be treated with metronidazole 2 g orally in a single dose, *plus* erythromycin base 500 mg PO qid for 7 days, *or* eythromycin ethylsuccinate 800 mg PO qid for 7 days.

Definition: *Pyuria* refers to presence of >10 leukocytes/mL of uncentrifuged urine. "Significant" *bacteriuria* generally has been defined as the presence of >100,000 bacteria/mL of urine (in urine cultures). Counts of 10,000/mL to 100,000/mL also can indicate UTI, especially in the presence of pyuria; the growth of $\geq 10^3$ colony-forming units per milliliter (CFU/mL) of a single predominant species reliably indicates true bacteriuria men, whereas counts $\geq 10^3$ CFU/mL or growth in any amount of three or more species, with none predominant, nearly always represents specimen contamination. The presence of bacteria on urinalysis implies bacterial counts >30,000/mL.

DIAGNOSIS

- Perform urinalysis (clean-catch specimen).
- Perform urine culture and colony count.
- Blood cultures are indicated only in suspected pyelonephritis or sepsis.
- Spiral CT, cystoscopy, and ultrasound are indicated in men with UTI and women with recurrent UTIs. Imaging is done to rule out obstruction, calculi, and papillary necrosis.

ETIOLOGY

- ***Escherichia coli:*** causes 75% of uncomplicated UTIs and often is found in complicated UTI
- ***Proteus:*** gram-negative rod that causes alkaline urine and promotes formation of struvite calculi
- ***Klebsiella:*** frequent cause of uncomplicated community-acquired UTI
- ***Enterococcus:*** most common gram-positive cause of UTI; often associated with prior antibiotic therapy, urologic instrumentation, or obstructive uropathy
- ***Pseudomonas:*** often associated with obstructive uropathy
- ***Staphylococcus* (in diabetic patients):** may indicate intrarenal abscess or a "spillover" from bacteremia rather than a true UTI

TREATMENT

- Conventional therapy is 7 to 10 days. Short-term therapy can be 3 days in uncomplicated UTI in a nondiabetic patient without history of recurrent UTI or urinary obstruction.
- Empiric agents include ciprofloxacin, trimethoprim-sulfamethoxazole, nitrofurantoin, amoxicillin/clavulanate, and cephalosporins

CLINICAL PEARL
- Treatment of asymptomatic bacteriuria in women with diabetes is not indicated and does not seem to reduce complications. Treatment is indicated, however, in pregnant patients, in patients who are about to undergo urologic surgery, and in recipients of renal transplants soon after transplantation.

Vaginitis, fungal

Definition: Vaginal infection usually caused by *Candida albicans*

DIAGNOSIS
- Vaginitis is characterized by a vaginal discharge (usually) or vulvar itching and irritation.
- *Candida* vaginitis is suggested clinically by pruritus in the vulvar area together with erythema of the vagina or vulva; a white discharge may be present.
- For diagnosis, examine a wet preparation or Gram stain of the vaginal discharge under a microscope at low-dry and high-dry power. The yeast or pseudohyphae of *Candida* are more easily identified when using 10% potassium hydroxide in wet preparation.
- Culture for *Trichomonas vaginalis* or *Candida* is more sensitive than microscopic examination, but the specificity of culture for *Candida* to diagnose vaginitis is less clear.

TREATMENT
- Fluconazole 150 mg PO tablet single dose *or*
- Clotrimazole 500 mg vaginal tablet 1 tablet single application, *or*
- Butoconazole 2% cream 5 g intravaginally for 3 days

Vaginitis, trichomonal

Definition: Vaginal infection caused by the protozoan *Trichomonas vaginalis*

DIAGNOSIS
- *T. vaginalis* typically causes a diffuse, malodorous, yellow-green discharge with vulvar irritation.
- The diagnosis of vaginitis is made by pH and microscopic examination of fresh samples of the discharge.

microscope at low-dry and high-dry power. The motile *T. vaginalis* usually are easily identified in the saline specimen.

TREATMENT
- **Recommended regimen:** metronidazole 2 g PO in a single dose
- **Alternative regimen:** metronidazole 500 mg bid for 7 days
- Treatment of the patient and sex partner results in relief of symptoms, microbiologic cure, and reduction of transmission.

Vaginosis, bacterial

Definition: Malodorous vaginal discharge that results from replacement of the normal hydrogen peroxide–producing *Lactobacillus* in the vagina with high concentrations of anaerobic bacteria (e.g., *Bacteroides, Mobiluncus*), *Giardia vaginalis,* and *Mycoplasma hominis*

DIAGNOSIS
- Bacterial vaginosis is diagnosed by the use of clinical or Gram stain criteria. Clinical criteria require three of the following symptoms or signs:
  - A homogeneous, white, noninflammatory discharge that smoothly coats the vaginal walls
  - Presence of clue cells on microscopic examination
  - pH of vaginal fluid >4.5.
  - A fishy odor of vaginal discharge before or after addition of 10% potassium hydroxide (whiff test)
- When Gram stain is used, determining the relative concentration of the bacterial morphologic types characteristic of the altered flora of bacterial vaginosis is an acceptable laboratory method for diagnosing bacterial vaginosis. Culture of *G. vaginalis* is not recommended as a diagnostic tool because it is not specific.

TREATMENT
- The principal goal of therapy is to relieve vaginal symptoms and signs. Only women with symptomatic disease require treatment.
- **Recommended regimen:** metronidazole 500 mg PO bid for 7 days, *or* metronidazole gel 0.75% 1 full applicator (5 g) intravaginally bid for 5 days, *or* clindamycin cream 2% 1 full applicator (5 g) intravaginally at bedtime for 7 days
- **Alternative regimens:** metronidazole 2 g PO in a single dose or clindamycin 300 mg PO bid for 7 days

CLINICAL PEARL

Patients should be advised to avoid using alcohol during treatment with metronidazole and for 24 hours thereafter. Clindamycin cream is oil based and may weaken latex condoms and diaphragms.

von Willebrand's disease

Definition: A congenital disorder of hemostasis characterized by defective or deficient von Willebrand factor (vWF). There are several subtypes of von Willebrand's disease. The most common type (80% of cases) is type I, which is caused by a quantitative decrease in vWF; type IIA and type IIB are the result of qualitative protein abnormalities; type III is a rare autosomal recessive disorder characterized by a near-complete quantitative deficiency of vWF. *Acquired von Willebrand's disease* is a rare disorder that usually occurs in elderly patients and usually presents with mucocutaneous bleeding abnormalities and no clinically meaningful family history. It is often accompanied by a hematoproliferative or autoimmune disorder. Successful treatment of the associated illness can reverse the clinical and laboratory manifestations.

DIAGNOSIS

- Initial testing includes partial thromboplastin time (increased), platelet count (normal), and bleeding time (prolonged).
- Subsequent tests include vWF level (decreased), factor VIII:C (decreased), and ristocetin agglutination (increased in type IIB).
- Type IIA can be distinguished from type I by absence of ristocetin cofactor activity and abnormal multimer.
- Type IIB is distinguished from type I by abnormal multimer.

TREATMENT

- The mainstay of treatment in von Willebrand's disease is the replacement of the deficient protein at the time of spontaneous bleeding or before invasive procedures are performed.
- Desmopressin acetate (DDAVP) is used to release stored vWF from endothelial cells. It is used to cover minor procedures and traumatic bleeding in mild type I von Willebrand's disease. Dose is 0.3 μg/kg in 100 mL of normal saline solution infused intravenously >20 minutes. DDAVP also is available as a nasal spray (dose of 150 μg spray administered to each nostril) as a preparation for minor surgery and management of minor bleeding episodes. DDAVP is not effective in type

- In patients with severe disease, replacement therapy in the form of cryoprecipitate is the method of choice. The standard dose is 1 bag of cryoprecipitate per 10 kg of body weight.
- Factor VIII concentrate rich in vWF (Humate-P) is useful to correct bleeding abnormalities.
- Life-threatening hemorrhage unresponsive to therapy with cryoprecipitate or factor VIII concentrate may require transfusion of normal platelets.

■ Wegener's granulomatosis

Definition: Multisystem disease generally consisting of the classic triad of:

- Necrotizing granulomatous lesions in the upper or lower respiratory tracts
- Generalized focal necrotizing vasculitis involving arteries and veins
- Focal glomerulonephritis of the kidneys
- "Limited" forms of the disease also can occur and may evolve into the classic triad; Wegener's granulomatosis can be classified using the *ELK* classification, which identifies the three major sites of involvement: *E*, ears, nose, and throat or respiratory tract; *L*, lungs; *K*, kidneys.

DIAGNOSIS
- **Clinical presentation:**
  - Clinical manifestations often vary with the stage of the disease and degree of organ involvement.
  - **Frequent manifestations:**
    - **Upper respiratory tract:** chronic sinusitis, chronic otitis media, mastoiditis, nasal crusting, obstruction and epistaxis, nasal septal perforation, nasal lacrimal duct stenosis, saddle nose deformities (resulting from cartilage destruction)
    - **Lung:** hemoptysis, multiple nodules, diffuse alveolar pattern
    - **Kidney:** renal insufficiency, glomerulonephritis
    - **Skin:** necrotizing skin lesions
    - **Nervous system:** mononeuritis multiplex, cranial nerve involvement
    - **Joints:** monarthritis or polyarthritis (nondeforming), usually affecting large joints

- **Mouth:** chronic ulcerative lesions of the oral mucosa, "mulberry" gingivitis
- **Eye:** proptosis, uveitis, episcleritis, retinal and optic nerve vasculitis
- Positive test for cytoplasmic pattern of antineutrophilic cytoplasmic antibody
- **Laboratory tests:** Anemia, leukocytosis, hematuria, red blood cell casts, proteinuria, elevated serum creatinine, decreased creatinine clearance, increased erythrocyte sedimentation rate, positive rheumatoid factor, and elevated C-reactive protein may be found.
- Chest x-ray may reveal bilateral multiple nodules, cavitated mass lesions, and pleural effusion (20%).
- Pulmonary function tests are useful in detecting stenosis of the airways.
- Biopsy of one or more affected organs should be attempted; the most reliable source for tissue diagnosis is the lung. Lesions in the nasopharynx (if present) can be easily biopsied.

TREATMENT

- Prednisone 60-80 mg/day and cyclophosphamide 2 mg/kg are generally effective and are used to control clinical manifestations; when the disease comes under control, prednisone is tapered, and cyclophosphamide is continued.
- Trimethoprim-sulfamethoxazole (TMP-SMZ) therapy may represent a useful alternative in patients with lesions limited to the upper or lower respiratory tracts in the absence of vasculitis or nephritis. Treatment with TMP-SMZ (160 mg/800 mg bid) also reduces the incidence of relapses in patients with Wegener's granulomatosis in remission.

Wernicke's encephalopathy

Definition: Syndrome of acute extraocular muscle dysfunction, confusion, and ataxia, resulting from thiamine deficiency

DIAGNOSIS

- Disturbance of extraocular motility, including nystagmus, abducens nerve palsy, and disorders of conjugate gaze
- Encephalopathy
- Ataxia of gait
- Peripheral neuropathy may be seen in addition to the above-listed typical findings.

- Serum chemistries
- Serum pyruvate elevated
- Whole blood or erythrocyte transketolase decreased; rapid resolution to normal in 24 hours with thiamine repletion
- **Imaging:**
  - MRI may show diencephalic and mesencephalic lesions acutely, but there is no definitive radiologic study for diagnosis.
  - CT scan may show cerebral atrophy from chronic alcoholism.

ETIOLOGY
- Thiamine deficiency from alcohol abuse or other malnourished state

TREATMENT
- Give thiamine 100 mg IV or IM immediately. Typically, give thiamine intravenously for 3-5 days, then change to oral administration.
- Avoid dextrose-containing fluids until thiamine is repleted.
- Give prophylactic treatment for delirium tremens if alcoholic.
- Attempt to treat alcoholism or underlying malnourished state.
- Dose for long-term oral thiamine repletion is typically 5 mg/day.
- Case reports suggest donepezil may help chronic memory problems.

Wolff-Parkinson-White (WPW) syndrome

Definition: ECG abnormality associated with earlier than normal ventricular depolarization after the atrial impulse and predisposing the affected person to tachyarrhythmias

DIAGNOSIS
- Three basic features characterize the ECG abnormalities in WPW syndrome (Fig. 15):
  - P-R interval <120 msec
  - QRS complex >120 msec with a slurred, slowly rising onset of QRS in some lead (delta wave)
  - ST-T wave changes

ETIOLOGY
- Existence of accessory pathways (Kent bundles)

WPW Preexcitation

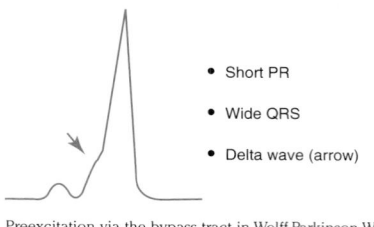

- Short PR

- Wide QRS

- Delta wave (arrow)

FIGURE 15. Preexcitation via the bypass tract in Wolff-Parkinson-White (WPW) syndrome is associated with the triad of findings shown here. (From Goldberger AL, Goldberger E: Clinical Electrocardiography: A Simplified Approach, 5th ed. St Louis, Mosby, 1994.)

TREATMENT
- No treatment in the absence of tachyarrhythmias
- Symptomatic tachyarrhythmias
- **Acute episode:** adenosine, verapamil, or diltiazem can be used to terminate an episode of reciprocal tachycardia.
- Digitalis should not be used because it can reduce refractoriness in the accessory pathway and accelerate the tachycardia. Cardioversion should be used in the presence of hemodynamic impairment.